AF411862

Bone Marrow Transplantation Across Major Genetic Barriers

Bone Marrow Transplantation Across Major Genetic Barriers

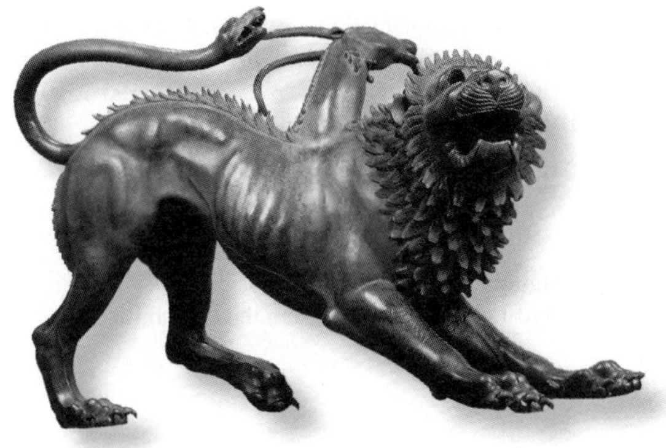

Editors

Yair Reisner
Weizmann Institute of Science, Israel

Massimo F Martelli
Perugia University, Italy

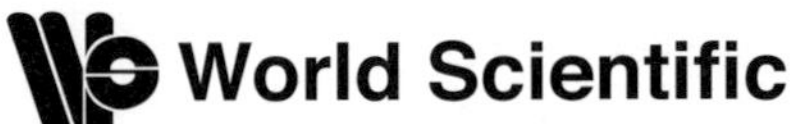

World Scientific

NEW JERSEY · LONDON · SINGAPORE · BEIJING · SHANGHAI · HONG KONG · TAIPEI · CHENNAI

Published by

World Scientific Publishing Co. Pte. Ltd.

5 Toh Tuck Link, Singapore 596224

USA office: 27 Warren Street, Suite 401-402, Hackensack, NJ 07601

UK office: 57 Shelton Street, Covent Garden, London WC2H 9HE

Library of Congress Cataloging-in-Publication Data
Bone marrow transplantation across major genetic barriers / editors, Yair Reisner,
    Massimo F. Martelli.
        p. ; cm.
    Includes bibliographical references and index.
    ISBN-13: 978-9814271264 (hardcover : alk. paper)
    ISBN-10: 9814271268 (hardcover : alk. paper)
    1. Bone marrow--Transplantation. 2. Hematopoietic stem cells. 3. Graft versus host disease--
Prevention. 4. Graft rejection--Prevention. 5. Human immunogenetics. I. Reisner, Yair.
II. Martelli, M. F.
    [DNLM: 1. Bone Marrow Transplantation--methods. 2. Genetic Variation. 3. HLA Antigens--
genetics. 4. Hematopoietic Stem Cell Transplantation--methods. 5. Hematopoietic Stem Cells--
immunology. 6. T-Lymphocytes--immunology. WH 380 B71193 2010]
    RD123.5.B6475 2010
    617.4'410592--dc22

                                                                                    2010025734

British Library Cataloguing-in-Publication Data
A catalogue record for this book is available from the British Library.

Typeset by Stallion Press
Email: enquiries@stallionpress.com

Printed in Singapore by Mainland Press Pte Ltd.

This book is dedicated to Robert A. Good, father of modern clinical immunology and cellular engineering whose vision paved the way to haploidentical bone marrow transplantation.

Preface

The importance of bone marrow transplantation for patients who do not have a matched sibling donor cannot be overestimated. The availability of matched volunteer donors in the public at large is limited by the remarkable genetic diversity of humans. Thus, although registries of such volunteers now include more than eight million individuals, we still face the problem of finding a matched donor for about 30% of patients in need. To address this burning issue, extensive clinical and investigational use of haploidentical hematopoietic stem cell transplantation is increasing rapidly in leading institutes around the world. This book summarizes the state of the art of these transplants in children and in adults, emphasizing future directions. Prevention of GVHD and graft rejection are clearly satisfactory and disease-free survival rates in acute leukemia patients in remission are similar to rates in transplants from unrelated donors or with cord blood. Since enhancing immune post-transplant reconstitution will improve survival even further, a major part of this book is dedicated to pre-clinical studies investigating how to boost thymus output or use adoptive transfer of immunity against infectious agents or malignant cells. We also present the exciting possibility of durable immune tolerance to donor tissues and organs by means of bone marrow transplantation.

We wish to thank our esteemed colleagues for presenting here their most up to date experience in various aspects of haploidentical stem cell transplantation. We also extend our thanks to Doreen Rosenberg and Geraldine Anne Boyd for their invaluable assistance in bringing this book to fruition.

Yair Reisner   Massimo F. Martelli

Contents

Chapter 1

Crossing HLA Barriers by "Megadose" Stem Cell Transplants

Yair Reisner[*,‡], *Massimo F. Martelli*[†]
and Esther Bachar-Lustig[*]

Introduction

Bone marrow transplantation (BMT) offers a curative treatment of choice for many patients with leukemia or other hematological disorders.[1–5] Despite the world registry network, which includes more than 8 million HLA-typed volunteers, the odds of finding a matched unrelated donor in the registries vary with the patient's race and range from approximately 60–80% for Caucasians to under 10% for ethnic minorities. Moreover, months are often required to identify the donor from a potential panel, establishing eligibility and harvesting of the BM cells. One must remember that age restrictions are extremely stringent for patients utilizing an unrelated donor, as morbidity and mortality rise with age in this type of transplant. Furthermore, with the development of molecular analysis, close matching has itself become more accurate over the years in an attempt to reduce the risk of graft failure and graft-versus-host disease (GvHD), decreasing even more the chance of finding a suitable matched

[*]Department of Immunology, Weizmann Institute of Science, Rehovot, Israel.
[†]Haematopoietic Stem Cell Transplant Unit, Section of Haematology and Immunology, University of Perugia, Perugia, Italy.
[‡]Corresponding author. Tel.: +972-8-9344023 Fax: +972-8-9344145. E-mail: Yair. Reisner@weizmann.ac.il.

donor. For all these reasons allogeneic BMT is not available for many candidates. On the other hand, virtually all patients have a readily available haploidentical family member. Using full haplotype mismatched related donors offers several advantages:

(1) Immediate donor availability for all transplant candidates;
(2) Ability to select the donor of choice from several available relatives on the basis of age, infectious disease status and NK cell alloreactivity;
(3) Controlled cell harvest and graft composition;
(4) Immediate access to donor-derived cellular therapies if required after transplantation.

However, the use of haploidentical donors has presented a major challenge over the past three decades, due to life-threatening immunological problems, namely GvHD and graft rejection.[6]

Crossing the HLA Barrier in SCID Patients

Numerous murine and clinical studies during the past three decades have demonstrated that effective T cell depletion of BM preparations can completely prevent the development of both acute and chronic GvHD, in the absence of any posttransplant prophlyaxis.[7–15] The proof of principle was initially established in the clinical setting during the early 1980s when it was demonstrated that effective T cell depletion can completely prevent GvHD in SCID patients, even when haploidentical three-locus HLA-mismatched BM is used.[11,12,14,15] The T cell depletion procedure used in these early studies comprised differential agglutination with soybean agglutinin followed by E-rossetting with sheep red blood cells.[10,16,17] The procedure was time-consuming but it yielded a 3.5-log depletion of T cells, which was adequate for the prevention of GvHD in our first 3 patients reported in *Blood* in 1983.[11] By now more than 200 patients have been treated by this approach and, as can be seen from the long term results of O'Reilly[18] (Sloan Kettering) and Buckly[19] (Duke), the two major groups using it, long term survival is around 80% (Fig. 1).

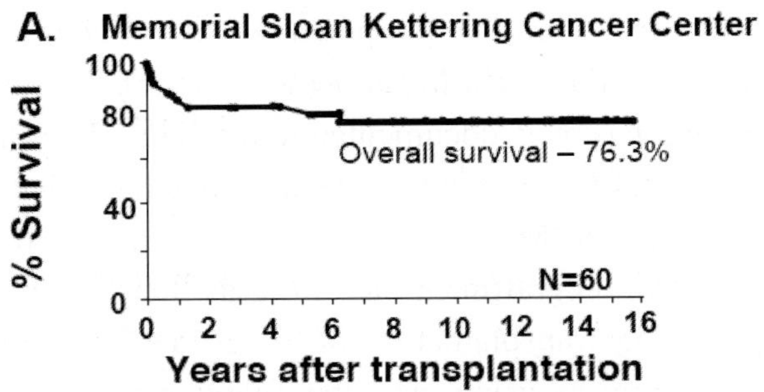

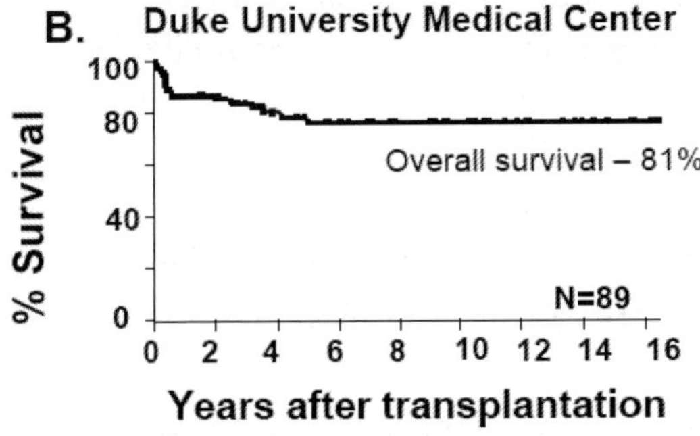

Fig. 1. Long term survival of SCID patients treated by transplantation of human T cell-depleted BM: results of O'Reilly *et al.* (A) (Sloan Kettering)[18] and Buckley *et al.* (B) (Duke University Medical Center).[19]

The Experimental Basis for "Megadose" Transplants in Leukemia Patients

Following the encouraging results in SCID patients, it was reasonable to assume that in leukemia patients pretreated with supralethal radiochemotherapy, the remaining immunity at the day of transplant would be dramatically reduced, reaching levels similar to those found in SCID patients. This led us to believe that graft rejection should not represent a major problem. However, early results suggested that this was not the case and a high rate of graft rejection was documented.[20–22]

Subsequently, using limit dilution analysis, we demonstrated the presence of residual alloreactive CTL-p in mice[23,24] or primates[25] conditioned with radiochemotherapy, similar to that employed in the treatment of leukemia patients. Likewise, the potential role of stem cell competition mediated by residual host hematopoietic stem cells surviving such lethal conditioning has been documented in mice.[26,27] Thus, further ablation of these residual stem cells by selective myeloablative agents such as dimethylmyleran (DMM)[26] or after thiotepa[28] was found to markedly enhance short term engraftment, as well as long term donor type chimerism following transplantation of T cell-depleted BM allografts (Fig. 2). Furthermore, by using the latter agents it is possible to dissect stem cell competition from T cell-mediated rejection, so as to develop appropriate mouse models for the assessment of new modalities addressing these two barriers separately. In particular, based on these studies the conditioning protocol previously based on lethal TBI, in conjunction with antilympocyte agents such as ATG and cyclophosphamide, was supplemented with thiotepa. In addition, myeloablated mice exhibiting minimal stem cell competition were used successfully to construct an

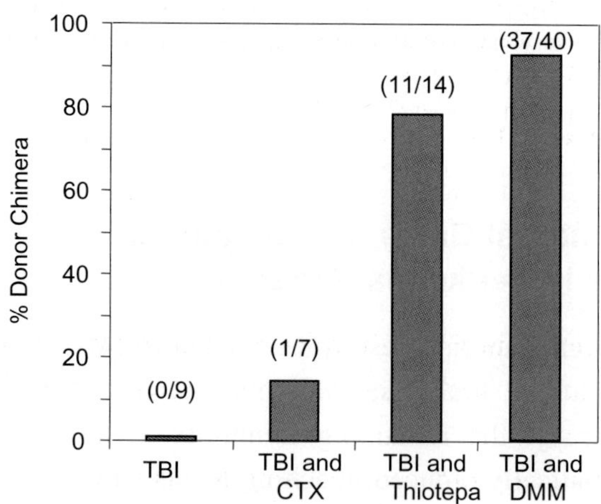

Fig. 2. Effect of conditioning with cyclophosphamide, thiotepa and DMM on the chimerism status of recipients. C3H/HeJ mice received 8 Gy TBI. Experimental groups were treated with cyclophosphamide (120 mg/kg body weight), thiotepa (10 mg/kg) and DMM 0.2 mg. T cell-depleted BM 3×10^6 from C57/BL donors was administered 1 or 2 days post-TBI. Chimerism status was evaluated 30 days posttransplant.[26,28]

Table 1. **Addition of PNA⁻ Thymocytes Prior to Bone Marrow Transplantation: Effect on Survival and Hematological Parameters 12 Days After Allogeneic Bone Marrow Transplantation**[26]

Addition of PNA⁻ Thymocytes ($\times 10^6$)	Transplanted Cells ($\times 10^6$)	Survival*	Hematological Parameters[†]		
			Leukocytes ($\times 10^{-3}$/mL)	Hemoglobin g/dL	Platelets ($\times 10^{-3}$/mL)
5	3	0/8	–	–	–
5	20	0/8	–	–	–
1	3	0/8	–	–	–
1	20	0/8	–	–	–
0.3	3	3/8	1.5 ± 0.2	4.7 ± 1.2	78 ± 28
0.3	20	6/8	17.0 ± 13.9	12.0 ± 1.7	506 ± 159
–	3	7/8	4.5 ± 1.3	12.5 ± 2.1	211 ± 54
–	20	3/3	4.4 ± 0.5	14.9 ± 0.7	605 ± 30

Female C3H/HeJ mice were conditioned with 8 Gy TBI (day 0) and DMM (0.2 mg/mouse, day +1). Thymocytes from C3H/HeJ mice were fractionated by differential agglutination with PNA and the immunocompetent (PNA⁻) cells were injected IV (day +2). Transplantation of T cell-depleated bone marrow from C57BL/6 donors was performed on day +3.

* Chimerism analysis shows that all mice surviving were donor type chimeras 30 days posttransplant.

[†] Hematological parameters are presented as average values ±SD. All surviving mice were tested on day 12.

experimental model in which T cell-mediated rejection is reconstituted selectively by addition of graduated numbers of syngeneic mature thymocytes (PNA⁻).[26]

As can be seen in Table 1, the reconstituted mice strongly reject BM allografts. A BM graft of 3×10^6 cells results in severe anemia, which is fatal even when the lowest number of 0.3×10^6 thymocytes are added. Graft rejection following this thymocyte dose can be overcome by a transplant of 20×10^6 BM cells, but it cannot be avoided by this large BM dose in recipients of 1.0×10^6 thymocytes.

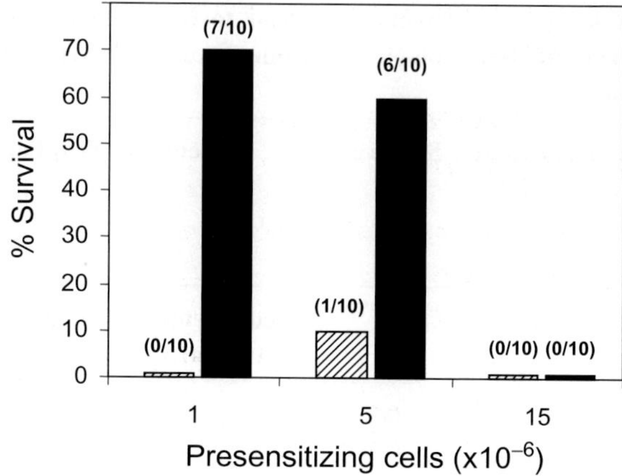

Fig. 3. Effect of the BM cell dose on survival 30 days after transplantation of T cell-depleted BM in presensitized mice. C3H/HeJ mice were presensitized with different numbers of irradiated (40 Gy) spleen cells from C57BL/6 mice 1 week prior to TBI (8 Gy). One day after TBI, the mice received either 3×10^6 (striped bars) or 20×10^6 (black bars) T-cell-depleted BM cells from C57BL/6 donors. Each group included 10 mice. Chimerism analysis showed that all mice surviving 30 days posttransplant were donor type chimeras.[26]

A similar ability to overcome rejection by cell dose escalation of T cell-depleted BM was observed in mice presensitized with irradiated donor type spleen cells (Fig. 3). Taken together, the quantitative relationship between residual host T cells and the number of T cell-depleted BM cells required to neutralize the resistance of these cells has been established and has led to several attempts to significantly increase the BM cell dose in humans. Initially, we hoped to achieve this goal by *ex vivo* expansion. However, with the advent of granulocyte–colony stimulating factor (G-CSF) mobilization in autologous transplants,[29,30] in 1993 it became possible to test the concept of dose escalation in humans by supplementing BM with peripheral blood progenitor cells (PBPCs) collected after administration of G-CSF to the donor. This pilot study carried out between 1993 and 1995 demonstrated for the first time that in humans, as in mice, cell dose escalation can facilitate engraftment of T cell-depleted mismatched transplants.[31,32]

How "Megadose" Transplants Overcome the Immune Barrier

Initial Evidence for Tolerance Induction by Human CD34[+] Hematopoietic Progenitor Cells

Our results for the first series of leukemia patients receiving a larger inoculum of T cell-depleted transplants could be attributed to several types of accessory cells which are not removed by the lectin separation, as previously shown in murine models employing lethally irradiated recipients.[27,33–41]

However, beginning in 1995, T cell depletion was substituted by positive selection of CD34 cells using magnetic beads. Further modification of the positive selection procedure in Perugia using Miltenyi magnetic beads and the clinical experience of 1999 are summarized by Aversa in this book. Importantly, this positive selection procedure in which all kinds of hypothetical facilitating cells are removed was not associated with any reduction in the engraftment rate, nor did it affect the speed of hematopoietic recovery. Thus, it seemed that cells within the highly CD34-enriched fraction might possess a marked capacity to overcome resistance to engraftment.

The intriguing question of how the CD34 cells overcome the barrier presented by host T cells was first addressed by Rachamim *et al.*[42] who demonstrated that cells within the CD34 fraction are endowed with potent veto activity (Fig. 4).

Veto activity was defined in 1980 by Miller[43] as the capacity to specifically suppress CTL precursors (CTLp), directed against Ags recognized by the veto cells themselves, but not against third party Ags (Fig. 5). Thus, the recognizing T cell, with specificity directed against the veto cell, is killed upon binding to its veto target. This inherent specificity of veto cells, eliminating only host CTLp directed against the donor Ags, while sparing other CTLp, which can further persist and fight infectious pathogens, has suggested that veto cells could offer a specific and effective modality for the induction of transplantation tolerance.

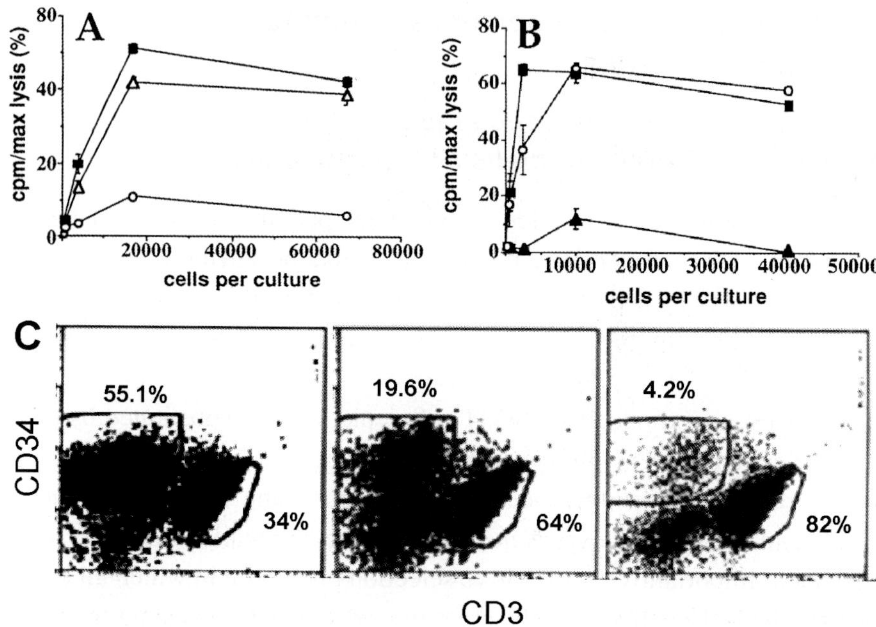

Fig. 4. The tolerizing effect of CD34[+] cells is abrogated by irradiation and requires cell-to-cell contact. (A) Responder cells (1.2×10^6/ml) were incubated with 1.2×10^6/ml irradiated (30 Gy) stimulator cells (black square) for 5 days. Irradiated (30 Gy) (white triangle) or nonirradiated (circle) CD34[+] cells from the same donor (1.2×10^6/ml) were added to some of the cultures, as indicated. After 5 days, the cells were isolated and the CTL-p frequency was measured. (B) Responder and irradiated simulator cells were combined in the lower chamber of a Transwell culture system, which contains an upper and a lower chamber. Purified CD34[+] cells were added to either the lower (black triangle) or the upper (circle) chamber, or were not added to the cultures (black square), as indicated. After 5 days of incubation, the cells were isolated and a limiting dilution assay for CTL-p was carried out. (C) Cellular composition after 5-day MLC. Equal numbers of responder T cells from donor C (84% purity) and irradiated allogeneic stimulator cells from either donor A (top panels) or donor B (bottom panels) were cocultured for 5 days, as described in *Materials and Methods*. Purified CD34[+] cells (87% purity) from donor A were also added to the cultures, in different numbers, as follows: 5×10^6 (left column), 5×10^5 (middle column) and 5×10^4 (right column). After 5 days, the cells were analyzed by two-color flow cytometry, utilizing fluorescence-labeled monoclonal antibodies against CD34 and CD3. Percentages of CD34[+] cells and of T cells are shown.[42]

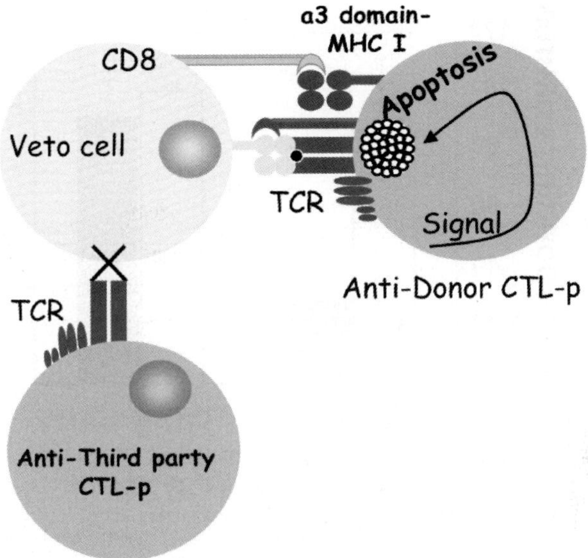

Fig. 5. The veto "concept." A CTL-p specifically recognizes the veto cell by the binding of its T cell receptor (TCR) to the MHC class I molecule on the veto cell. Once the cells interact, instead of triggering stimulation and expansion of the CTL-p, the veto cell induces the transduction of a death signal (apoptosis) in the CTL-p. The veto activity is specific, as a CTL-p, which bears its TCR against the third party MHC molecule, does not recognize the veto cell, and thus survives. In CD8[+] veto cells, the binding of the CD8 molecule to the α3 domain of the MHC class I molecule on the CTL-p, plays a role in the apoptosis signal.[83]

Several important attributes of the CD34[+] veto cells were shown by Gur *et al.*,[44] including the importance of the CD34[+] HLA class I recognition for their activity and their specific inhibition of effector T cells expressing IL-2 and IFN-γ. The latter could provide a useful surrogate assay for the regulatory activity of CD34[+] cells. This could be of importance considering the relatively low frequency of alloreactive CTL-p in the blood of normal individuals, which necessitates the use of indirect assays to monitor *in vitro* the fate of these cells upon interaction with a given immune regulatory population. Thus, it is possible to measure the inhibition of effector activity by functional assays, such as limit dilution analysis (LDA) for CTL-p (Fig. 6), or by a surrogate assay of effector cells expressing IL-2 and IFN-γ (Fig. 7).

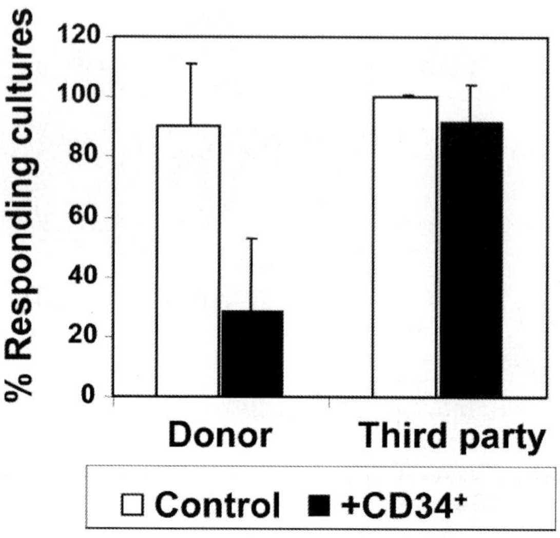

Fig. 6. The regulatory activity of CD34 cells: evidence for target specificity. The average CTL response (SD) in the presence (black bars) or absence (white bars) of CD34$^+$ cells at a veto-to-responder cell ratio of 0.5. The veto effect was tested by a limiting dilution assay as follows: equal numbers (1 × 106/mL) of responder cells and irradiated allogeneic stimulator cells from the donor of the CD34 cells and a third party donor were cocultured for 5 days. The responder cells were then cultured again for 7 days under limiting dilution, and the CTL activity was determined by ^{51}Cr release assay. Data represent the average ± standard deviation of 11 independent experiments using different donor and third party pairs. A significant difference ($P < 0.001$ on the t-test compared with control cultures without CD34 cells) between control cultures and those including CD34 cells was found upon stimulation against donor cells.[44]

This veto activity of CD34$^+$ progenitor cells may be mediated by cells other than the most primitive pluripotential hematopoietic stem cells and, therefore, while it is still very difficult to expand the latter cells *ex vivo*, it has been possible, recently, to expand the veto cells within the CD34$^+$ cell fraction and increase their number by 20–80-fold simply by short term culture along the myeloid differentiation.[44]

More recently, a major mechanism for tolerance induction exerted by several drugs or cell subpopulations involves anergy induction in the responder T cells. Thus, anergy can be induced by a costimulation

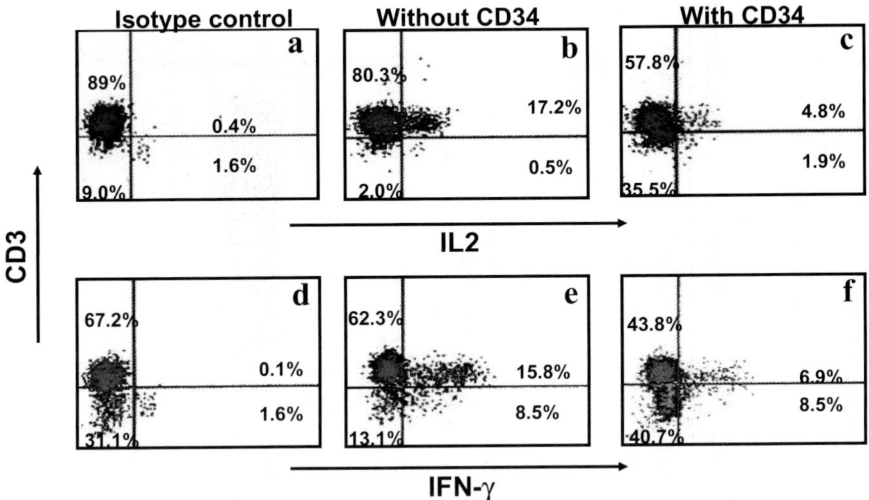

Fig. 7. Regulatory activity of CD34[+] cells: effect on intracellular staining of IL-2 and IFN-γ in the effector T cells. Responder cells and irradiated allogeneic stimulator cells from the CD34[+] cell donor were cocultured for 6 days in the absence or presence of CD34[+] cells (0.5:1 CD34[+] to responder cell). The cells were subjected to an additional 7-day limiting dilution culture. They were then incubated with phorbal myristate acetate, ionomycin and monensin. After that, they were fixed and stained to enable detection of the intracellular IL-2 (a–c) and IFN-γ (d–f). Lymphocytes were gated based on their FSC/SSC profile. The percentage of the gated double positive cells is indicated.[44]

blockade with CTLA4-Ig,[45,46] anti-CD40L,[47,48] or anti-B7[49] antibodies by cytokines such as IL-10[50,51] or by suppressor T cells such as CD4[+]CD25[+] cells.[52–56] In addition, stimulation with APCs of a DC2 subset[57,58] or skewing the T cell response into a Th2 type by the appropriate cytokines, such as IL-4 or IL-10,[59] creates an unfavorable setting for the development of alloreactive CTLs. Our studies, using anti-CD28 mAb or the addition of exogenous IL-2 to bypass the requirement for costimulation via B7, as well as using anti-IL-10-blocking mAbs, have ruled out the possibility that CD34[+] cells induce tolerance by such mechanisms (Table 2).

Furthermore, Gur *et al.*[60] showed that the only effective way to reverse the inhibitory activity of CD34[+] cells was afforded by a caspase

Table 2.   Effect of Different Regulatory Agents on the Inhibitory Activity of CD34[+] Cells[60]

Treatment[*]	MLR Cultures[†]	Number of Responding/ Nonresponding Cultures[‡]		Statistical Significance[§]		
		Responding	Nonresponding	P Value	P Range	Significance
Anti-HLA-1	A	16	0	ND	ND	ND
	B	9	7	0.0004	$P < 0.001$	S
	A[#]	16	0	ND	ND	ND
	D	15	1	0.3016	$P > 0.1$	NS
Anti-IL-10	A	16	0	ND	ND	ND
	B	7	9	5.7E-06	$P < 0.001$	S
	C	16	0	ND	ND	ND
	D	3	13	8.3E-17	$P < 0.001$	S
Anti-CD28[‖]	A	37	11	ND	ND	ND
	B	9	39	3.9E-25	$P < 0.001$	S
	C	30	2	ND	ND	ND
	D	5	43	1.4E-37	$P < 0.001$	S
Anti-CD2	A	6	10	ND	ND	ND
	B	2	14	0.0024	$0.01 > P > 0.001$	S
	C	10	6	ND	ND	ND
	D	1	15	1.4E-20	$P < 0.001$	S
IL-2[¶]	A	27	5	ND	ND	ND
	B	13	19	4.6E-07	$P < 0.001$	S
	C	28	4	ND	ND	ND
	D	10	22	6.6E-12	$P < 0.001$	S

(Continued)

Table 2 *(Continued)*

Treatment[*]	MLR Cultures[†]	Number of Responding/ Nonresponding Cultures[‡]		Statistical Significance[§]		
		Responding	Nonresponding	P Value	P Range	Significance
IL-12[¶]	A	12	20	ND	ND	ND
	B	3	29	4.8E-08	$P < 0.001$	S
	C	31	0	ND	ND	ND
	D	7	25	3.8E-25	$P < 0.001$	S

ND — not done; S — significant; NS — not significant.

[*]The tested regulatory agents were added at the initiation of the MLR to the culture medium, at their optimal concentration, according to the manufacturer's recommendation and to preliminary titration experiments, except for anti-HLA-1. This agent was preincubated with the CD34$^+$ cells and washed prior to their addition to the MLR culture.

[†]MLR cultures in which responder cells were stimulated against allogeneic PBMCs from the CD34$^+$ cells' donor, in the absence (A and C) or presence (B and D) of CD34$^+$ cells, were established.

[‡]The potential of different agents to reverse the inhibitory regulatory activity of CD34$^+$ cells was evaluated by comparing the inhibition in the presence (C and D) and in the absence (A and B) of the specific agent. Briefly, a five-day MLR was established in which the responder cells were then recultured for seven more days under limiting dilution in microtiter plates. For each experiment, the number of positive and of negative cultures, tested at the highest effector cell concentration (40,000 cells per well), are shown. Wells were scored positive for CTL activity when Cr release exceeded the mean spontaneous release value by at least three standard deviations of the mean. The regulatory activity of CD34$^+$ cells was evaluated by their capacity to inhibit alloreactive CTL-p clones in the MLR to which they were added at a ratio of 0.5:1 CD34$^+$/responder cell. The addition of CD34$^+$ cells to the MLR against third-party stimulators did not lead to a significant inhibition ($P > 0.1$). Thus, in a total of five experiments carried out in the absence of CD34$^+$ cells, 3 of 96 anti-third-party MLR culture wells were scored negative while 6 of 96 were scored negative in the presence of CD34$^+$ cells.

[§]The results were statistically analyzed by the x^2 test.

[‖]The results represent a total of three experiments.

[¶]The results represent a total of two experiments.

[#]The role of anti-HLA-1 antibody was tested by incubating the antibody with CD34$^+$ cells prior to their addition to the MLR. Thus, for the statistical analysis of results in culture D we used as a reference the results of culture A.

inhibitor such as BD-FMK, which induces resistance to apoptosis in effector T cells.[60] Collectively, these results strongly supported a deletion-based mechanism similar to that reported for veto CD8 T cells.[61–64]

Two types of veto cells that have been widely characterized are the CD8[+] CTL[64–66] and CD8[+] BM cells.[67–69] In both instances it has been shown that FasL is likely involved in the killing of the effector cells by the veto cells. However, our failure to reverse CD34[+] cell-mediated regulatory activity by anti-Fas antibody led us to investigate the role of other death ligands, such as TNF-α and TGF-β. In contrast to other studies showing that CD2[+]CD3[−]CD8[+]CD16[+] veto cells in the monkey BM mediate their effect through TGF-β, our study indicates that the regulatory activity of CD34[+] cells is likely mediated by TNF-α and not by TGF-β (Fig. 8).

Previous insights into the veto mechanism of CD8[+] veto T cells have indicated that both CD8 and FasL on the veto cells might be required to

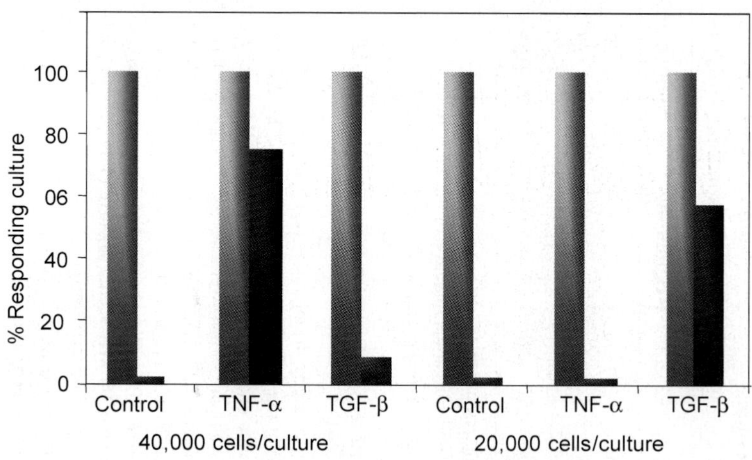

Fig. 8. CD34[+]-cell-mediated suppression of CTL responses is blocked by the addition of anti–TNF-α but not by the addition of anti–TGF-β1. A 5-day MLR was established in which responder cells were stimulated against allogeneic cells from the CD34[+] cell donor, in the presence (*gray*) or absence (*black*) of CD34 cells. Anti–TNF-α or TGF-β1 neutralizing mAbs were added at the beginning of the MLR at a concentration of 5 μg/mL. The CTL activity was determined by the end of 7-day limiting dilution cultures. The data show the percentage of responding cultures at cell concentrations of 4×10^4 and 2×10^4 cells per well.[60]

induce specific deletion of the effector cells.[64,70] Such a mechanism involves initial recognition of the veto cell by the TCR of the effector cell, leading to expression of Fas upon activation and thereby allowing Fas–FasL apoptosis to take place, once inhibitory molecules such as FLICE-inhibitory protein (FLIP) or XIap are downregulated in the effector cell (Fig. 9). The extra affinity required to maintain the interaction between the effector cell and the veto cell might be provided through binding between CD8 on the veto cell and the class I α3 domain on the effector cell, but some form of signaling via this interaction might also occur.[64,70,71]

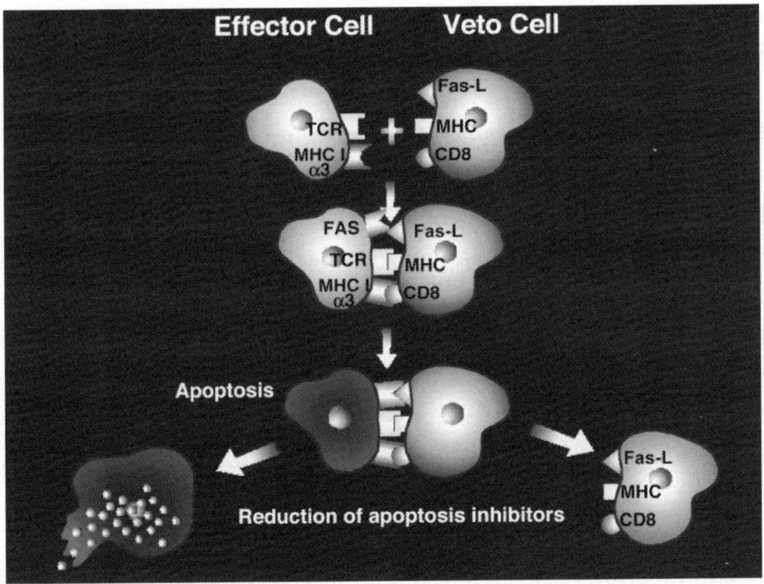

Fig. 9. Veto CTLs induce apoptosis in the effector T cells by the Fas–FasL mechanism. Upon engagement between the TCR of the effector cell and class I of the veto cell, the effector cell is activated and Fas is upregulated. However, the presence of FasL on the veto CTL is not sufficient to trigger apoptosis, as FLIP is also upregulated. The high affinity interaction between the CD8 on the veto cell and the α3 domain on the effector cell likely maintains the contact long enough (60–72 h) for FLIP and other inhibitory molecules to be downregulated, and for Fas–FasL killing to be completed.[71]

Considering that human CD34[+] cells do not express CD8 molecules, our results indicate that the extra affinity afforded by CD8 on CD8[+] veto cells could be provided by other adhesion molecules on the CD34[+] cells. Preliminary results suggest that LFA1–ICAM1 might be involved in this context.

This veto activity of CD34[+] progenitor cells may be mediated by cells other than the most primitive pluripotential hematopoietic stem cells and, therefore, while it is still very difficult to expand the latter cells *ex vivo*, it has been possible, recently, to expand the veto cells within the CD34[+] cell fraction and increase their number by 20–80-fold simply by short term culture along the myeloid differentiation.[44] Furthermore, Gur *et al.* demonstrated that during *ex vivo* differentiation of myeloid cells from CD34[+]CD33[−] hematopoietic stem cells, the veto activity is also exhibited by immature CD34[+]CD33[+] as well as CD34[−]CD3433[+] cells. The veto potential is apparently lost upon completion of maturation at the level of CD14[+] monocytes or CD13[+] neutrophils.

Preliminary results suggest that immature dendritic cells, previously shown to induce immune tolerance (L. Zangi *et al.*, unpublished results), exhibit marked veto activity on CD8 T cells while suppressing CD4 T cells through an MHC-independent mechanism mediated by the NO system.

Finally, NK cells which were shown to exhibit veto activity upon activation with IL-2 were also shown to appear rather early during the posttransplant period.[72,73] Collectively, based on these observations, the following working hypothesis can be suggested. After transplantation of purified CD34 cells, the likelihood of activation of antidonor CTLp is proportional to the level of residual host T cells and is inversely correlated with the number of veto cells. Veto activity can be contributed initially by the CD34 cells infused and subsequently by the CD33 progeny of these cells which grow exponentially within the first few days posttransplant and also include CD11c[+] immature dendritic cells. In addition, when using donors of HLA genotypes, which allow the generation of alloreactive NK cells, such cells can also be generated during the first few days after transplant and eradicate mature CTLs which were able to escape the veto cells and to differentiate into antidonor CTLs. The establishment of the haploidentical graft is therefore greatly dependent not only on the ability of the initial inoculum of the CD34 cells to veto antidonor CTLp, but also on their ability to seed the BM and to generate as rapidly as possible the second or third derivatives which are required to complete the eradication of host antidonor T cells. Clearly, this working hypothesis is consistent with the role of agents that enhance homing of donor stem cells, as well lymphotoxic or myeloablative agents used in preparative regimens prior to transplantation.

A Major Remaining Challenge: Enhancing Immune Reconstitution

The reliable engraftment, in the absence of GvHD, attained by "Megadose" purified CD34 transplants has led to the use of mismatched haploidentical donor cells in thousands of patients with high-risk acute leukemia who urgently need a transplant and who do not have, or cannot find, a matched donor. Indeed, our observed transplant-related mortality (TRM) and event-free survival (EFS) are comparable to those described in patients at the same stage of disease who received transplants from matched unrelated donors.

A major remaining clinical problem is the slow immune recovery of the antimicrobial and antiviral responses. In fact, about 40% of the non-leukemic deaths in more than 250 patients transplanted in Perugia since 2002 were due mainly to bacterial or fungal infections. The incidence of infection-related deaths was linked to the delay in immune reconstitution and to the fact that most patients had a long history of disease, had been heavily pretreated and/or were in relapse at the time of transplant. Indeed, multivariate analyses showed that a history of infections and colonization at transplant were the most significant factors in infection-related deaths. Relatively high infection-related mortality rates and similar patterns of immune reconstitution are common to other T cell-depleted transplants, such as T cell-depleted matched unrelated transplants.[74]

Several mechanisms are responsible for the posttransplant immune deficiency. Tissue damage by conditioning regimens prevents T cell homing to peripheral lymphoid tissues, where generation and maintenance of T cell memory take place. In adults, because thymic function is in decay, early immune recovery stems from expansion of the mature T cells in the graft and, months later, from *de novo* production of naïve T cells. In unmanipulated transplants, peripheral T cell expansion is antagonized by the immune suppressive therapy for GvHD prophylaxis. In T cell-depleted transplants, without any postgrafting immune suppression, homeostatic expansion of the T cells in the graft proceeds undisturbed. However, as the number of T cells has to be extremely low in order to prevent GvHD, immune recovery is inevitably slow.

Current research is focusing on two major approaches, namely investigating potential new agents that can boost thymic function in transplant recipients and adoptive transfer of host nonreactive T cells. The former includes KGF,[75–78] IL7[79] and biochemical ablation of the male sex hormone. The latter can be further divided into *ex vivo*-expanded pathogen-specific T cells[80] or polyclonal expansion of host nonreactive T cells.[71,81–83] Two promising methods currently in clinical trials for generating such cells are photodepletion of T cells found to respond in MLR of donor cells against the host[84] and generation of anti-third-party CTLs under IL2 starvation.[71,81–83]

Another most promising approach based on the preclinical mouse studies of Negrin *et al.*[85–90] is based on the capacity of Treg cells to neutralize the GvH reactivity associated with infusion of donor type T cells. Thus, promising preliminary clinical results have been obtained recently in more than 17 leukemia patients receiving "megadose" CD34 stem cell haploidentical transplants, in conjunction with infusion of 1×10^6 per kg body weight purified T cells and 2×10^6 per kg body weight Treg cells. In particular, these results indicate that the speed of recovery of peripheral donor CD4 and CD8 T cells is markedly enhanced following the infusion of donor T cells, reaching levels similar to those found in matched sibling transplants under a similar time frame. Most importantly, as expected from the mouse studies, GvHD is effectively prevented by the "umbrella" of the Treg cells.

If indeed a long term followup of this approach will confirm these promising results, the road will be open for wide use of haploidentical transplants in acute leukemia patients.

References

1. Thomas ED. (1983) Marrow transplantation for malignant diseases. *J Clin Oncol* **1**: 517–531.
2. Kernan NA, Bartsch G, Ash RC *et al.* (1993) Analysis of 462 transplantations from unrelated donors facilitated by the national marrow donor program. *N Engl J Med* **328**: 593.
3. Champlin R. (1993) Bone marrow transplantation for leukemia utilizing HLA-matched unrelated donors. *Bone Marrow Transplant* **11**(Suppl 1): 74–77.
4. Beatty PG, Mori M, Milford E. (1995) Impact of racial genetic polymorphism on the probability of finding an HLA-matched donor. *Transplantation* **60**: 778–783.
5. Anasetti E, Etzioni R, Petersdorf EW *et al.* (1995) Marrow transplantation from unrelated volunteer donors. *Annu Rev Med* **46**: 169–179.
6. Anasetti C, Beatty PG, Storb R *et al.* (1990) Effect of HLA incompatibility on graft-versus-host disease, relapse, and survival after marrow transplantation for patients with leukemia or lymphoma. *Hum Immunol* **29**: 79–91.
7. Dicke KA, Van Bekkum DW. (1971) Allogeneic bone marrow transplantation after elimination of immunocompetent cells by means of density gradient centrifugation. *Transplant Proc* **3**: 666.
8. Yunis EJ, Good RA, Smith J, Stutman O. (1974) Protection of lethally irradiated mice by spleen cells from neonatally thymectomized mice. *Proc Natl Acad Sci USA* **71**: 2544.
9. Boehmer H, Sprent JMN. (1975) Tolerance to histocompatibility determinants in tetraparental bone marrow chimeras. *J Exp Med* **141**.
10. Reisner Y, Kapoor N, Kirkpatrick D *et al.* (1981) Transplantation for acute leukaemia with HLA-A and B non-identical parental marrow

cells fractionated with soybean agglutinin and sheep red blood cells. *Lancet* **ii**: 327–331.

11. Reisner Y, Kapoor N, Kirkpatrick D *et al.* (1983) Transplantation for severe combined immunodeficiency with HLA-A, B, D, DR incompatible parental marrow cells fractionated by soybean agglutinin and sheep red blood cells. *Blood* **61**: 341–348.

12. Friedrich W, Goldmann SF, Vetter U *et al.* (1984) Immunoreconstitution in severe combined immunodeficiency after transplantation of HLA-haploidentical, T cell-depleted bone marrow. *Lancet* **1**: 761–764.

13. O'Reilly RJ, Brochstein J, Collins N *et al.* (1986) Evaluation of HLA-haplotype disparate parental marrow grafts depleted of T lymphocytes by differential agglutination with a soybean lectin and E-rosette depletion for the treatment of severe combined immunodeficiency. *Vox Sang* **51**(Suppl 2): 81–86.

14. Buckley RH, Schiff SE, Sampson HA *et al.* (1986) Development of immunity in human severe primary T cell deficiency following haploidentical bone marrow stem cell transplantation. *J Immunol* **136**: 2398–2407.

15. Fischer A, Durandy A, de Villartay JP *et al.* (1986) HLA-haploidentical bone marrow transplantation for severe combined immunodeficiency using E rosette fractionation and cyclosporine. *Blood* **67**: 444–449.

16. Reisner Y, Kapoor N, O'Reilly RJ, RA. G. (1980) Allogeneic bone marrow transplantation using stem cells fractionated by lectins: VI. *In vitro* analysis of human and monkey bone marrow cells fractionated by sheep red blood cells and soybean agglutinin. *Lancet* **ii**: 1320.

17. Reisner Y, Kapoor N, Pollack S *et al.* (1983) Use of lectins in bone marrow transplantation. In: Gale RP (ed), *Recent Advances in Bone Marrow Transplantation*. Allan R. Liss, New York, pp. 355–387.

18. O'Reilly RJ. (2004) *Hematopoietic Cell Transplantation* (2nd ed). Blackwell, Malden.

19. Buckley RH, Schiff SE, Schiff RI *et al.* (1999) Hematopoietic stem-cell transplantation for the treatment of severe combined immunodeficiency. *N Engl J Med* **340**: 508–516.

20. Gale RP, Reisner Y. (1986) Graft rejection and graft-versus-host disease: Mirror images. *Lancet* **1**: 1468–1470.

21. Kernan NA, Flomenberg N, Dupont B, O'Reilly RJ. (1987) Graft rejection in recipients of T cell-depleted HLA-nonidentical marrow transplants for leukemia: Identification of host-derived antidonor allocytotoxic T lymphocytes. *Transplantation* **43**: 842–847.

22. Martin PJ. (1990) The role of donor lymphoid cells in allogeneic marrow engraftment. *Bone Marrow Transplant* **6**: 283.

23. Schwartz E, Lapidot T, Gozes D *et al.* (1987) Abrogation of bone marrow allograft resistance in mice by increased total body irradiation correlates with eradication of host clonable T cells and alloreactive cytotoxic precursors. *J Immunol* **138**: 460–465.

24. Terenzi A, Aversa F, Albi N *et al.* (1993) Residual clonable host cell detection for predicting engraftment of T cell depleted BMTs. *Bone Marrow Transplant* **11**: 357–361.

25. Reisner Y, Ben-Bassat I, Douer D *et al.* (1986) Demonstration of clonable alloreactive host T cells in a primate model for bone marrow transplantation. *Proc Natl Acad Sci USA* **83**: 4012–4015.

26. Lapidot T, Terenzi A, Singer TS *et al.* (1989) Enhancement by dimethyl myleran of donor type chimerism in murine recipients of bone marrow allografts. *Blood* **73**: 2025.

27. Lapidot T, Lubin I, Terenzi A *et al.* (1990) Enhancement of bone marrow allografts from nude mice into mismatched recipients by T cells void of graft-versus-host activity. *Proc Natl Acad Sci USA* **87**: 4595–4599.

28. Terenzi A, Lubin I, Lapidot T *et al.* (1990) Enhancement of T cell-depleted bone marrow allografts in mice by thiotepa. *Transplantation* **50**: 717–720.

29. Sheridan WP, Glenn-Begley C, Juttner CA *et al.* (1992) Effect of peripheral-blood progenitor cells mobilised by filgrastin (G-CSF) on platelet recovery after high-dose chemotherapy. *Lancet* **339**: 640–644.

30. Bensinger W, Singer J, Appelbaum F *et al.* (1993) Autologous transplantation with peripheral blood mononuclear cells collected after

administration of recombinant granulocyte stimulating factor. *Blood* **81**: 3158–3163.

31. Aversa F, Tabilio A, Terenzi A *et al.* (1994) Successful engraftment of T cell-depleted haploidentical "three-loci" incompatible transplants in leukemia patients by addition of recombinant human granulocyte colony-stimulating factor-mobilized peripheral blood progenitor cells to bone marrow inoculum. *Blood* **84**: 3948–3955.

32. Reisner Y, Martelli MF. (1995) Bone marrow transplantation across HLA barriers by increasing the number of transplanted cells. *Immunol Today* **16**: 437–440.

33. Lapidot T, Faktorowich Y, Lubin I, Reisner Y. (1992) Enhancement of T cell-depleted bone marrow allografts in the absence of graft-versus-host disease is mediated by $CD8^+$ $CD4^-$ and not by $CD8^-$ $CD4^+$ thymocytes. *Blood* **80**: 2406–2411.

34. Cobbold SP, Martin G, Qin S, Waldmann H. (1986) Monoclonal antibodies to promote marrow engraftment and tissue graft tolerance. *Nature* **323**: 164–166.

35. Strober S, Palathumpat V, Schwadron R, Hertel-Wulff B. (1987) Cloned natural suppressor cells prevent lethal graft-vs-host disease. *J Immunol* **138**: 699–703.

36. Kikuya S, Inaba M, Ogata H *et al.* (1988) Wheat germ agglutinin-positive cells in a stem cell-enriched fraction of mouse bone marrow have potent natural suppressor activity. *Proc Natl Acad Sci USA* **85**: 4824–4826.

37. Tscherning T, Claesson M. (1991) Veto-like down-regulation of T helper cell reactivity *in vivo* by injection of semi-allogeneic spleen cells. *Immunol Lett* **29**: 223–228.

38. Kiyoshi H, Hiruma K, Nakamura H *et al.* (1992) Clonal deletion of postthymic T cells: Veto cells kill precursor cytotoxic T lymphocytes. *J Exp Med.* **175**: 863–868.

39. Pierce GE, Watts LM. (1993) Thy 1+ donor cells function as veto cells in the maintenance of tolerance across a major histocompatibility complex disparity in mixed-lymphoid radiation chimeras. *Transplant Proc* **25**: 331–333.

40. Pierce GE, Watts LM. (1993) Do donor cells function as veto cells in the induction and maintenance of tolerance across an MHC disparity in mixed lymphoid radiation chimeras? *Transplantation* **55**: 882–887.

41. Kaufman CL, Colson YL, Wren SM *et al.* (1994) Phenotypic characterization of a novel bone marrow-derived cell that facilitates engraftment of allogeneic bone marrow stem cells. *Blood* **84**: 2436–2446.

42. Rachamin N, Gan J, Segall H *et al.* (1997) Potential role of CD34 stem cells in tolerance induction. Third International Congress of the Cell Transplant Society. **29**(4): 2255–2256.

43. Miller RG. (1980) An immunological suppressor cell inactivating cytotoxic T-lymphocyte precursor cells recognizing it. *Nature* **287**: 544–546.

44. Gur H, Krauthgamer R, Berrebi A *et al.* (2002) Tolerance induction by megadose hematopoietic progenitor cells: Expansion of veto cells by short-term culture of purified human CD34(+) cells. *Blood* **99**: 4174–4181.

45. Lenschow DJ, Zeng Y, Thistlethwaite JR *et al.* (1992) Long-term survival of xenogeneic pancreatic islet grafts induced by CTLA4lg. *Science* **257**: 789–792.

46. Wekerle T, Kurtz J, Ito H. (2000) Allogeneic bone marrow transplantation with co-stimulatory blockade induces macrochimerism and tolerance without cytoreductive host treatment. *Nat Med* **6**: 464–469.

47. Honey K, Cobbold SP, Waldmann H. (1999) CD40 ligand blockade induces CD4[+] T cell tolerance and linked suppression. *J Immunol* **163**: 4805–4810.

48. Parker DC, Greiner DL, Phillips NE *et al.* (1995) Survival of mouse pancreatic islet allografts in recipients treated with allogeneic small lymphocytes and antibody to CD40 ligand. *Proc Natl Acad Sci USA* **92**: 9560–9564.

49. Judge TA, Wu Z, Zheng XG *et al.* (1999) The role of CD80, CD86, and CTLA4 in alloimmune responses and the induction of long-term allograft survival. *J Immunol* **162**: 1947–1951.

50. Groux H, O'Garra A, Bigler M *et al.* (1997) A CD4$^+$ T cell subset inhibits antigen-specific T cell responses and prevents colitis. *Nature* **389**: 737–742.

51. Groux H, Bigler M, de Vries JE, Roncarolo MG. (1998) Inhibitory and stimulatory effects of IL-10 on human CD8$^+$ T cells. *J Immunol* **160**: 3188–3193.

52. Sakaguchi S, Sakaguchi N, Asano M *et al.* (1995) Immunologic self-tolerance maintained by activated T cells expressing IL-2 receptor alpha-chains (CD25): Breakdown of a single mechanism of self-tolerance causes various autoimmune diseases. *J Immunol* **155**: 1151–1164.

53. Thornton AM, Shevach EM. (1998) CD4$^+$CD25$^+$ immunoregulatory T cells suppress polyclonal T cell activation *in vitro* by inhibiting interleukin 2 production. *J Exp Med* **188**: 287–296.

54. Cederbom L HH, Ivars F. (2000) CD4$^+$CD25$^+$ regulatory T cells down-regulate co-stimulatory molecules on antigen-presenting cells. *Eur J Immunol* **30**: 1538–1543.

55. Levings MK SR, Roncarolo MG. (2001) Human CD25(+)CD4(+) T regulatory cells suppress naive and memory T cell proliferation and can be expanded *in vitro* without loss of function. *J Exp Med* **193**: 1295–1302.

56. Taylor PA, Lees CJ, Blazar BR. (2002) The infusion of *ex vivo* activated and expanded CD4(+)CD25(+) immune regulatory cells inhibits graft-versus-host disease lethality. *Blood* **99**: 3493–3499.

57. Rissoan MC, Soumelis V, Kadowaki N *et al.* (1999) Reciprocal control of T helper cell and dendritic cell differentiation. *Science* **283**: 1183–1186.

58. Arpinati M, Green CL, Heimfeld S *et al.* (2000) Granulocyte-colony stimulating factor mobilizes T helper 2-inducing dendritic cells. *Blood* **95**: 2484–2490.

59. He XY, Chen J, Verma N *et al.* (1998) Treatment with interleukin-4 prolongs allogeneic neonatal heart graft survival by inducing T helper 2 responses. *Transplantation* **65**: 1145–1152.

60. Gur H, Krauthgamer R, Bachar-Lustig E *et al.* (2005) Immune regulatory activity of CD34$^+$ progenitor cells: Evidence for a deletion-based mechanism mediated by TNF-alpha. *Blood* **105**: 2585–2593.

61. Sambhara SR, Miller RG. (1991) Programmed cell death of T cells signaled by the T cell receptor and the alpha 3 domain of class I MHC. *Science* **252**: 1424–1427.

62. Sambhara SR, Miller RG. (1994) Reduction of CTL antipeptide response mediated by CD8$^+$ cells whose class I MHC can bind the peptide. *J Immunol* **152**: 1103–1109.

63. Hiruma K, Nakamura H, Henkart PA, Gress RE. (1992) Clonal deletion of postthymic T cells: Veto cells kill precursor cytotoxic T lymphocytes. *J Exp Med* **175**: 863–868.

64. Reich-Zeliger S, Zhao Y, Krauthgamer R *et al.* (2000) Anti-third party CD8$^+$ CTLs as potent veto cells: Coexpression of CD8 and FasL is a prerequisite. *Immunity* **13**: 507–515.

65. Claesson MH, Miller RG. (1984) Functional heterogeneity in allospecific cytotoxic T lymphocyte clones. I. CTL clones express strong anti-self suppressive activity. *J Exp Med* **160**: 1702–1716.

66. Fink PJ, Rammensee HG, Benedetto JD *et al.* (1984) Studies on the mechanism of suppression of primary cytotoxic responses by cloned cytotoxic T lymphocytes. *J Immunol* **133**: 1769–1774.

67. Verbanac KM, Carver FM, Haisch CE, Thomas JM. (1994) A role for transforming growth factor-beta in the veto mechanism in transplant tolerance. *Transplantation* **57**: 893–900.

68. George JF, Sweeney SD, Kirklin JK *et al.* (1998) An essential role for Fas ligand in transplantation tolerance induced by donor bone marrow. *Nat Med* **4**: 333–335.

69. Goldstein DR, Chang T, Sweeney SD *et al.* (2000) A differential requirement for CD8$^+$ donor cells in the augmentation of allograft survival by posttransplantation administration of donor spleen cells and donor bone marrow cells. *Transplantation* **70**: 1068–1073.

70. Reich-Zeliger S, Gan J, Bachar-Lustig E, Reisner Y. (2004) Tolerance induction by veto CTLs in the TCR transgenic 2C mouse model.

II. Deletion of effector cells by Fas–Fas ligand apoptosis. *J Immunol* **173**: 6660–6666.

71. Reisner Y, Reich-Zeliger S, Bachar-Lustig E. (2006) The role of veto cells in bone marrow transplantation. *Curr Opin Organ Transplant* **11**: 366–372.

72. Reich-Zeliger S, Bachar-Lustig E, Gan J, Reisner Y. (2004) Tolerance induction by veto CTLs in the TCR transgenic 2C mouse model. I. Relative reactivity of different veto cells. *J Immunol* **173**: 6654–6659.

73. Chrobak P, RE G. (2001) Veto activity of activated bone marrow does not require perforin and Fas ligand. *Cell Immunol* **208**: 80.

74. Small TN, Papadopoulos EB, Boulad F *et al.* (1999) Comparison of immune reconstitution after unrelated and related T cell-depleted bone marrow transplantation: Effect of patient age and donor leukocyte infusions. *Blood* **93**: 467–480.

75. Rossi SW, Jeker LT, Ueno T *et al.* (2007) Keratinocyte growth factor (KGF) enhances postnatal T cell development via enhancements in proliferation and function of thymic epithelial cells. *Blood* **109**: 3803–3811.

76. Seggewiss R, Lore K, Guenaga FJ *et al.* (2007) Keratinocyte growth factor augments immune reconstitution after autologous hematopoietic progenitor cell transplantation in rhesus macaques. *Blood* **110**: 441–449.

77. Seggewiss R, HE. (2007) Hematopoietic growth factors including keratinocyte growth factor in allogeneic and autologous stem cell transplantation. *Semin Hematol* **44**: 203–211.

78. Kelly RM, Highfill SL, Panoskaltsis-Mortari A *et al.* (2008) Keratinocyte growth factor and androgen blockade work in concert to protect against conditioning regimen-induced thymic epithelial damage and enhance T cell reconstitution after murine bone marrow transplantation. *Blood* **111**: 5734–5744.

79. Magri M, Yatim A, Benne C *et al.* (2009) Notch ligands potentiate IL-7-driven proliferation and survival of human thymocyte precursors. *Eur J Immunol* **39**: 1231–1240.

80. Li Pira G, Ivaldi F, Tripodi G *et al.* (2008) Positive selection and expansion of cytomegalovirus-specific CD4 and CD8 T cells in sealed systems: Potential applications for adoptive cellular immunoreconstitution. *J Immunother* **31**: 762–770.

81. Bachar-Lustig E, Reich-Zeliger S, Reisner Y. (2003) Anti-third-party veto CTLs overcome rejection of hematopoietic allografts: Synergism with rapamycin and BM cell dose. *Blood* **102**: 1943–1950.

82. Reich-Zeliger S, Bachar-Lustig E, Bar-Ilan A, Reisner Y. (2007) Tolerance induction in presensitized bone marrow recipients by veto CTLs: Effective deletion of host anti-donor memory effector cells. *J Immunol* **179**: 6389–6394.

83. Ophir E, Reisner Y. (2009) Induction of tolerance in organ recipients by hematopoietic stem cell transplantation. *Int Immunopharmacol* **9**: 694–700.

84. Perruccio K, Topini F, Tosti A *et al.* (2008) Photodynamic purging of alloreactive T cells for adoptive immunotherapy after haploidentical stem cell transplantation. *Blood Cells Mol Dis* **40**: 76–83.

85. Edinger M, Hoffmann P, Ermann J *et al.* (2003) CD4(+)CD25(+) regulatory T cells preserve graft-versus-tumor activity while inhibiting graft-versus-host disease after bone marrow transplantation. *Nat Med* **9**: 1144–1150.

86. Ermann J, Hoffmann P, Edinger M *et al.* (2005) Only the CD62L$^+$ subpopulation of CD4$^+$CD25$^+$ regulatory T cells protects from lethal acute GvHD. *Blood* **105**: 2220–2226.

87. Nguyen VH, Shashidhar S, Chang DS *et al.* (2008) The impact of regulatory T cells on T-cell immunity following hematopoietic cell transplantation. *Blood* **111**: 945–953.

88. Negrin RS, Hou JZ. (2007) Promise and challenges of human regulatory T cells in the clinic. *Biol Blood Marrow Transplant* **13**: 12–16.

89. Negrin RS. (2008) Immune regulatory networks in the post-transplant setting. *Blood Cells Mol Dis* **40**: 117–118.

90. Zeiser R, Nguyen VH, Hou JZ *et al.* (2007) Early CD30 signaling is critical for adoptively transferred CD4$^+$CD25$^+$ regulatory T cells in prevention of acute graft-versus-host disease. *Blood* **109**: 2225–2233.

Chapter 2

The Haploidentical Option for High-Risk Hematological Malignancies

Franco Aversa,†, Yair Reisner‡ and Massimo F. Martelli†*

Hematopoietic stem cell transplantation (HSCT) from one-haplotype mismatched donors (HMD) is increasingly being used to treat patients with high-risk acute leukemia who do not have a matched donor. The graft is a megadose of positively/negatively T-cell depleted or unmanipulated progenitor cells. Although haploidentical transplant modalities are based mainly on high intensity conditioning regimens, recently introduced reduced intensity regimens (RIC) showed promise in extending the opportunity of HSCT to an elderly population with more comorbidities. Besides the conditioning regimen and the megadose of stem cells, donor natural killer cell (NK) alloreactivity also plays a role in facilitating engraftment, in reducing graft-vs-host disease (GvHD) and in preventing relapse. Post-transplant immune reconstitution is highly predictive of outcome following T cell-depleted transplantation.

Mismatched/haploidentical transplant provides an alternative approach for patients with high-risk acute leukemia. Overall survival and clinical outcome continue to improve. Future challenges lie in determining the safest preparative conditioning regimen; minimizing GvHD while preserving effective graft-vs-leukemia (GvL) and promoting rapid immune reconstitution.

Introduction

Despite advances in chemotherapy, most adults with acute lymphoblastic leukemia (ALL) or acute myeloid leukemia (AML) relapse and few

*Corresponding author.

†Haematopoietic Stem Cell Transplant Unit, Section of Haematology and Immunology, University of Perugia, Perugia, Italy. E-mail: aversa@unipg.it.

‡Department of Immunology, Weizmann Institute of Science, Rehovot, Israel.

survive, especially when they have unfavorable cytogenetics at diagnosis, when they do not achieve complete remission (CR) after the first induction cycle, and when they are in second or later remission.[1–3]

Under these circumstances, an allogeneic HSCT is preferred as a post-remission therapy.[4–7] However, as only 30% of patients will have a matched sibling to act as a donor, the only other option is transplantation from an alternative donor.

Phenotypically matched unrelated donors are the most widely sought and adopted for allogeneic transplant even though the lapse in time from registering to identifying a donor can lead to disease progression in patients who urgently need a transplant.[8–10]

Unrelated umbilical cord blood transplantation (UCBT) has emerged as a viable option, at least in pediatric patients.[11] It offers the advantages of immediate availability of cryopreserved samples, easy procurement with no risk to the donor, and acceptance of mismatches at two of the six antigens. For adults, however, UCBT are seldom considered because the great divergency between body weight and number of hematopoietic cells in a standard cord blood unit, particularly if associated with a two-antigen mismatch, increases the risk of graft failure and delays hematopoietic reconstitution.[12–14]

Another alternative source of stem cells is the family donor with whom the patient shares one HLA haplotype for HLA-A, B, C and DR but not the other.[15] This donor is immediately available for all transplant candidates, and unlike transplants from other alternative stem cell sources, the haploidentical transplant offers the advantage of another family member who is immediately available as an alternative donor, or even a second graft from the original donor for nearly all patients who reject the graft. Furthermore, any engrafted patients may potentially benefit from future attempts to modulate the cellular environment by delayed infusions of donor cell populations.[16,17]

Unfortunately, in full haplotype mismatched transplants, the high frequency of alloreactive donor T cells in unmanipulated grafts that recognize major histocompatibility (MHC) antigens, is associated with an extremely high incidence of severe, acute GvHD.[18] Although extensive

T cell depletion prevents GvHD the rejection rates rise steeply[19] because the balance between competing host and donor T cells shifts in favor of the unopposed host-vs-graft reaction.

Overcoming HLA-Histocompatibility Barriers

Resistance to engraftment is mainly mediated by recipient anti-donor cytotoxic T-lymphocyte precursors (CTL-p) which survive standard pre-transplant cytoreduction[20,21] and which, donor T cells in unmanipulated transplants eliminate or inactivate. In T cell depleted animal transplant models, the standard dose of total body irradiation (TBI) combined with anti-T monoclonal antibodies or alternatively, a greater dose of TBI, suppresses the residual recipient immune system, thus ensuring engraftment.[21–23] Engraftment is also enhanced when myeloablative drugs (dimethyl-myleran, busulfan or thiotepa) are associated with TBI.[24,25] However, enhancing immunosuppression and myeloablation by adding anti-thymocyte globulin (ATG) and thiotepa to single dose TBI and cyclophosphamide (CY), as we did in leukemia patients in 1992, still did not ensure engraftment of full-haplotype mismatched T cell-depleted bone marrow cells (Aversa *et al.*, unpublished observations).

In the late 1980s, Reisner *et al.* reported escalating doses of T cell-depleted mismatched bone marrow cells were associated with full donor type engraftment in mice that had been presensitized with donor lymphocytes;[9,10,38] in mice whose immune system had been partially reconstituted with graduated numbers of host T cells before the transplant;[38] and in mice pretreated with doses of TBI that spared a substantial number of recipient T lymphocytes.[26–28]

In 1993, we transplanted for the first time a megadose of stem cells in patients with acute leukemia.[29] We added T cell-depleted granulocyte-colony-stimulating-factor (G-CSF)-mobilized peripheral blood progenitor cells (PBPCs) to T cell-depleted bone marrow cells, to increase the number of stem cells in the inoculum to a median of 10.8×10^6 CD34$^+$ cells/kg recipient body weight, which was 10 times the number of CD34$^+$ cells in T cell-depleted bone marrow cells. After T cell depletion with soybean agglutination and E-rosetting, which was the only prophylaxis for GvHD, patients received a median of 2×10^5 CD3$^+$ cells/kg recipient body weight. This first pilot study included 36 mostly adult patients with advanced end-stage acute leukemia who were conditioned with a highly immunosuppressive and myeloablative regimen. Eighty percent achieved primary sustained engraftment and only 18% of evaluable patients developed grade II to IV acute GvHD.

The barrier to engraftment of T cell-depleted mismatched transplants was first overcome in clinical studies through the application of this principle of the megadose of stem cells in combination with an immuno-myelo-ablative pre-transplant conditioning regimen.

A feasible hypothesis is that a megadose of purified CD34$^+$ cells reduces the frequency of occurrence of host anti-donor cytoxic T lymphocyte precursors (CTL-p$_s$) *in vivo.*[30,31] *In vitro* studies show that cells within the CD34$^+$ cell population exhibit "veto" activity, i.e. in bulk mixed lymphocyte reactions they are able to neutralize specific CTL-p$_s$ directed against their antigens but not against a third party.[30–32] Furthermore, early myeloid CD33$^+$ cells (CD34$^+$ and CD34$^-$), harvested 7–12 days after *ex vivo* expansion of CD34$^+$ cells are also endowed with marked veto activity, which is not found in late myeloid cells expressing CD14 or CD11b. Therefore, soon after transplantation, infused CD34$^+$ cells and their CD33$^+$ progeny, which expand exponentially, could inhibit residual anti-donor CTL-p$_s$ in recipients.[30–33]

Since our haplo transplant program started, 112 patients with ALL and 164 with AML have been transplanted from haploidentical donors. Overall, the ages ranged from 2 to 68 years. All these patients were at high risk for post-transplant relapse because 112 were actually in relapse at transplant, 93 were in second or later CR and even the 71 patients in first hematological remission were at high risk because of unfavorable cytogenetics in 36, secondary leukemia in 13, primary induction failure in 14 and high blast count in the remaining 8.

All the patients received a TBI-based conditioning regimen. TBI was given in a single fraction of 8 Gy at an instantaneous dose-rate of 16 cGy per min, with the lungs shielded to receive 4 Gy. Radiation was followed by thiotepa (5 mg/kg for 2 consecutive days) and rabbit anti-thymocyte globulin (ATG) was given at either 25 mg/kg if ATG-Fresenius or 6 mg/kg if Thymoglobuline, always over 5 days. Immunosuppression was enhanced by using cyclophosphamide (40 mg/kg for two consecutive days) in the first 36 patients and fludarabine (40 mg/m^2 for 5 days) in the others. After it had been observed in a murine model that the immunosuppressive effect of TBI + in fludarabine[34] (a drug that was safe widespread use for treatment of lymphoproliferative disorders) was found in a murine model, to be similar to TBI + CY. Consequently, in an attempt to reduce extra-hematological toxicity, fludarabine was substituted for CY in the conditioning protocol in October 1995. No immune suppression was given after transplantation and since 1999, no post-transplant G-CSF was administered[35] (Table 1).

To achieve the ideal graft composition, in 1995, the authors started to positively select CD34$^+$ cells. One-round E-rosetting was followed by positive immunoselection of the CD34$^+$ cells using the Ceprate–SC system (Cell Pro, Bothell, Washington).[36] Since January 1999, CD34$^+$ cells

Table 1.   Haploidentical HSCT Program.

Years	1993–1995	1995–1998	1999→
Patients	36	44	196
Stem cell source	BM and PBPCs	PBPCs only in 29	PBPCs
Graft processing	SBA/E-rosette	CD34$^+$ selection by Cellpros	CD34$^+$ selection by Clinimacs
Conditioning	sTBI-TT-CY-ATG	sTBI-TT-F-ATG	sTBI-TT-F-ATG
G-CSF post-Tx	Yes	Yes	No
Age in years Median (range)	25 (2–51)	24 (4–53)	34 (6–68)
Diseases			
AML	12	21	131
ALL	24	23	65
Disease status			
CR1	—	7	63
CR ≥ 2	18	22	64
Relapse	18	15	69

have been selected in a one-step procedure using the Clinimacs (Miltenyi Biotec, Bergisch Gladbach, Germany) device.[37,38] Automated peripheral blood CD34[+] cell immunoselection for graft processing is time and labor saving and ensures a high CD34[+] cell recovery rate. Besides providing 4.5 log T cell depletion of the graft, it guarantees a 3.5 log B cell depletion, which helps prevent EBV-related lymphoproliferative disorders and autoimmune phenomena.[39]

Clinical Outcomes

a) *Engraftment and GvHD*

Recipients of positively-selected grafts received a median of 12×10^6 CD34[+] cells/kg (range 8–30) and 1.0×10^4 CD3[+] cells/kg (range 0.0–3.0). The donor T cells were significantly higher in the 36 recipients of lectin-separated grafts (medianly 2.2×10^5 CD3[+] cells/kg). The use of bone marrow as a source of stem cells was abandoned in 1996 as sufficent numbers of CD34[+] cells could be collected from G-CSF-mobilized peripheral blood.

Under the protocol that included fludarabine, primary full-donor engraftment was achieved in 96% of patients, which was significantly better as compared with the authors' initial report (Fig. 1a). The shape of the curves changes depending on whether or not G-CSF was given. Rejection was reversed in all but one via transplanting CD34[+] cells from either the same or different donors after immunosuppression with cyclophosphamide (40 mg/kg × 2), rabbit ATG (2.5 mg/kg × 4) and flu-darabine ($40\ \text{mg/m}^2 \times 4$). Thus, 98% of the evaluable patients engrafted with full donor-type chimerism in peripheral blood and in bone marrow were achieved.

ATG in the conditioning regimen persists in plasma for several days after administration[40] and exerts *in vivo* T cell depletion. Together with this, positive selection of peripheral blood cells ensured the number of infused donar T cells was below the threshold dose for GvHD, thus preventing acute and chromic GvHD (Fig. 1b).

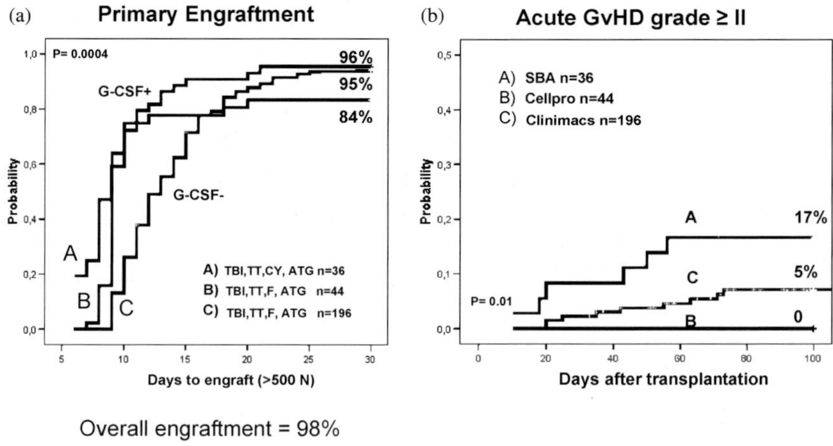

Figure 1. Engraftment and GvHD.

b) *Leukemia Relapse*

The risk of leukemia relapse could be higher in T cell-depleted transplants because of the lack of GvHD-related GvL effect.[41] As the GvL effect is conventionally achieved through T cell-mediated alloreactions directed against histocompatibility antigens displayed on recipient leukemia cells, in the haploidentical transplant setting the need for extensive T cell depletion might have been expected to result in a weak or no GvL effect.

Actually, in the authors' series of high-risk patients, in whom cumulative incidence estimates were used for relapse and TRM (as they are competing risks), relapse rates were lower than might have been expected given the transplant setting and the risk factors. In patients transplanted in remission (Fig. 2a), cumulative incidence of relapse was 0.17 (95% C.I. 0.10–0.26) and 0.27 (95% C.I. 0.17–0.38) in the 97 AML and 67 ALL sub-groups respectively. In the 67 AML and 45 ALL patients who were already in relapse at the transplant (Fig. 2b), the cumulative incidence of relapse rose to 0.34 (95% C.I. 0.22–0.45) and 0.56 (95% C.I. 0.40–0.69), respectively. In this setting, a relapse rate ranging from 0.17 to 0.56 is more than satisfactory and the authors are of the view that the intensely

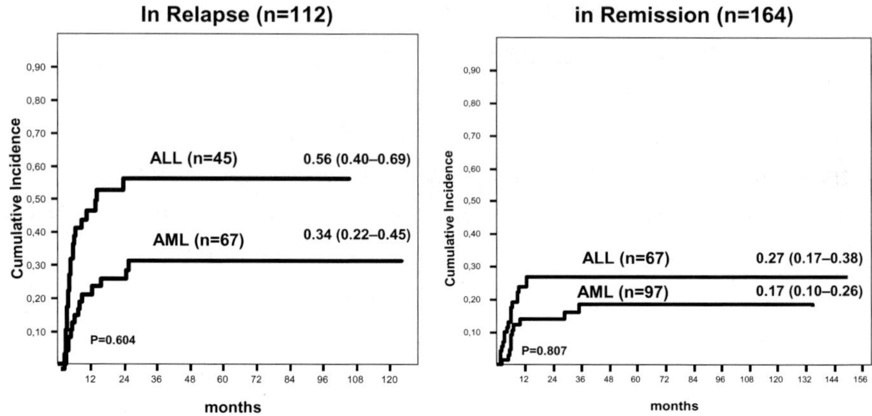

Figure 2. Leukemia relapse.

myeloablative conditioning regimen might have compensated for the lack of T cell-mediated GvL effect. Furthermore, unlike matched transplants, haploidentical transplants can rely on another type of alloreactivity, mediated by natural killer (NK) cells, which is triggered by MHC mismatches between killer cell Ig-like receptors (KIR) on donor NK cells and HLA class I molecules on recipient cells.[42–44]

NK cells have recently been recognized as an effector system which by-passes the obstacles inherent to T cell alloreactivity.[45] Although NK cells were first identified by their ability to kill certain tumor cell lines in the absence of deliberate stimulation *in vitro* or *in vivo*, their nature and the functional mechanisms allowing them to discriminate between tumor and normal cells remained elusive until recent years.[45,46]

NK cells are negatively regulated by clonally distributed inhibitory receptors that are specific for self MHC class I molecules.[47] The lack of engagement of such MHC-specific receptors may result in target cell lysis. Consequently, NK cells kill target cells that have no, or low levels, of MHC class I molecules. In HLA haplotype-mismatched hematopoietic transplantation with a potential for GvH NK-mediated reactions, the engrafted stem cells give rise to an NK cell wave of donor origin which regenerates the same repertoire as the donor's, and so includes high-frequencies of donor-vs-recipient alloreactive NK cells.[42–50] Experimental evidence confirmed NK cells were directly involved in controlling relapse of AML. *In vitro* studies showed myeloid leukemias were killed by alloreactive NK cells but only a minor fraction of common phenotype acute lymphoblastic leukemias were lysed.[43] Indeed, donor-vs-recipient NK cell alloreactivity is associated with a powerful graft-vs-AML effect in patients transplanted in remission, who had an only 3% cumulative incidence of relapse (Fig. 3b). No benefits from NK alloreactivity emerged in patients who were already in relapse at transplantation (Fig. 3a).

One consequence of the haploidentical transplant studies is revision of the current criteria for donor selection. Donor selection for AML now involves a search for the donor who is able to mount donor-vs-recipient NK cell alloreactivity.

NK alloreactivity is determined by HLA-C high-resolution molecular typing and KIR genotyping as well as by functional assessment of donor NK clone repertoire in cytotoxicity assays.[43,51,52] The search for NK alloreactive donors may require extension from the immediate family

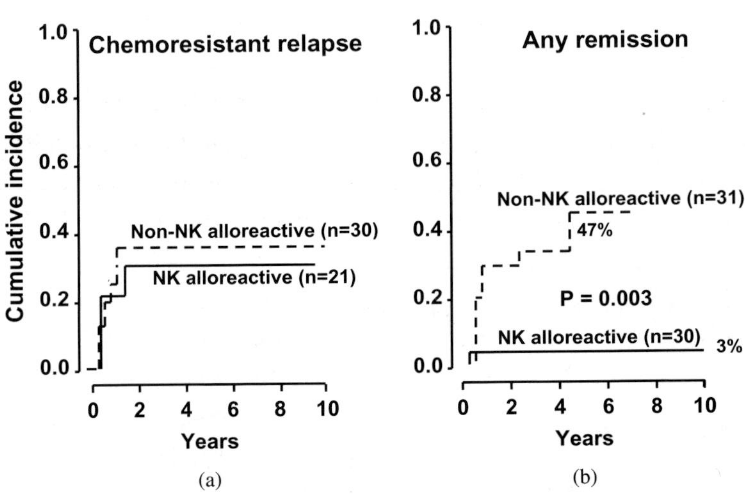

Figure 3.   Leukemia relapse and NK alloreactivity in AML.

(parents and siblings) to other family members such as aunts, uncles and cousins. An extended search raises the chance of finding an NK alloreactive donor from the random 30% to >60%. This approaches the maximum, because one-third of the population blocks NK cells from every donor as they express all three class I groups recognized by KIRs (HLA-C group 1, HLA-C group 2, and HLA-Bw4 alleles).

c) *Non-Leukemic Mortality*

Despite rapid neutrophil recovery, recipients of mismatched transplants tend to remain susceptible to opportunistic infections and, in fact, 75 of the 118 non-leukemic deaths were caused by infections, mainly CMV and aspergillus. The cumulative-incidence estimate of death without relapse was 0.48 (95% C.I. 0.39–0.52) for 164 patients in any CR at transplant; it rose to 0.55 (95% C.I. 0.49–0.62) for 112 patients transplanted in relapse (Fig. 4).

Transplant-related mortality, a major problem in all transplants from alternative sources, depends mainly on slow immunological recovery which increases susceptibility to life-threatening infections.[53] For up to one year after transplant, early immune recovery in adults with

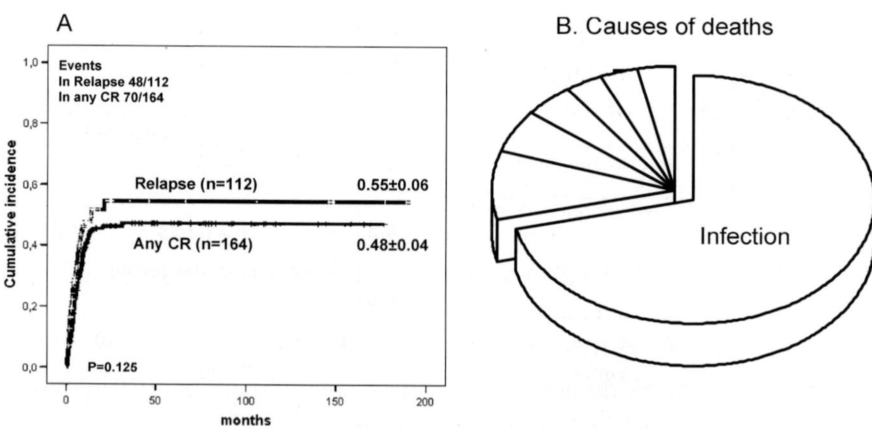

Figure 4.   Transplant-related mortality.

their decayed thymic function, stems from expansion of mature T cells in the graft, and months later, from *de novo* production of naïve T cells. Unfortunately, conditioning-induced tissue damage prevents T cell homing to peripheral lymphoid tissues, where T cell memory is generated and maintained.[54,55] In unrelated donor and cord blood transplants GvHD prophylaxis, GvHD itself and its therapy antagonize T cell expansion and function. In haploidentical transplants, extensive T cell depletion is required to prevent GvHD, so the T cell repertoire is limited and the ATG in the conditioning could delay T cell homeostatic expansion. Another aspect of the post-transplant immune deficiency, which has emerged from recent studies, is the impact of G-CSF in transplant recipients. G-CSF promotes Th-2 immune deviation which, unlike Th-1 responses, does not protect against fungi, bacteria and viruses. As G-CSF blocks IL12 production in antigen presenting cells, it decreases pathogen-specific responses.[56] Patients who do not receive G-CSF after transplant recover $CD4^+$ cell-count faster and most post-transplant $CD4^+$ cell clones exhibit usual Th1-Th0 features.[35]

Any further reduction in TRM will only be achieved by hastening post-transplant immune recovery and several strategies are currently under investigation. Our group in Perugia has initially developed a strategy for transferring donor pathogen-specific immune responses safely across the HLA barrier.[57] Large numbers of donor T cell clones raised against *Aspergillus fumigatus* and *CMV* antigens were screened for cross-reactivity to host alloantigens by MLR. Non-host-reactive clones, presumably devoid of GvHD potential, were pooled and infused into recipients soon after transplant. Untreated patients developed Aspergillus- and CMV-specific T cell responses *in vitro* more than nine months post-transplant. All patients who had received the infusions exhibited Aspergillus- and CMV-specific responses within three weeks, i.e. five weeks post-grafting and no patient developed GvHD. This strategy is labor intensive, and is currently unsuitable for routine clinical use, as cloning and screening procedures do not always satisfy quality controls. Furthermore, as it does not provide wide immune reconstitution, the authors are currently focussing on photoallodepletion of post-transplant T cell infusions.

To date, low doses seem to be safe but inefficacious. With a higher dose, a marked increase in CD4 responses to fungi, starting as early as one month after infusion, has been observed. Also, there was no GvHD.[58]

Another promising approach which was developed in Milan, is post-transplant infusion of TK-transduced donor lymphocytes which are designed to provide wide spectrum immunological reconstitution. The preliminary results of this on-going study show immune recovery is good when TK transduced donor cells engraft. Engrafted TK-cells promote an early immune reconstitution of a wide T cell repertoire and provide protection against CMV reactivation and disease.[59–61]

The London group treated 16 patients with cytomegalovirus lysate-pulsed, monocyte-derived dendritic cells. In eight cases viral titers decreased within five days and antiviral drug therapy was not required. A low incidence of late CMV reactivation (2/14 evaluable patients vs 45/72 historical controls, $p = 0.001$) and no significant toxicities were observed. HCMV-specific cytotoxic T lymphocytes (3–5 log) expanded *in vivo* within days of adoptive transfer and T-cell receptor CDR3 lengths were identical to those of the transferred cells.[62]

Encouraging results were achieved in other centers using *ex vivo*-expanded EBV-specific allogeneic CTL clones to prevent or manage EBV-associated diseases, including post-transplant lymphoproliferative disorders.[63]

All these approaches show that cell therapy is feasible after haploidentical transplantation and that it may help re-build immunity to infections.

d) *Event-Free Survival*

Estimates of EFS obtained by the authors show that outcomes are extremely poor in patients who are transplanted in chemoresistant relapse. However, 18% EFS for advanced AML patients that has been achieved is really quite good, considering that there were no other options beyond the haplo-transplant.

The 4-year EFS ranged from 30% in ALL to 43% in AML in patients who were transplanted in any CR (Fig. 4). These results compare favorably with the register reports on the same categories of patients.[64–68]

In AML patients, EFS improved significantly when the patients with the same disease status at transplant received grafts from NK alloreactive donors. It rose to a remarkable 67% when the recipients of grafts from NK alloreactive donors were in remission at transplant (Fig. 5a). Even patients with AML in chemo-resistant relapse benefit from haploidentical transplantation from NK alloreactive donors. Although the relapse rates and the incidence of GvHD were similar whether donors were NK alloreactive or not, the 30% event-free survival in relapsing patients transplanted from NK alloreactive donors was much better than the 6% survival in the others (Fig. 5b).

Multivariate analysis confirmed that transplantation from an NK alloreactive donor is a strong independent good prognosis factor. In analyzing all AML patients transplanted from non-NK alloreactive vs NK alloreactive donors, while no effect of transplantation from an NK alloreactive donor could be discerned in the first six months post-transplant (relative risk vs non-NK alloreactive donor: 0.95 [95% CI 0.61–1.92],

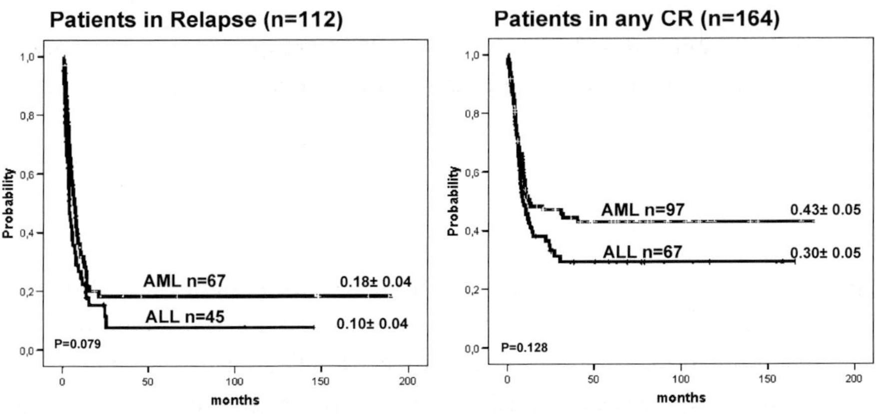

Figure 5. Event-free survival.

$P = N.S.$), patients surviving longer than six months after transplant had a highly reduced risk of relapse or death when transplanted from an NK alloreactive donor (relative risk vs non-alloreactive donor 0.07 [95% CI 0.02–0.26], $P < 0.001$). The only other prognostically significant pre-transplant variable emerging from multivariate analyses was disease status at time of transplant, with a relative risk of 2.37 for patients transplanted in relapse vs patients transplanted in remission.

In the survivors, the quality of life is excellent as all have a 100% PS from 8 to 12 months post-transplant onwards. The major factor determining such good quality of life is lack of immunosuppressive therapy and the minimal incidence of chronic GvHD.

Haploidentical SCT Based on Feto-Maternal Microchimaerism

Several groups have developed haploidentical stem cell transplant strategies based on the principle of tolerance induction as the result of *in utero* exposure to maternal antigens and the development of long-lasting fetomaternal microchimerism.[69–71] A large International Bone Marrow Transplantation Registry analysis by van Rood *et al.*[72] showed that the incidence of grades II–IV acute GvHD following non-T-cell-depleted haploidentical SCT was related to haplotype inheritance. Transplants from a non-inherited maternal antigen (NIMA) mismatched sibling were associated with significantly less acute GvHD.

In a retrospective analysis, we investigated the probability of event free survival (EFS), and the cumulative incidences of relapse mortality, TRM, GvHD and rejection in 118 consecutive patients transplanted, after T cell depletion of the graft, from either the father or the mother, in two centers (Division of Hematology, University of Perugia and Pediatric Hematology/Oncology, University of Pavia) between 1993 and 2006 for acute myeloid and lymphoblasitc leukemia (AML, ALL).[73] A cohort of 79 patients receiving transplantation from a haploidentical sibling donor during the same period of time, using the same transplantation protocol, served as controls.

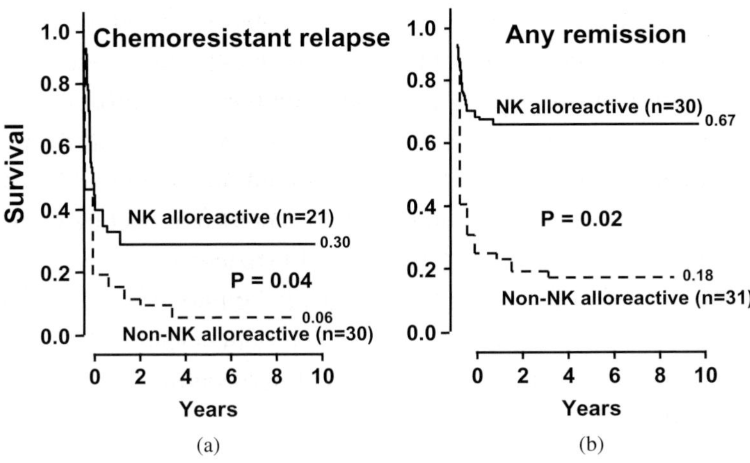

Figure 6. EFS and NK alloreactivity in AML.

The probability of EFS at five years of patients transplanted from maternal donors was 50.6% ±7% as compared to 11.1% ± 4% for patients transplanted from paternal donors ($p < 0.0001$, Fig. 6a), the unadjusted hazard ratio being 2.56 (95% confidence interval 1.60–4.00). The survival advantage in maternal transplant recipients was observed in both ALL ($N = 67$, 5-year EFS of 45.8% ± 10% vs 13.1% ± 6% [$p = 0.10$]) and AML ($N = 51$, 5-year EFS 55.3% ± 11% vs 7.5% ± 5% [$p < 0.001$], respectively). The benefit of having the mother as donor was more evident for patients transplanted in remission ($N = 67$, 5-year EFS 62.0% ± 9% vs 12.6% ± 7%, $p = 0.004$) than for those in chemoresistant disease ($N = 51$, 5-year EFS 24.2% ± 12% vs 9.6% ± 5%, $p = 0.38$).

These data strongly suggest further studies are warranted to determine whether donor gender should be incorporated into donor selection criteria in haplotype mismatched parent-to-child HSCT.

Conclusions

The high rejection rate and incidence of severe GvHD which prevented the haploidentical transplant from being clinically feasible have been overcome through a combination of high intensity conditioning and a megadose of stem cells. In adult patients with high risk acute leukemia, outcomes after mismatched transplant from family members are better than after conventional maintenance chemotherapy as long as the patients are transplanted before their disease becomes refractory. Exploiting donor-vs-recipient NK cell alloreactivity has helped to capture an optimal GvL effect without GvHD. The only drawback at present with the haploidentical transplant is the high incidence of infection-related mortality and in fact, all current on-going experimental studies are aimed at improving post-transplant immunological reconstitution. There is no doubt that once this aim is achieved, physicians will be less hesitant to recommend the mismatched hematopoietic stem cell transplant as a routine option rather than a last resort, in the early stages of high risk acute leukemia patients.

Unfortunately, the choice of the best alternative source of stem cells for individual patients without matched sibling donors is hampered by the lack of randomized studies supplying data on outcomes after MUD, UCB, and haploidentical transplants.

Designing such a study is difficult because, at present, allocation of a patient to one of these three options could reflect a transplant center's preferential use of a particular transplant modality rather than selection of the best donor for each individual patient.

References

1. Byrd JC, Mrozek K, Dodge RK *et al.* (2002) Pretreatment cytogenetic abnormalities are predictive of induction success, cumulative incidence of relapse, and overall survival in adult patients with *de novo* acute myeloid leukemia: results from Cancer and Leukemia Group B (CALGB 8461). *Blood* **100**: 4325–4336.
2. Hoelzer D, Gokbuget N, Ottmann O *et al.* (2002) Acute lymphoblastic leukemia. *Hematology* (Am Soc Hematol Educ Program), pp. 162–192.

3. Litzow MR. (2007) Progress and strategies for patients with relapsed and refractory acute myeloid leukemia. *Curr Opin Hematol* **14**(2): 130–137.

4. Burnett AK, Wheatley K, Goldstone AH *et al.* (2002) The value of allogeneic bone marrow transplant in patients with acute myeloid leukaemia at differing risk of relapse: Results of the UK MRC AML 10 trial. *Br J Haematol* **118**: 385–400.

5. Biggs JC, Horowitz MM, Gale RP *et al.* (1992) Bone marrow transplants may cure patients with acute leukemia never achieving remission with chemotherapy. *Blood* **80**: 1090–1093.

6. Forman SJ, Schmidt GM, Nademanee AP *et al.* (1991) Allogeneic bone marrow transplantation as therapy for primary induction failure for patients with acute leukemia. *J Clin Oncol* **9**: 1570–1574.

7. Lodewyck T, Cornelissen JJ. (2008) Allogeneic stem cell transplantation in acute myeloid leukemia: A risk-adapted approach. *Blood Rev* **22**(6): 293–302.

8. Petersdorf EW. (2008) Optimal HLA matching in hematopoietic cell transplantation. *Curr Opin Immunol* **20**(5): 588–593.

9. Madrigal A, Shaw BE. (2008) Immunogenetic factors in donors and patients that affect the outcome of hematopoietic stem cell transplantation. *Blood Cells Mol Dis* **40**(1): 40–43.

10. Lee SJ, Klein J, Haagenson M *et al.* (2007) High-resolution donor-recipient HLA matching contributes to the success of unrelated donor marrow transplantation. *Blood* **110**(13): 4576–4583.

11. Takahashi S. (2007) Leukemia: Cord blood for allogeneic stem cell transplantation. *Curr Opin Oncol* **19**(6): 667–672. Review.

12. Sanz MA, Sanz GF. (2002) Unrelated donor umbelical cord blood transplantation in adults. *Leukemia* **16**: 1984–1991.

13. Rocha V, Labopin M, Sanz G *et al.* (2004) Transplants of umbilical cord blood or bone marrow from unrelated donors in adult with leukemia. *N Engl J Med* **351**: 2276–2285.

14. Brunstein CG, Setubal DC, Wagner JE. (2007) Expanding the role of umbilical cord blood transplantation. *Br J Haematol* **137**(1): 20–35.

15. Henslee-Downey PJ, Abhyankar SH, Parrish RS *et al.* (1987) Use of partially mismatched related donors extends access to allogeneic marrow transplant. *Blood* **89**: 3864–3872.

16. Kang Y, Chao NJ, Aversa F. (2008) Unmanipulated or CD34 selected haplotype mismatched transplants. *Curr Opin Hematol* **15**(6): 561–567. Review.

17. Symons HJ, Fuchs EJ. (2008) Hematopoietic SCT from partially HLA-mismatched (HLA-haploidentical) related donors. *Bone Marrow Transplant* **42**(6): 365–377.

18. Anasetti C, Beatty PG, Storb R *et al.* (1990) Effect of HLA incompatibility on graft-versus-host disease, relapse, and survival after marrow transplantation for patients with leukemia or lymphoma. *Hum Immunol* **29**: 79–91.

19. Kernan NA, Flomenberg N, Dupont B, O'Reilly RJ. (1987) Graft rejection in recipients of T-depleted HLA-nonidentical marrow transplants for leukemia: Identification of host-derived anti-donor allocytotoxic T lymphocytes. *Transplantation* **43**: 842–847.

20. Reisner Y, Ben-Bassat I, Douer D *et al.* (1986) Demonstration of clonable alloreactive host T cells in a primate model for bone marrow transplantation. *Proc Natl Acad Sci USA* **83**: 4012–4015.

21. Schwartz E, Lapidot T, Gozes D *et al.* (1987) Abrogation of bone marrow allograft resistance in mice by increased total body irradiation correlates with eradication of host clonable T-cells and alloreactive cytotoxic precursors. *J Immunol* **138**: 460–465.

22. Lapidot T, Singer TS, Salomon O *et al.* (1988) Booster irradiation to the spleen following total body irradiation: A new immunosuppressive approach for allogeneic bone marrow transplantation. *J Immunol* **141**: 2619–2624.

23. Cobbold SP, Martin G, Quin S, Waldman H. (1986) Monoclonal antibodies to promote marrow engraftment and tissue graft tolerance. *Nature* **323**: 164–166.

24. Lapidot T, Terenzi A, Singer TS *et al.* (1989) Enhancement by dimethyl myleran of donor type chimerism in murine recipients of bone marrow allografts. *Blood* **73**: 2025–2032.

25. Terenzi A, Lubin I, Lapidot T *et al.* (1990) Enhancement of T-cell-depleted bone marrow allografts in mice by thiotepa. *Transplantation* **50**: 717–720.

26. Reisner Y. (1990) Engraftment of T-cell-depleted bone marrow in murine models for allogeneic bone marrow transplantation. *Cancer Treat Res* **50**: 9–25.

27. Bachar-Lusting E, Rachamim N, Li HW *et al.* (1995) Megadose of T cell-depleted bone marrow overcomes MHC barriers in sublethally irradiated mice. *Nat Med* **1**: 1268–1273.

28. Reisner Y, Martelli MF. (1999) Stem cell escalation enables HLA-disparate haematopoietic transplants in leukaemia patients. *Immunol Today* **20**(8): 343–347. Review.

29. Aversa F, Tabilio A, Terenzi A *et al.* (1994) Successful engraftment of T-cell-depleted haploidentical "three-loci" incompatible transplants in leukemia patients by addition of recombinant human granulocyte colony-stimulating factor-mobilized peripheral blood progenitor cells to bone marrow inoculum. *Blood* **84**: 3948–3955.

30. Rachamin N, Gan J, Segall R *et al.* (1998) Tolerance induction by "megadose" hematopoietic transplants: Donor-type human CD34 stem cells induce potent specific reduction of host anti-donor cytotoxic T lymphocyte precursors in mixed lymphocyte culture. *Transplantation* **65**: 1386–1393.

31. Martelli MF, Aversa F, Bachar-Lusting E *et al.* (2002) Transplants across human leukocyte antigen barriers. *Semin Hematol* **39**(1): 48–56.

32. Gur H, Krauthgamer R, Berrebi A *et al.* (2002) Tolerance induction by megadose hematopoietic progenitor cells: Expansion of veto cells by short-term culture of purified human CD34(+) cells. *Blood* **99**: 4174–4181.

33. Gur H, Krauthgamer R, Bachar-Lustig E *et al.* (2005) Immune regulatory activity of CD34+ progenitor cells: Evidence for a deletion-based mechanism mediated by TNF-alpha. *Blood* **105**(6): 2585–2593.

34. Terenzi A, Aristei C, Aversa F *et al.* (1996) Efficacy of fludarabine as an immunosuppressor for bone marrow transplantation conditioning: Preliminary results. *Transplant Proc* **28**: 3101.

35. Volpi I, Perruccio K, Tosti A *et al.* (2001) Post-grafting granulocyte colony-stimulating factor administration impairs functional immune recovery in recipients of HLA haplotype-mismatched hematopoietic transplants. *Blood* **97**: 2514–2521.

36. Aversa F, Tabilio A, Velardi A *et al.* (1998) Treatment of high risk acute leukemia with T-cell-depleted stem cells from related donors with one fully mismatched HLA haplotype. *N Engl J Med* **339**: 1186–1193.

37. Aversa F. (2002) Hematopoietic stem cell transplantation from full-haplotype mismatched donors. *Transfus Apher Sci* **27**(2): 175–181. Review.

38. Aversa F, Terenzi A, Tabilio A *et al.* (2005) Full-haplotype mismatched hematopoietic stem cell transplantation: A phase II study in patients with acute leukemia at high risk or relapse. *J Clin Oncol* **23**: 3447–3454.

39. Liu D, Tammik C, Zou JZ *et al.* (2004) Effect of combined T- and B-cell depletion of allogeneic HLA-mismatched bone marrow graft on the magnitude and kinetics of Epstein-Barr virus load in the peripheral blood of bone marrow transplant recipients. *Clin Transplant* **18**(5): 518–524.

40. Waller EK, Langston AA, Lonial S *et al.* (2003) Pharmacokinetics and pharmacodynamics of anti-thymocyte globulin in recipients of partially HLA-matched blood hematopoietic progenitor cell transplantation. *Biol Blood Marrow Transplant* **9**(7): 460–471.

41. Marmont AM, Horowitz MM, Gale RP *et al.* (1991) T-cell depletion of HLA-identical transplants in leukemia. *Blood* **78**: 2120–2130.

42. Ruggeri L, Capanni M, Casucci M *et al.* (1999) Role of natural killer cell alloreactivity in HLA-mismatched hematopoietic stem cell transplantation. *Blood* **94**: 333–339.

43. Ruggeri L, Capanni M, Urbani E *et al.* (2002) Effectiveness of donor natural killer cell alloreactivity in mismatched hematopoietic transplants. *Science* **295**: 2097–2100.

44. Velardi A, Ruggeri L, Moretta A, Moretta L. (2002) NK cells: A lesson from mismatched hematopoietic transplantation. *Trends Immunol* **23**: 438–444.

45. Parham P. (2005) MHC class I molecules and KIRs in human history, health and survival. *Nat Rev Immunol* **5**: 201–214.

46. Yawata M, Yawata N, Draghi M *et al.* (2006) Roles for HLA and KIR polymorphisms in natural killer cell repertoire selection and modulation of effector function. *J Exp Med* **203**: 633–645

47. Moretta L, Moretta A. (2004) Killer immunoglobulin-like receptors. *Curr Opin Immunol* **16**: 626–633.

48. Ruggeri L, Mancusi A, Capanni M *et al.* (2007) Donor natural killer cell allorecognition of missing self in haploidentical hematopoietic transplantation for acute myeloid leukemia: Challenging its predictive value. *Blood* **110**: 433–440.

49. Ruggeri L, Aversa F, Martelli MF, Velardi A. (2006) Haploidentical transplantation and natural killer cell recognition of missing self. *Immunol Rev* **214**: 202–218.

50. Ruggeri L, Mancusi A, Burchielli E *et al.* (2007) Natural killer cell alloreactivity in allogeneic hematopoietic transplantation. *Curr Opin Oncol* **19**(2): 142–147.

51. Ruggeri L, Capanni M, Mancusi A *et al.* (2004) Natural killer cells as a therapeutic tool in mismatched transplantation. *Best Pract Res Clin Haematol* **17**(3): 427–38.

52. Leung W, Iyengar R, Turner V *et al.* (2004) Determinants of antileukemia effects of allogeneic NK cells. *J Immunol* **172**: 644–650.

53. Ochs L, Ou Shu X, Miller J *et al.* (1995) Late infections after allogeneic bone marrow transplantation: Comparison of incidence in related and unrelated donor transplant recipients. *Blood* **86**: 3979–3986.

54. Dumont-Girard F, Roux E, van Lier RA *et al.* (1998) Reconstitution of the T-cell compartment after bone marrow transplantation: Restoration of the repertoire by thymic emigrants. *Blood* **92**: 4464–4471.

55. Heitger A, Greinix H, Mannhalter C *et al.* (2000) Requirement of residual thymus to restore normal T-cell subsets after human allogeneic bone marrow transplantation. *Transplantation* **69**: 2366–2373.

56. Pan L, Delmonte J Jr, Jalonen CK *et al.* (1995) Pretreatment of donor mice with granulocyte colony-stimulating factor polarizes donor T lymphocytes toward type-2 cytokine production and reduces severity of experimental graft-versus-host disease. *Blood* **86**: 4422–4429.

57. Perruccio K, Tosti A, Burchielli E *et al.* (2005) Transferring functional immune responses to pathogens after haploidentical hematopoietic transplantation. *Blood* **106**: 4397–4406.

58. Perruccio K, Topini F, Tosti A *et al.* (2008) Photodynamic purging of alloreactive T cells for adoptive immunotherapy after haploidentical stem cell transplantation. *Blood Cells Mol Dis* **40**(1): 76–83.

59. Marktel S, Magnani Z, Ciceri F *et al.* (2003) Immunologic potential of donor lymphocytes expressing a suicide gene for early immune reconstitution after hematopoietic T-cell-depleted stem cell transplantation. *Blood* **101**(4): 1290–1298.

60. Ciceri F, Bonini C, Gallo-Stampino C, Bordignon C. (2005) Modulation of GvHD by suicide-gene transduced donor T lymphocytes: Clinical applications in mismatched transplantation. *Cytotherapy* **7**(2): 144–149.

61. Traversari C, Marktel S, Magnani Z *et al.* (2007) The potential immunogenicity of the TK suicide gene does not prevent full clinical benefit associated with the use of TK-transduced donor lymphocytes in HSCT for hematologic malignancies. *Blood* **109**(11): 4708–4715.

62. Peggs KS, Mackinnon S. (2004) Augmentation of virus-specific immunity after hematopoietic stem cell transplantation by adoptive T-cell therapy. *Hum Immunol* **65**(5): 550–557.

63. Comoli P, Basso S, Zecca M *et al.* (2007) Preemptive therapy of EBV related lymphoproliferative disease after pediatric haploidentical stem cell transplantation. *Am J Transplant* **7**(6): 1648–1655.

64. Sierra J, Storer B, Hansen JA *et al.* (2000) Unrelated donor marrow transplantation for acute myeloid leukemia: An update of the Seattle experience. Bone Marrow Transplant **26**: 397–404.

65. Cornelissen JJ, Carston M, Kollman C *et al.* (2001) Unrelated marrow transplantation for adult patients with poor-risk acute lymphoblastic leukemia: Strong graft-versus-leukemia effect and risk factors determining outcome. *Blood* **97**: 1572–1577.

66. Laughlin MJ, Barker J, Bambach B *et al.* (2001) Hematopoietic engraftment and survival in adult recipients of umbilical-cord blood from unrelated donors. *N Engl J Med* **344**: 1815–1822.

67. Ottinger HD, Ferencik S, Beelen DW *et al.* (2003) Hematopoietic stem cell transplantation: Contrasting the outcome of transplantations from HLA-identical siblings, partially HLA-mismatched related donors, and HLA-matched unrelated donors. *Blood* **102**: 1131–1137.

68. Cairo MS, Rocha V, Gluckman E *et al.* (2008) Alternative allogeneic donor sources for transplantation for childhood diseases: Unrelated cord blood and haploidentical family donors. *Biol Blood Marrow Transplant* **14**(1 Suppl 1): 44–53.

69. Ichinohe T, Uchiyama T, Shimazaki C *et al.* (2004) Feasibility of HLA-haploidentical hematopoietic stem cell transplantation between noninherited maternal antigen (NIMA)-mismatched family members linked with long-term fetomaternal microchimerism. *Blood* **104**: 3821–3828.

70. Yoshihara T, Morimoto A, Inukai T *et al.* (2004) Non-T-cell-depleted HLA haploidentical stem cell transplantation based on feto-maternal microchimerism in pediatric patients with advanced malignancies. *Bone Marrow Transplant* **34**: 373–375.

71. Obama K, Takemoto Y, Takatsuka Y, Utsunomiya A. (2004) Successful reduced-intensity HLA-haploidentical stem cell transplantation based

on the concept of feto-maternal tolerance for an elderly patient with myelodysplastic syndrome. *Bone Marrow Transplant* **33**: 253.

72. van Rood JJ, Loberiza FR Jr, Zhang MJ *et al.* (2002) Effect of tolerance to noninherited maternal antigens on the occurrence of graft-versus-host disease after bone marrow transplantation from a parent or an HLA-haploidentical sibling. *Blood* **99**(5): 1572–1577.

73. Stern M, Ruggeri L, Mancusi A *et al.* (2008) Survival after T cell-depleted haploidentical stem cell transplantation is improved using the mother as donor. *Blood* **112**(7): 2990–2995.

Haploidentical Allogeneic Hematopoietic Cell Transplantation in Adults Using CD3/CD19 Depletion and Reduced Intensity Conditioning

*Wolfgang A. Bethge**

Introduction

Allogeneic hematopoietic cell transplantation (HCT) is the only curative treatment modality for a variety of hematological and non-hematological diseases. However, only for 25% of patients, a suitable matched related donor, and for up to 70% of patients, a matched unrelated donor, respectively, can be found.[1] In ethnical minorities or if the aggressive course of the disease requires fast identification of a suitable donor, donor search can be even more difficult. A successful strategy for haploidentical HCT would eliminate the "lacking donor" problem, since virtually every patient has a potentially suitable haploidentical related donor among parents, children or relatives.

Historically, haploidentical HCT was complicated by a high incidence of engraftment failure, GVHD, and infectious complications, resulting in an unacceptably high treatment-related morbidity and mortality.[2] Graft rejection and GVHD are primarily mediated by host and donor T cells. Attempts to overcome the HLA-barrier were therefore

---

*Medical Center University of Tuebingen, Hematology/Oncology, Otfried-Mueller Str. 10, 72076 Tuebingen, Germany, e-mail: wolfgang.bethge@med.uni-tuebingen.de.

focused on strategies of effective host and graft T cell depletion. But even after effective T cell depletion, the success rate of haploidentical HCT remained dismal. This changed with the observation of a group of investigators in Italy and Israel that successful engraftment over major HLA-barriers is feasible using high doses of T cell-depleted peripheral blood stem cells. In 1995, Bachar-Lustig *et al.* showed in mice[3] that the rejection of T cell-depleted bone marrow cells can be overcome by increasing the stem cell dose four- or five-fold to a "megadose" of $CD34^+$ cells. Simultaneously, first clinical trials evaluating such an approach were started 1993 by Aversa *et al.* in Perugia after the harvest of megadoses (i.e. $>10 \times 10^6$ $CD34^+$ cells/kg) of stem cells in man was made possible due to the availability of hematopoietic growth factors.[4] In 1998, Aversa *et al.* reported their experience with HCT in 43 patients transplanted with stem cells from haploidentical sibling donors for treatment of advanced acute leukemia.[5] In Chapter 1 of this book, Aversa *et al.* give an udpated account of their experience with haploidentical HCT in patients with advanced acute leukemia. Intensive conditioning with total-body irradiation, thiotepa, fludarabine, and antithymocyte globulin was used, followed by a graft of a megadose of $CD34^+$ immunoselected peripheral blood progenitor cells. The strategy allows successful haploidentical HCT with a low rate of GVHD (<10%) and a promising event-free survival of 47% at two years for patients transplanted in complete remission. For patients transplanted in relapse, however, EFS remained at only a dismal 4%, mainly due to relapse.[6] The Perugia group was also able to demonstrate the important role of NK cells in the haploidentical setting. Ruggeri *et al.* described the potency of NK-alloreactivity determined by the "missing-self" recognition in a mouse model and also in the clinical setting of haploidentical HCT.[7] In a recent update of their experience of haploidentical HCT in AML, they demonstrated an increase from 18% to 67% EFS if a haploidentical graft from a NK-alloreactive donor is used.[8] Therefore, NK-alloreactive haploidentical HCT might be especially suited for patients with high risk AML even in case of relapse after a preceding HCT.

Since then, promising data have been published by several groups using "megadoses" of CD34-selected stem cells, together with high dose conditioning for haploidentical HCT.[4–7,9–15] In order to overcome the engraftment barrier, most regimens for haploidentical HCT are based on intensive myeloablative conditioning regimens with either single fraction total body irradiation combined with fludarabine or cyclophosphamide and thiothepa or other TBI or busulfan-based protocols. These toxic conditioning regimens exclude elderly, comorbid or heavily pretreated patients from this treatment strategy. Non relapse mortality (NRM) with 35–40% is high, even in younger, fit patients. The main reasons for NRM are infections or regimen-related toxicities.[6] Improvements are also warranted for the high incidence of relapse in patients not in CR at the time of HCT.[6,16,17] As a crucial prerequisite for successful haploidentical HCT, a "megadose" ($>10 \times 10^6$ CD34$^+$ cells/kg) of CD34-selected stem cells was postulated, which can easily be achieved in children but can be a major obstacle in adults. At doses below 10×10^6 CD34$^+$ cells/kg rate of rejection increases and kinetics of engraftment and immune-reconstitution are delayed. Slow engraftment was particularly observed in patients receiving less than 8×10^6 CD34$^+$/kg.[16]

Haplo RIC Using CD3/CD19-depleted Grafts

Studies at the University of Tübingen Medical Center are therefore aimed at strategies to improve engraftment in order to allow successful haploidentical HCT in adults, even with CD34-doses below 8×10^6 CD34$^+$/kg. To enable haploidentical HCT in elderly, comorbid or heavily pretreated patients, a reduced-intensity conditioning regimen was chosen. Based on the notion that grafts depleted of T- and B cells, in contrast to CD34 selection, may contain significantly more graft facilitating cells such as NK cells, monocytes and granulocytes in addition to CD34$^+$ stem cells, it was hypothesized that this may improve engraftment and immune reconstitution. Recent studies have revealed the existence of CD34$^-$ stem cells with repopulating capacity which are likely precursors of CD34$^+$ stem cells.[18] Graft facilitating cells such as CD8$^+$ T cells, but also NK cells, monocytes and antigen-presenting cells (APCs) have been defined.[19–24] It was also shown that $CD34^+$ stem cells themselves have immunoregulatory properties.[25,26] However, profound T cell and B cell depletion is thought to be a fundamental prerequisite for haploidentical HCT to avoid severe GVHD and EBV-related lymphoproliferative disease. Graft CD3/CD19 depletion was performed with anti-CD3- and anti-CD19-coated microbeads on a CliniMACS device. This approach of immunomagnetic depletion allows the transplantation of an "untouched" graft product in contrast to CD34-selected stem cells which are coated with CD34-specific microbeads, potentially altering the characteristics of the stem cells transplanted.

Table 1 illustrates the difference between CD34-selected and CD3/CD19-depleted grafts. CD34 selection results in grafts which are highly enriched in $CD34^+$ cells, with a mean purity of $CD34^+$ cells of 97%.[27,28] T cell depletion is profound with >4 log reduction in $CD3^+$ cells. The resulting graft contains $CD34^+$ cells of high purity with a median recovery of 71%. The graft contains virtually no NK cells, monocytes or granulocytes. In contrast, after CD3/CD19 depletion, the graft contains high numbers of $CD34^-$ cells, encompassing also cells with engraftment facilitating properties such as NK cells, monocytes and antigen presenting cells. T- and B cell depletion

Table 1.   Graft Composition after CD3/CD19 Depletion[a]

Cell Population	CD34 Selection ($n = 17$)	CD3/CD19 Depletion ($n = 19$)
Total cell number pre	5.8×10^{10}	5.0×10^{10}
Total cell number post	0.03×10^{10}	1.5×10^{10}
T-cells	0.11%	0.003%
T-cell depletion	4.6 log	4.4 log
CD19+ cells	Not done	0.003%
Stem cell purity	97.5%	0.97%
Stem cell recovery	78%	59%
NK-cells/kg BW	0.003×10^6	35×10^6
Monocytes/kg BW	0.3×10^6	130×10^6
Granulocytes/kg BW	0.3×10^6	38×10^6

[a] Values were determined by flow cytometry pre and post each immunomagnetic selection/depletion procedure. Numbers present medians of all evaluable procedures.

is profound with 4.4 log. The grafts comprise only 0.97% CD34$^+$ cells due to the high content of non-CD34$^+$ cells. Recoveries of CD34$^+$ cells are comparable, allowing sufficient numbers of CD34$^-$ cells to be collected after a median of two leukaphereses per patient using both methods.

In order to improve on the high treatment-related toxicity of the high dose conditioning used for CD34-selected grafts, a dose-reduced conditioning regimen consisting of fludarabine (150–200 mg/m²), thiotepa (10 mg/kg), melphalan (120 mg/m²) and OKT-3 (5 mg/day, day −5 to +14) (Fig. 1) was used.[29] All the patients received cryopreserved peripheral blood stem cells processed with CD3/CD19 depletion on day 0. The patients received no support with G-CSF post-transplant. For purpose of postgrafting immunosuppression, mycophenolate mofetil (MMF, 15 mg/kg bid) was used if the T cell content in the graft exceeded 5×10^4 CD3$^+$ cells/kg.

In addition to chemotherapy, the anti-CD3 mAb OKT-3 is applied in this regimen in order to deplete remaining host-T cells, to avoid graft rejection. In contrast to anti-thymocyte globulin (ATG), OKT-3 spars incoming engraftment-facilitating cells such as NK cells, which are targeted by polyclonal agents such as ATG.

This regimen is of low toxicity, allowing its use even in an older or heavily pretreated patient population, including patients having received allogeneic or autologous HCTs previously.

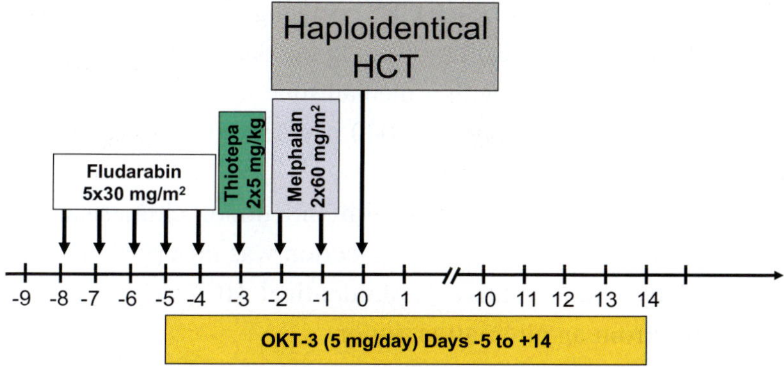

Figure 1.

Between 2003 and 2007, haploidentical HCT were carried out in 29 patients with hematologic malignancies (AML ($n = 16$); ALL ($n = 7$); NHL ($n = 3$); MM ($n = 2$); and CML ($n = 1$)). The patients received CD3/CD19-depleted grafts from haploidentical family donors at the University Hospitals of Tübingen, Dresden, Würzburg, Münster and Essen, all in Germany.[30]

All the patients had high risk disease, with either relapse after a preceding HCT (auto = 4, allo = 11) or treatment refractory disease. The median age of the patients was 42 (range, 21–59) years, which is about a decade older than previously reported in adult patients receiving haploidentical HCT with CD34-selected grafts.[6,17]

The donors were either siblings ($n = 10$), mothers ($n = 7$), children ($n = 8$) or cousins ($n = 4$) of the patients. All donor-recipient pairs had at least a two-loci mismatch. Peripheral blood mononuclear cells (PBMCs) were mobilized with human G-CSF at a dose of $2 \times 5\ \mu g/kg/day$ for 5 days and peripheral blood stem cell collection was performed on days 5 and 6. A CD34 content of the graft of at least 6×10^6 CD34$^+$ cells/kg recipient body weight was targeted. CD3/CD19 depletion was performed by negative selection using the automated CliniMACS device as described (Miltenyi Biotec, Bergisch-Gladbach, Germany).[28,31]

The CD3/CD19-depleted grafts contained a median of 7.6×10^6 (range, 3.4–17×10^6) CD34$^+$ cells/kg, 4.4×10^4 (range, 0.006–44×10^4) CD3$^+$ T-cells/kg and 7.2×10^7 (range, 0.02–37.3×10^7) CD56$^+$ cells/kg. One graft contained with 44×10^4 CD3$^+$ cells/kg, an unusually high number of T cells due to technical problems in the depletion procedure.

Engraftment was rapid with a median time to >500 granulocytes/μL of 12 (range, 10–21) days, and >20 000 platelets/μL of 11 (range, 7–38) days (Fig. 2).

All but one patient engrafted with full donor chimerism by day 14–26 after HCT. One case of graft rejection was observed. The patient was rescued by a consecutive haploidentical HCT with CD3/CD19-depleted cells from an alternative donor.

The positive influence of graft composition and conditioning regimen on engraftment kinetics is illustrated by the comparison of the fast

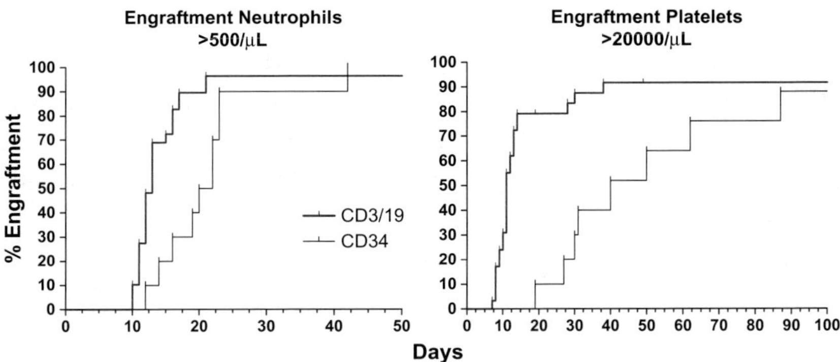

Figure 2. Time to recovery of neutrophils and platelets. Percentage of patients engrafted by time from the day of transplantation in a cumulative curve for neutrophils >500/μL and platelets >20 000/μL. Thin black line indicates recovery of historical patients after intensive conditioning and CD34 selection.

engraftment observed in patients receiving CD3/CD19-depleted grafts as compared to our historical experience after CD34-selected grafts (Fig. 2). This also translated into low transfusional requirements in the CD3/CD19 patients. These engraftment kinetics data are similar to the data reported by Aversa *et al.* after haploidentical HCT with CD34-selected grafts (median 11 days to ANC>1000/μL and 15 days to PLT>25 000/μL).[6] Of note, the CD3/CD19-depleted cohort received a much lower median CD34-dose with 7.6×10^6 CD34$^+$/kg versus 13.8×10^6 CD34$^+$/kg in the Aversa study. The fast engraftment seen in the CD3/CD19 group with CD34-doses as low as 3.4×10^6 CD34$^+$ cells/kg demonstrates that successful haploidentical HCT may be feasible even without megadoses of CD34$^+$ stem cells.

Detailed T cell, B cell and NK cell reconstitution data was evaluated in up to 16 patients. The median CD3$^+$ count on day 50 (+/−20 days) was 16 (range, 0–412) and on day 100 (+/−20 days) 227 (range, 15–1416) cells/μL. Median day 50 (+/−20 days) CD56$^+$ count was 891 (range, 13–6554) cells/μL, median day 100 (+/−20 days) CD56$^+$ count was 634 (range, 186–3698) cells/μL (Fig. 3).

Eleven patients were evaluable for B-cell reconstitution. Median day 100 (+/−20 days) CD19$^+$ count was 18 (range, 0–226) cells/μL.

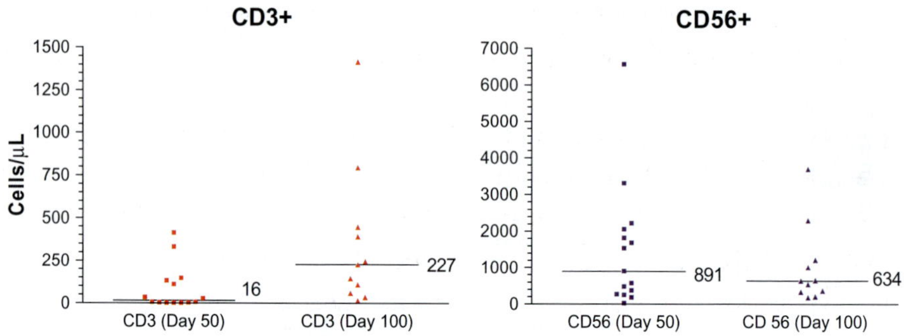

Figure 3. Count of CD3$^+$ T cells and CD56$^+$ NK cells on days +50 and +100. Absolute CD3 and CD56$^+$ count in 16 evaluable patients on days +50 and +100 (+/−20 days) after HCT.

CMV-reactivation was observed in 12 out of 24 patients at risk. Seven infectious deaths occurred (Sepsis = 1, Pneumonia = 4, CMV = 1, HHV-6/CMV = 1). In patients with active but controlled pulmonary infiltrates of invasive fungal infections, no progression of infiltrates during therapy but rapid resolution upon neutrophile engraftment was observed. Evaluation of the immune reconstitution shows fast reconstitution of NK cells in the CD3/CD19 patients (Fig. 3). The fast NK cell reconstitution might be directly related to the high NK cell content of CD3/CD19 depleted grafts.

NK cells may be of similar importance in the haploidentical setting as T cells in HLA-matched transplants. NK cells may confer important engraftment facilitating and graft-versus-tumor effects after haploidentical transplantation, especially in the setting of KIR-mismatch. Ruggeri *et al.* was able show significant positive impact of the presence of a KIR-mismatch on engraftment.[20] Furthermore, patients who received transplants from a KIR-mismatched donor for AML showed significantly fewer relapses and better survival.[7] NK cells may play important role in the defense against bacterial, viral and fungal infections. Cook *et al.* were able to demonstrate that transplantation from KIR-mismatched donors results in a significantly lower incidence of CMV-reactivation.[32] There is also increasing evidence for the important role of NK cells in the defense against fungal infections.[33] Compared to the haploidentical HCT with CD34-selected grafts and high dose conditioning, the CD3/CD19-depleted group seemed to show less infectious complications, potentially related to a better and faster NK cell reconstitution. Even patients with active but controlled invasive fungal infections and transplanted with CD3/CD19-depleted cells, showed rapid clearance of their pulmonary infiltrates upon engraftment, albeit virtually no T cells were detectable at that time.

T cell reconstitution after haploidentical HCT with CD3/CD19-depleted grafts seemed to be faster compared to historical data on CD34-selected grafts. T cell reconstitution was nevertheless, slow, reflecting the still low numbers of residual T cells in the graft. In the pediatric population, an even faster T cell reconstitution was seen after CD3/CD19-depleted haploidentical HCT.[34] This may be explained by the presence of an still functional thymus in children. B cell reconstitution is slower in the CD3/CD19 group, reflecting the low number of $CD19^+$ B cells found in the graft after immunomagnetic CD19-depletion. However, comparing the immune reconstitution of patients transplanted with CD3/CD19-depleted or CD34-selected grafts, one has to consider the different conditioning regimens used. Dose-reduced conditioning regimens as used in the CD3/CD19 patients may allow faster immune recovery.

The regimen was well tolerated, with maximum acute toxicity being grade 2–3 mucositis. Initially, using 200 mg/m^2 fludarabine, severe neurotoxicity in four patients was observed. In consequence, the fludarabine dose was reduced to 150 mg/m^2. TRM in the first 100 days was 6/29 (20%), with deaths due to idiopathic pneumonia syndrome ($n = 1$), mucormycosis ($n = 1$), pneumonia ($n = 3$) or GVHD ($n = 1$). The incidence of grade II–IV° GVHD was 48%, with grade II° = 10, III° = 2 and IV° = 2. One patient, who received the highest T cell dose, developed lethal grade IV GVHD. Three cases of limited chronic GVHD were observed to date. Twenty patients died, 12 due to relapse, 7 due to infections and one patient due to GVHD. Overall survival was 9/29 patients

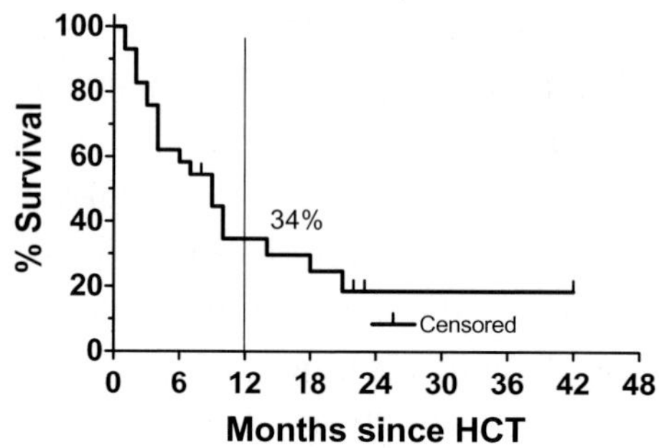

Figure 4.

(31%) with a median follow-up of 241 days (range, 112–1271). The Kaplan-Meier estimate of event-free and overall survival was 34% at 12 month (Fig. 4).

In the group transplantated with CD3/CD19-depleted grafts, a higher incidence and degree of GVHD after haploidentical HCT was observed as compared to the reported low incidence of <10% in patients receiving haploidentical HCT with CD34-selected grafts.[6] This may reflect the higher median T cell dose transplanted in these patients. The acute GVHD observed was mainly moderate skin GVHD, readily responsive to steroid therapy. The single case of lethal grade 4 GVHD in the CD3/CD19 group was the result of an excessive accidental CD3-dose of more than 40×10^4 $CD3^+$ cells/kg. With this regimen, doses of $<5 \times 10^4$ $CD3^+$ cells/kg seem safe even without GVHD prophylaxis; doses of $>5 \times 10^4$ $CD3^+$ cells/kg require MMF or a calcineurin inhibitor as GVHD-prophylaxis; and doses of $>15 \times 10^4$ $CD3^+$ cells/kg should be avoided.

The estimated overall survival of 34% at one year seems promising, given the high risk profile of the patient treated, with more than half receiving a second or third HCT. This survival rate is at least similar to what has been reported after haploidentical HCT with CD34-selected grafts and what could be expected after matched related HCT in a similar high risk cohort of patients.

In conclusion, haploidentical HCT with CD3/CD19-depleted grafts and dose-reduced conditioning is feasible in adults, resulting in fast engraftment and immune reconstitution. The regimen described allow haploidentical HCT in an older or heavily pretreated patient population even without a megadose of CD34$^+$ stem cells.

Literature

1. Martin PJ. (2004) Overview of marrow transplantation immunology. In: Blume KG, Forman SJ, Appelbaum FR (eds.). *Thomas' Hematopoietic Cell Transplantation*. Blackwell Science, Inc. Malden, MA, pp. 16–30.

2. Anasetti C *et al.* (1990) Effect of HLA incompatibility on graft-versus-host disease, relapse, and survival after marrow transplantation for patients with leukemia or lymphoma. *Hum Immunol* **29**: 79–91.

3. Bachar-Lustig E, Rachamim N, Li HW, Lan F, Reisner Y. (1995) Megadose of T cell-depleted bone marrow overcomes MHC barriers in sublethally irradiated mice. *Nat Med* **1**: 1268–1273.

4. Aversa F *et al.* (1994) Successful engraftment of T-cell-depleted haploidentical "three-loci" incompatible transplants in leukemia patients by addition of recombinant human granulocyte colony-stimulating factor-mobilized peripheral blood progenitor cells to bone marrow inoculum. *Blood* **84**: 3948–3955.

5. Aversa F *et al.* (1998) Treatment of high-risk acute leukemia with T-cell-depleted stem cells from related donors with one fully mismatched HLA haplotype. *N Engl J Med* **339**: 1186–1193.

6. Aversa F *et al.* (2005) Full haplotype-mismatched hematopoietic stem-cell transplantation: A phase II study in patients with acute leukemia at high risk of relapse. *J Clin Oncol* **23**: 3447–3454.

7. Ruggeri L *et al.* (2002) Effectiveness of donor natural killer cell alloreactivity in mismatched hematopoietic transplants. *Science* **295**: 2097–2100.

8. Ruggeri L *et al.* (2007) Donor natural killer cell allorecognition of missing self in haploidentical hematopoietic transplantation for acute myeloid leukemia: Challenging its predictive value. *Blood* **110**: 433–440.

9. Aversa F *et al.* (2002) Haploidentical stem cell transplantation for acute leukemia. *Int J Hematol* **76**(1): 165–168.

10. Handgretinger R *et al.* (2001) Megadose transplantation of purified peripheral blood CD34(+) progenitor cells from HLA-mismatched parental donors in children. *Bone Marrow Transplant* **27**: 777–783.

11. Handgretinger R, Klingebiel T, Lang P, Gordon P, Niethammer D. (2003) Megadose transplantation of highly purified haploidentical stem cells: Current results and future prospects. *Pediatr Transplant* 7(3): 51–55.

12. Martelli MF *et al.* (2002) Transplants across human leukocyte antigen barriers. *Semin Hematol* **39**: 48–56.

13. Bunjes D *et al.* (2002) CD34+ selected cells in mismatched stem cell transplantation: A single centre experience of haploidentical peripheral blood stem cell transplantation. *Bone Marrow Transplant* **25**(2): S9–11.

14. Klingebiel T, Handgretinger R, Lang P, Bader P, Niethammer D. (2004) Haploidentical transplantation for acute lymphoblastic leukemia in childhood. *Blood Rev* **18**: 181–192.

15. Marks DI *et al.* (2006) Haploidentical stem cell transplantation for children with acute leukaemia. *Br J Haematol* **134**: 196–201.

16. Lang P *et al.* (2004) Transplantation of a combination of CD133+ and CD34+ selected progenitor cells from alternative donors. *Br J Haematol* **124**: 72–79.

17. Nguyen S *et al.* (2005) NK-cell reconstitution after haploidentical hematopoietic stem-cell transplantations: Immaturity of NK cells and inhibitory effect of NKG2A override GvL effect. *Blood* **105**: 4135–4142.

18. Zanjani ED, Almeida-Porada G, Livingston AG, Zeng H, Ogawa M. (2003) Reversible expression of CD34 by adult human bone marrow long-term engrafting hematopoietic stem cells. *Exp Hematol* **31**: 406–412.

19. Bornhauser M *et al.* (1999) Stable engraftment after megadose blood stem cell transplantation across the HLA barrier: The case for natural killer cells as graft-facilitating cells. *Transplantation* **68**: 87–88.

20. Ruggeri L *et al.* (1999) Role of natural killer cell alloreactivity in HLA-mismatched hematopoietic stem cell transplantation. *Blood* **94**: 333–339.

21. Jacquet EG, Schanie CL, Fugier-Vivier I, Willer SS, Ildstad ST. (2003) Facilitating cells as a venue to establish mixed chimerism and tolerance. *Pediatr Transplant* **7**: 348–357.

22. Grimes HL *et al.* (2004) Graft facilitating cells are derived from hematopoietic stem cells and functionally require CD3, but are distinct from T lymphocytes. *Exp Hematol* **32**: 946–954.

23. Tanaka J, Imamura M, Kasai M, Asaka M, Torok-Storb B. (1999) The role of accessory cells in allogeneic peripheral blood stem cell transplantation. *Int J Hematol* **69**: 70–74.

24. Fugier-Vivier IJ *et al.* (2005) Plasmacytoid precursor dendritic cells facilitate allogeneic hematopoietic stem cell engraftment. *J Exp Med* **201**: 373–383.

25. Gur H *et al.* (2002) Tolerance induction by megadose hematopoietic progenitor cells: Expansion of veto cells by short-term culture of purified human CD34(+) cells. *Blood* **99**: 4174–4181.

26. Gur H *et al.* (2005) Immune regulatory activity of CD34+ progenitor cells: Evidence for a deletion-based mechanism mediated by TNF-{alpha}. *Blood* **105**: 2585–2593.

27. Lang P *et al.* (1999) Clinical scale isolation of highly purified peripheral CD34+ progenitors for autologous and allogeneic transplantation in children. *Bone Marrow Transplant* **24**: 583–589.

28. Schumm M *et al.* (1999) Isolation of highly purified autologous and allogeneic peripheral CD34+ cells using the CliniMACS device. *J Hematother* **8**: 209–218.

29. Bethge WA *et al.* (2006) Haploidentical allogeneic hematopoietic cell transplantation in adults with reduced-intensity conditioning and CB3/CD19 depletion: Fast engraftment and low toxicity. *Exp Hematol* **34**: 1746–1757.

30. Bethge WA *et al.* (2008) Haploidentical allogeneic hematopoietic cell transplantation in adults using CD3/CD19 depletion and reduced intensity conditioning: An update. *Blood Cells Mol Dis* **40**: 13–19.

31. Barfield RC *et al.* (2004) A one-step large-scale method for T- and B-cell depletion of mobilized PBSC for allogeneic transplantation. *Cytotherapy* **6**: 1–6.

32. Cook M *et al.* (2005) Donor KIR genotype has a major influence on the rate of cytomegalovirus reactivation following T-cell replete stem cell transplantation. *Blood.*

33. Morrison BE, Park SJ, Mooney JM, Mehrad B. (2003) Chemokine-mediated recruitment of NK cells is a critical host defense mechanism in invasive aspergillosis. *J Clin Invest* **112**: 1862–1870.

34. Lang P *et al.* (2005) A comparison between three graft manipulation methods for haploidentical stem cell transplantation in pediatric patients: Preliminary results of a pilot study. *Klin Padiatr* **217**: 334–338.

Chapter 4

Unmanipulated HLA-Mismatched/Haploidentical Blood and Marrow Hematopoietic Stem Cell Transplantation

*Xiao-Jun Huang**

Introduction

Human leukocyte antigen (HLA)–mismatched/haploidentical hematopoietic stem cell transplantation (HSCT) has been proceeding for more than 20 years.[1–8] Early practice by Fred Hutchinson Cancer Research Center demonstrated the promise and limitation of haploidentical HSCT for leukemia.[9] The overall survival for patients with acute leukemia in remission was not significantly different following HLA-matched and one-antigen-mismatched donor HSCT, while the outcome of patients receiving HLA-2- or three-locus-mismatched transplant was poor. Compared to HLA-identical sibling donor transplantation, haploidentical transplantation had a significantly higher incidence of severe graft-vs-host disease (GvHD), delayed engraftment and graft failure, which carried a high mortality rate. This result suggested that transplants involving patients who had two- or three-antigen-mismatched related donors should be avoided routinely in patients with hematological malignancies, and that haploidentical HSCT using the conventional myeloablative conditioning

*Peking University Institute of Hematology. Tel.: +861088326006, Fax: +861088324577
E-mail: xjhrm@medmail.com.cn.

regimen and pharmacological (cyclosporine-based) GvHD prophylaxis was a problem.[3]

Aversa *et al.*[7,8,10] employed extensive *ex vivo* T cell depletion and the megadose stem cell that had successfully overcome the HLA barrier to engraftment in mice. Although extensive T cell depletion or CD34 cell selection improves engraftment and reduces GvHD, the manipulation is associated with prolonged immune deficiencies and increased risks of infectious complications.[4] To overcome the above-mentioned shortcomings, unmanipulated allografts and posttransplant immune suppression were focused on by researchers from Johns Hopkins University,[11,12] Peking University[5,6,13] and other transplant centers.[14–16]

In Japan, Ogawa *et al.*[14] demonstrated that the incidence of severe GvHD was reduced to an acceptable level using pharmacological GvHD prophylaxis with tacrolimus, methotrexate, mycophenolate mofetil and high-dose steroids in 30 unmanipulated HSCTs. Eleven patients (36.7%) developed grade II–III acute GvHD, seven (23.3%) died from transplant-related mortality (TRM) and 39% relapsed. These outcomes indicated that additional strategies are needed in order to effectively prevent/treat GvHD in unmanipulated haploidentical transplant settings. Recently, a jointed phase I/II trial in 68 patients with advanced hematological malignancies ($n = 67$) or paroxysmal nocturnal hemoglobinuria ($n = 1$) who received nonmyeloablative, unmanipulated haploidentical marrow transplant, followed by 50 mg/kg per day of cyclophosphamide administered at day 3 or days 3 and 4 after transplant, was performed at Johns Hopkins University and Fred Hutchison Cancer Research Center.[11] Luznik *et al.*[11] found that graft rejection occurred in 9/66 evaluable patients (13%). Nonrelapse mortality and relapse at 1 year were 15% and 51%, respectively. The incidence of extensive chronic GvHD at 1 year was 5% in patients who received two doses of posttransplant cyclophosphamide. Actuarial overall survival (OS) and event-free survival (EFS) at 2 years after transplantation were 36% and 26%, respectively. These transplant outcomes are encouraging, although more patients and a longer followup are needed for confirmation. At Peking University, Huang *et al.*[5] reported that 171 patients underwent transplantation from haploidentical family donors and the disease-free survival (DFS) at 2 years was 68% for standard-risk leukemia and 42% in high-risk patients. The transplant outcomes of patients who underwent unmanipulated HLA-mismatched/haploidentical blood and marrow transplantation at Peking University Institute of Hematology are shown in Table 1.[5,6,13,17–19] The basic and clinical research on unmanipulated HLA-mismatched/haploidentical blood and marrow transplantation at our center are discussed below.

Clinical Results of HLA-Mismatched/Haploidentical HSCT

Establishment of the GIAC Protocol

In contrast to CD34-selected haplotype-mismatched transplants,[4,8,20] Peking University researchers developed a novel approach to HLA-mismatched/haploidentical transplantation without *in vitro* T cell depletion.[5,6,13,19] This strategy — (the GIAC protocol) — sequentially applies, *in vivo* modulation of the recipient, the donor T cell function, and the dose of donor hematopoietic stem cells. The protocol entails the following: treating donors with G-CSF to induce donor immunological tolerance; intensified immunological suppression to both promote engraftment and prevent GvHD; inclusion of ATG for the prophylaxis of GvHD and graft rejection; and a combination of G-CSF-primed bone marrow harvest (G-BM) and G-CSF-mobilized peripheral blood stem cell harvest (G-PB) as the source of stem cell grafts.

The conditioning regimen of the GIAC protocol consists of cytosine arabinoside (4 g/m^2/d, i.v.) on days −10 and −9, busulfan (12 mg/kg p.o. or 0.8 mg × 12/kg, i.v. in 12 doses) on days −8, −7 and −6, cyclophosphamide (1.8 g/m^2/d, i.v.) on days −5 and −4, simustine (250 mg/m^2, orally on day −3), and ATG (thymoglobulin, 2.5 mg/kg/d, i.v. of the Sangstat product) on days −5 to −2. GvHD prophylaxis included cyclosporine A (CsA), mycophenolate mofetil (MMF), and short-term methotrexate. The dosage of CsA was 2.5 mg/kg/d, i.v. from day 9 before transplantation until bowel function returned to normal. At that point, the

Table 1. Unmanipulated HLA-Mismatched/Haploidentical Blood and Marrow Transplantation.

Patients (n)	Disease	Conditioning	GvHD Prophylaxis	GR	aGvHD	cGvHD Limited Extensive	TRM	Relapse	LFS	References
58	ALL/AML/ CML/MDS	Bu/Cy/Ara-C/ MeCCNU+ ATG or TBI	CsA/MTX/MMF	0	37.9%		7/58	9/58	69.3% @ 2 yrs	Huang *et al.* (2004)
171	ALL/AML/ CML/MDS	Bu/Cy/Ara-C/ MeCCNU+ATG	CsA/MTX/MMF	0	55%		19% SR @ 2 yrs 31% HR @ 2 yrs	SR 12% HR 39%	SR 68% @ 2 yrs HR 42% @ 2 yrs	Huang *et al.* (2006)
135	ALL/AML/ CML/MDS	Bu/Cy/Ara-C/ MeCCNU+ATG	CsA/MTX/MMF	1.5%	(II–IV) 40%		22%	18%	64% @ 2 yrs	Lu *et al.* (2006)
8	AML/ALL	Cy/TBI/ATG/ MeCCNU ($n = 4$) Flu/TBI/ATG/ MeCCNU ($n = 4$)	CsA/MTX/MMF	0	5/8		0/8	1/8	7/8	Han *et al.* (2007)
42	AML/ALL/ CML	Bu/Cy/Ara-C/ MeCCNU+ATG	CsA/MTX/MMF	0	57.2%		20.4 ± 6.5% @ 1 yr	21.43%	57.3 ± 8% @ 3 yrs	Liu *et al.* (2008)

(*Continued*)

Table 1. *(Continued)*

Patients (n)	Disease	Conditioning	GvHD Prophylaxis	GR	aGvHD	cGvHD Limited Extensive	TRM	Relapse	LFS	References
93	CML	Bu/Cy/Ara-C/ MeCCNU+ATG	CsA/MTX/MMF	0	64.25%		28.3% @ 1 yr 16.92% @ 1 yr 13.33% @ 1 yr 7.69% @ 1 yr	CP1 3.77% CP2 0% AP 13.94% BC 38.46%	76.5% @ 1 yr 74.5% @ 4 yrs	Huang *et al.* (2008)
250	AML/ALL	Bu/Cy/Ara-C/ MeCCNU+ATG	CsA/MTX/MMF	0	45.8%		SR AML 11.9% @ 3 yrs ALL 24.3% @ 3 yrs HR AML 20.2% @ 3 yrs ALL 48.5% @ 3 yrs	SR AML 19.4% @ 3 yrs ALL 21.2% @ 3 yrs HR AML 29.4% @ 3 yrs ALL 50.8% @ 3 yrs	SR AML70.7% @ 3 yrs ALL 59.7% @ 3 yrs HR AML 55.9% @ 3 yrs ALL 24.8% @ 3 yrs	Huang *et al.* (2009)

Abbreviations: HLA = human leukocyte antigen; AML = acute myeloid leukemia; ALL = acute lymphoblastic leukemia; CML = chronic myeloid leukemia; MDS = myelodysplasic syndrome; Bu = busulfan; Cy = cyclophosphamide; ATG = antihuman thymocyte immunoglobulin; GvHD = graft-vs-host diease; CsA = cyclosporine A; MMF = mycophenolate mofetil; Flu = fludarabine; SR = standard risk; HR = high-risk; GR = graft failure; aGvHD = acute GvHD; cGvHD = chronic GvHD; TRM = transplant-related mortality; LFS = leukemia-free survival; CP = chronic phase; AP = accelerated phase; BC = blast crisis.

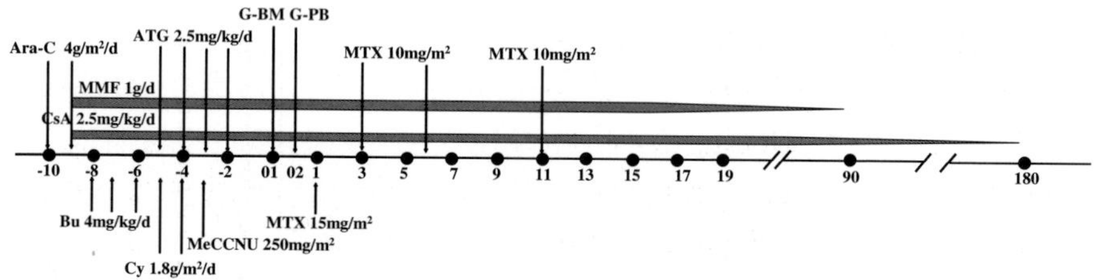

Fig. 1. Conditioning regimen for unmanipulated HLA-mismatched/haploidentical blood and marrow transplantation.

patient was switched to oral CsA. MMF was administered orally, 0.5 g every 12 h, from day 9 before transplantation to day 30 after transplantation, tapered to half on day +30, and discontinued around days +60 to +90. The dosage of methotrexate was 15 mg/m^2, administered i.v. on day 1, and 10 mg/m^2 on days 3, 6 and 11 after transplantation. Whole blood CsA concentration was monitored weekly using fluorescence polarization immunoassay and the dosage was adjusted to attain the blood concentration of 150–250 ng/ml. In cases where no evidence of GvHD was detected by days +40 to +50, the CsA dosage was reduced gradually and discontinued around days +180 to +270. In cases where occurrence of GvHD was detected, CsA was continued (Fig. 1). Via this GIAC protocol, promising results have been achieved at Peking University Institute of Hematology (Table 1).[5,6,13,19] Compared with unmanipulated mismatched stem cell transplantation in Japan,[14,15] and some transplant centers in the USA,[11] mixture grafts of G-BM and G-PB and myeloablative conditioning regimens were used at our center.

Clinical Results

Engraftment

In the GIAC protocol, G-BM and G-PB were used simultaneously as allografts. The median number of total nuclear cells, CD34$^+$ cells, CD3$^+$ cells, CD4$^+$ cells and CD8$^+$ cells infused into the patients was 7.33 × 10^8/kg (range 2.40–17.85), 2.19 × 10^6/kg (range 0.83–9.69),

1.64×10^8/kg (range 0.35–6.34), 0.85×10^8/kg (range 0.19–3.81) and 0.63×10^8/kg (range 0.13–2.99), respectively.[21] Huang *et al.*[5] reported that 171 patients, including 86 in the high-risk group, underwent transplantation involving HLA-mismatched/haploidentical family donors. The results showed that all patients achieved hematopoietic recovery after transplantation. The median time for myeloid engraftment was 12 days (range 9–26 days) and for platelets 15 days (range 8–151 days). In 42 pediatric patients, the median times of myeloid and platelet recovery were 14 (9–22) days and 22 (8–90) days after transplantation, respectively.[17] There was no significant association between the extent of HLA disparity and the time of myeloid or platelet recovery in HLA-mismatched/ haploidentical transplant settings.[5,17]

In 2006, the results for 293 patients with leukemia undergoing HLA-identical sibling ($n = 158$) or related HLA-mismatched/haploidentical ($n = 135$) HSCT performed during the same time period were compared.[6] Analyses of chimerism indicated that all patients achieved full donor chimerism by day 30 after HSCT. All patients engrafted to absolute neutrophil counts (ANCs) exceeding 0.5×10^9/L, with a median time to neutrophil engraftment of 15 days (range 10–25 days) in matched HSCT versus 12 days (range 10–25 days) in mismatched HSCT ($P < 0.001$). 156 and 128 patients achieved platelet engraftments in both matched and mismatched groups, respectively, at 15 days (range 2–108 days) versus 15 days (range 7–151 days), $P = 0.57$. Primary platelet engraftment failure or secondary thrombocytopenia occurred in 19 patients, with 8 patients in the matched HSCT group and 11 in the mismatched HSCT group. Among them, 8 patients finally received additional mobilized donor peripheral blood stem cell grafts (PBSCs), and 6 of them are alive and well. All these data confirmed that engraftment in unmanipulated HLA-mismatched/ haploidentical HSCT is comparable to HLA-matched sibling HSCT.[6]

In HLA-matched allogeneic or autologous transplant settings, multiple factors have been reported to be associated with hematopoietic reconstitution, such as sex pairing between donor and recipient, conditioning regimen, number of $CD34^+$ cells infused, ABO mismatch, $CD3^+$ cells, $CD8^+$ cells and subsets of $CD34^+$ cells in the allografts.[22–24] In a large sample retrospective study, Chang *et al.*[21] found that all patients reached an ANC of 500/μL in a median of 13 days (range 9–49 days). Univariate analysis showed a trend toward an association of sex (female vs. male) with neutrophil engraftment. Moreover, a trend toward association between time to transplantation after diagnosis (≤210 d vs. >210 d) and disease stage (advanced stage vs early stage) with neutrophil engraftment was demonstrated. 331 of 348 patients (95.11%) reached an untransfused platelet count of more than 20,000/μL in a median of 16 days (range 7–356 days). Six factors were found to be associated with platelet engraftment, including age of recipients, HLA match, disease stage ($P = 0.011$), infused nuclear cells/kg of recipient weight, infused CD34$^+$ cells/kg of recipient weight, and infused CD8$^+$ cells/kg of recipient weight. Multivariate analysis indicated that a low number of CD34$^+$ cells ($<2.19 \times 10^6$/kg) in allografts, and an advanced disease stage were independently associated with an increased risk of platelet engraftment, while, in pediatric patients,[25] only infused CD34$^+$ cells/kg of recipient weight were significantly associated with an increased risk of platelet engraftment. Patients receiving a CD34$^+$ cell dose of more than 2.42×10^6/kg had a short time [12 days (range 7–176 days)] to achieve an untransfused platelet engraftment, compared to 18 days (range 7–180 days) in patients receiving a lower dose. In summary, the factors in hematopoietic reconstitution are somewhat different from those in sibling HLA-identical transplantation and cord blood transplantation, as previously reported. Our results suggest that a higher number of CD34$^+$ cells in allografts should be preferred to ensure rapid platelet engraftment, especially in patients with advanced stage disease since this is also associated with delayed platelet recovery in our transplant setting.[21,25] Further studies to define the underlying mechanism of delayed platelet engraftment are clearly required for improving transplant outcomes.

Graft-vs-host disease

Graft-versus-host disease (GvHD) is the most frequent complication and is associated with considerable morbidity and mortality after allogeneic

HSCT. At Peking University, we combined G-BM and G-PB after myeloablative conditioning and posttransplant immune suppression with MMF and CsA. Among the 171 patients, 47 (27.5%) had no acute GvHD, 51 (29.8%) had grade I, 51 (29.8%) had grade II, 9 (5.3%) had grade III and 13 (7.6%) had grade IV. At 100 days after transplantation, the cumulative incidence was 55.0% for grade II–IV acute GvHD, and 23.1% for grade III–IV acute GvHD. The incidence of chronic GvHD was 44.67%, with 21.3% for limited and 23.3% for extensive, respectively.[5] We further reported that 42 children under 14 years old with hematological malignancies underwent haploidentical HSCT.[17] The cumulative incidence of acute GvHD of grade II–IV was 57.2%, and that of grade III–IV was 13.8%. The cumulative incidence of chronic GvHD was 56.7% for total and 29.5% for extensive. Apparently, the incidence of grade III–IV in pediatric patients was lower than that for adult patients. In 93 patients with CML following unmanipulated HLA-mismatched/haploidentical transplantation, the cumulative incidence of acute GvHD was 64.52%, and grade III–IV was 26.45%, 61.79% had chronic GvHD, and 28.93% had extensive chronic GvHD.[19] In contrast to previously published data, no association of HLA disparity with incidence and severity of acute and chronic GvHD was found in the GIAC protocol, except that the cumulative incidence of grade II–IV and III–IV acute GvHD in CML patients with HLA-B plus HLA-DR–mismatched donors was significantly higher than in those without ($P = 0.011$ and 0.015, respectively) after haploidentical transplantation.[19] These results indicate that the HLA barrier was overcome using the GIAC protocol.

Our results suggest that the incidences of grade III–IV aGvHD and extensive chronic GvHD were acceptable in patients after unmanipulated HLA-mismatched/haploidentical transplantation, although the T cell dose in grafts was more than 100×10^6/kg.[5,6,13,17,19,26] Moreover, comparable incidences of GvHD were found between patients who underwent haploidentical transplantation and those after HLA-identical sibling transplantation or unrelated allo-HSCT.[6,27] These findings may be related to (1) T cell hyporesponsiveness maintained after *in vitro* mixture of G-PB and G-BM in different proportions;[28,29] (2) the use of ATG before transplantation, which may induce depletion of infused donor T lymphocytes *in vivo* and thus lower the incidence of GvHD; (3) the possible effect of combination of CSP, MTX and MMF as postgrafting immunosuppression; (4) the application of G-CSF day +5 post transplant, which may further regulate T cell function;[5,17] (5) the immunomodulatory effect of mesenchymal stem cells (MSCs)/mesenchymal (stroma) progenitor cells (MPCs) from the G-CSF-mobilized marrow graft and PBSCs, respectively.[30]

The Japanese Collaborative Study Group examined the outcomes of 35 patients with advanced hematological malignancies who underwent HLA-2-antigen- or HLA-3-antigen-incompatible HSCT involving a microchimeric NIMA-mismatched donor.[15] The results showed that grade II/IV acute GvHD occurred in 19 (56%) of 34 evaluable patients, while extensive chronic GvHD developed in 13 (57%) of 23 evaluable patients. Multivariate analysis demonstrated that NIMA mismatch in the GvH direction was associated with a lower risk of severe grade III–IV acute GvHD when compared with NIPA mismatch ($P = 0.03$). Two hundred and sixty-nine patients receiving one or two HLA-A, –B, –DR antigen–mismatched sibling or parental non-T cell-depleted bone marrow transplants for AML, ALL or CML between 1985 and 1997 were reported to the International Bone Marrow Transplant Registry (IBMTR).[16] van Rood *et al.*[16] found that, after unmanipulated haploidentical HSCT, the incidence of grade II–IV acute GvHD was related to haplotype inheritance; acute GvHD was significantly less frequent after transplants from NIMA-mismatched siblings (41%) than that from NIPA-mismatched siblings (55%). However, in our unmanipulated HLA-mismatched/haploidentical transplant settings,[5,6,13,17,19,26] no effect of NIMA-mismatched siblings on GvHD was found. Several factors may account for this different result: (1) all patients except for one — who received bone marrow plus peripheral blood grafts — in Ichinohe or van Rood's studies received peripheral blood grafts or bone marrow grafts only;[15,16] (2) the application of G-CSF on day 5 posttransplant may have contributed to the different result; (3) the GIAC protocol was different from those reported by Ichinohe *et al.*[15] and von Rood *et al.*,[16] in particular, no ATG was included in their transplant settings.

Luo *et al.*[26] recently examined the absolute numbers and relative proportions of $CD4^+$, $CD8^+$, $CD14^+$ and $CD34^+$ cells contained in allografts and their impact on early engraftment and later clinical outcomes in 141 patients with hematological malignancies who underwent unmanipulated HLA-mismatched/haploidentical HSCT without *in vitro* T cell depletion. They demonstrated that a higher CD4/CD8 in G-BM was associated with a significantly increased risk of acute GvHD of grade II–IV, even after adjusting for an ABO major mismatch. In another study, the effects of natural killer (NK) cells in allografts on transplant outcomes in patients receiving G-PB and G-BM from HLA-haploidentical donors were investigated.[31] This study showed that factors correlating the high incidence of acute GvHD are KIR ligand mismatch and a higher dose of $CD56^{bright}$ NK cells (41.9×10^6/kg) in the allografts, while a higher $CD56^{dim}/CD56^{bri}$ NK cell ratio (more than 8.0) in allografts was correlated with a decreased risk of grade III–IV aGvHD after unmanipulated HLA-mismatched/haploidentical transplantation.[31]

Recently, a prospective study showed that a high cell dose of $CD4^+CD45RA^+CD62L^+$ cells in allografts increases the incidence of grade II–IV aGvHD after unmanipulated blood and marrow transplantation.[32] Moreover, a high number of $CD4^+$ naïve T cells increased the incidence of chronic GvHD. These findings are interesting and important, because selective depletion of $CD4^+CD62L^+$ naïve cells in allografts may decrease the development of GvHD in umanipulated HLA-mismatched/haploidentical transplant settings if our preliminary results can be confirmed in future studies.

Relapse and management

Relapse is one of the most important causes of mortality after HLA-matched sibling or unrelated transplantation as well as umbilical cord blood transplantation. Several factors, including disease status, recipient age, and dendritic cells in allografts, are associated with a high relapse rate following HLA-identical transplant. The Peking University study evaluated 250 GIAC recipients (AML 108, ALL 142). Of the 250 patients,

45 (AML 13, ALL 32) relapsed after transplantation; of these, 22 (AML 6, ALL 16) were from the high-risk group. The 3-year probability of relapse in the standard-risk group was 11.9% and 24.3% for AML and ALL, respectively, and that in the high-risk group was 20.2% and 48.5% for AML and ALL, respectively.[13] In 42 pediatric patients, all 9 of the patients who relapsed after HSCT were diagnosed with ALL before transplantation, and 5 were from the high-risk group. The probability of relapse for high-risk patients was 37 ± 0.2% at 2 years after transplantation.[17] Comparison analysis showed that there were no differences in the relapse rate between patients who underwent unmanipulated HLA-mismatched/ haploidentical transplantation and those who received HLA-identical or unrelated HSCT.[6] Three factors, including advanced disease status,[5,13,26] higher CD4/CD8 in G-BM,[26] and delayed lymphocyte recovery at day 30 posttransplantation (unpublished data), are correlated with increased relapse rates; while a higher CD56dim/CD56bri NK cell ratio (more than 8.0) was correlated with a decreased rate of relapse after haploidentical transplantation without *in vitro* T cell depletion.[31]

Ruggeri *et al.*[33,34] indicated that the probability of relapse for ALL patients was 85% at 5 years after CD34-selected haplotype identical transplantation. In contrast to their report, we found that the 3-year probability of relapse was 24.3% and 48.5% for ALL in the standard-risk and the high-risk group, respectively, following unmanipulated HLA-mismatched/haploidentical transplantation.[13] It seems that the relapse rate of ALL patients after unmanipulated HLA-mismatched/haploidentical transplantation is lower than that of those after CD34-selected haplotype-identical transplantation, although this is deficient in comparability. Several factors may be related to the result: (1) some differences, including compositions in allografts and the conditioning regimen, exist between CD34-selected haplotype-identical transplant and the GIAC protocol; (2) the kinetics of NK cell recovery and the role of NK cell alloreactivity are also different between these two haploidentical transplant protocols; (3) the use of modified donor lymphocyte infusion (DLI) for prophylaxis of relapse in some patients following GIAC protocol may be another reason.[35]

In HLA-matched, related or unrelated HSCT settings, DLI has been shown to exert a GVL effect and has been successfully used for treatment of leukemia relapse, although DLI could be followed by a high rate of severe GvHD and, sometimes, pancytopenia and infection.[36] To conquer these shortcomings, a modified DLI strategy was adopted at our center. This strategy includes[35,37–39]: (1) G-CSF-primed peripheral blood progenitor cells instead of steady-donor lymphocyte harvests; (2) the use of a short-term immunosuppressive agent (cyclosporine A or methotrexate 10 mg once per week for 2–4 weeks) for prevention of DLI-associated GvHD. Our preliminary results suggest that using immunosuppressive agents for 2–4 weeks may reduce DLI-associated acute GvHD without influencing relapse and survival after G-CSF-primed DLI in HLA-matched sibling HSCT.[39]

With respect to the safety and efficiency of modified DLI in HLA-identical transplant settings, modified DLI was used to treat relapse of patients after unmanipulated HLA-mismatched/haploidentical transplantation.[37] Twenty patients who underwent haploidentical T cell-replete HSCT between April 1, 2002 and May 1, 2005, and then relapsed, were included in this study. They were diagnosed with relapse of leukemia at a median of 4.5 (1.5–35) months after HLA-mismatched/haploidentical transplantation without *in vitro* T cell depletion. Nine patients received chemotherapies before DLI. Two patients — one with Ph$^+$ ALL and the other with CML in the blastic phase — were given imatinib (300–400 mg/day) for 22 and 89 days, respectively, and the patient with CML achieved complete remission. Nine patients received DLI without any prior intervention. After DLI, 11 patients received CsA (blood concentration of 150–250 ng/mL for 2–4 weeks) or a low dose of MTX (10 mg once per week for 2–4 weeks) for prophylaxis against GvHD, and 9 patients received no GvHD prophylaxis. The incidence of grade III–IV aGvHD was significantly lower in patients with GvHD prophylaxis than in those without (55.56% vs 9.09%; $P = 0.013$). Fifteen patients achieved CR at a median of 289 (40–1388) days after DLI, rarely accompanied by pancytopenia. Eight of 20 patients survived in CR for a median of 1118 (range 754–1468) days after HSCT and 808 (range 627–1388) days after modified DLI. The 1-year and 2-year LFS were 60% and 40%, respectively. These results suggest that G-CSF-primed DLI was a potentially effective therapeutic option for patients who relapsed after HLA-mismatched/haploidentical HSCT. Moreover, administering a short-term immunosuppressive agent, such as CsA, and MTX, may decrease the incidence of GvHD following DLI.[37]

Considering the higher relapse rate of high-risk leukemia, even after unmanipulated HLA-mismatched/hapolidentical HSCT, and the safety and efficiency of modified DLI in our transplant settings,[37] we further explored the possibility of applying the modified DLI strategy against leukemia recurrence from therapeutic DLI to prophylaxis DLI for patients with advanced hematological malignancies.[35] Twenty-nine patients received prophylactic modified DLI at a median 75 (33–120) days after unmanipulated HLA-mismatched/haploidentical HSCT. Grades III–IV acute GvHD occurred in 6 patients, and all cases were controlled. Eleven patients were alive and relapse-free with a probability of LFS of $37.3 \pm 9.6\%$ at 3 years. Chronic GvHD was associated with a lower relapse rate and a higher probability of LFS.[35] These results suggest that prophylactic modified DLI is feasible in preventing relapse in patients with advanced leukemia after HLA-mismatched/haploidentical HSCT.

IL-2 has been used as a single agent or in conjunction with adoptive immunotherapy posttransplant. In a study reported by Liu *et al.*,[40] 19 patients with acute lymphoblastic malignancy were considered candidates for IL-2 therapy, if they were evaluated as having a high probability of disease recurrence post-HSCT (HLA-identical sibling, $n = 6$; haploidentical sibling, $n = 11$; unrelated donor, $n = 2$). The criteria for high probability of disease relapse after HSCT included: (1) standard-risk patients with evidence of minimal residual disease (MRD) after HSCT detected by flow cytometry; (2) high-risk patients. All patients were scheduled to receive the first cycle of IL-2 at a dose of 1 million units per day subcutaneously for a period of 14 days. After a 14-day rest, another cycle started. The alternating protocol continued until the occurrence of one of the following conditions: (1) patients were unable to tolerate the treatment; (2) primary disease relapsed; (3) patients developed GvHD;

(4) IL-2 had been administered for 12–18 months after transplantation; (5) subjects decided to withdraw from the study. Liu *et al.*[40] found that fever was the major toxicity during the subcutaneous IL-2 therapy. Among 15 patients who survived over 100 days, 6 ps (40.0%) developed limited chronic GvHD, of skin rashes, during IL-2 therapy. Similar cGvHD occurrences were observed in the patients undergoing HLA-haploidentical HSCT (2/6 patients) and HLA-identical HSCT (3/7 patients) in this cohort. With the median followup of 6 months (range 3–19 months) after the first IL-2 therapy, 14 of 15 evaluable patients with acute lymphoblastic malignancies at "high risk" of disease recurrence were disease-free (93.3%). In conclusion, low-dose IL-2 subcutaneous administration from 100 days for a prolonged period could be a safe and effective strategy to prevent relapse in acute lymphoblastic malignancy patients with a high risk of recurrence after unmanipulated allo-HSCT.

Taken together, the encouraging preliminary results of the modified DLI strategy and low-dose IL-2 may at least provide the means of offering a therapeutic and/or prophylaxic graft-versus-tumor effect to a major portion of patients who relapse after transplantation.[35,37–40] One developmental challenge for the future is to determine the patients who will benefit from immune modulation therapy posttransplantation using a prognosis index, such as Wilms' tumor suppressor gene (WT1), and day +30 absolute lymphocyte counts.

Transplant-related mortality and survival

Under the GIAC protocol, Huang *et al.*[5] found that 39 of the 171 patients died from transplant-related complications. The causes of nonrelapse death included GvHD in 13 cases, infection in 21 cases, and other causes in 5 cases, such as heart failure and hepatic failure. In 42 pediatric patients, the TRM was 19% (8/42): 4 from infection, 2 from heart failure, 1 from severe acute GvHD, and 1 from lymphoproliferative disorders.[17] For CML patients, the nonrelapse mortality was 8.72% for 100 days, 20.72% for 1 year, and 20.72% for 2 years. The 100-day TRM of patients in CP1, CP2/CR2, AP and BC was 7.8%, 7.1%, 13.3% and 7.7%, respectively. The 1-year TRM of patients in CP1, CP2/CR2, AP and BC was 28.3%, 16.92%, 13.33% and 7.69%, respectively.[19] In a recent report, 250 acute leukemia patients received allografts from related donors. The TRM on day 100 after transplantation in the standard- and high-risk groups was 6.8% and 5.9% for AML and 6.9% and 25.9% for ALL, respectively. At 3 years, the TRM in the standard- and high-risk groups was 19.4% and 29.4% for AML and 21.2% and 50.8% for ALL, respectively.

Three factors, including advanced disease status,[13,26] higher CD4/CD8 in G-BM,[26] and time from diagnosis to transplant (>450 days for CML patients),[19] are correlated with increased TRM following unmanipulated haploidentical blood and marrow transplantation. Zhao *et al.*[31] found that a higher CD56^{dim}/CD56^{bri} NK cell ratio (more than 8.0) in allografts was correlated with a decrease risk of TRM (HR 0.072; $P = 0.012$). Therefore, further reduction in TRM after unmanipulated HLA-mismatched/ haploidentical transplantation should aim at this poor prognosis index by hastening posttransplant immune reconstitution, using the G/GM test and fungal PCR for early diagnosis of fungal infection, and improving anti-fungal and antiviral efficacy with pre-emptive management strategy. Peking University researchers demonstrated an interesting phenomenon; they found that CMV-specific cytotoxic T lymphocytes (CTLs) in the allografts were inversely correlated with CMV infection and CMV disease after unmanipulated HLA-mismatched/haploidentical transplantation, indicating that graft engineering could decrease CMV infection and improve transplant outcomes (unpublished data).

Superior LFS after unmanipulated HLA-mismatched/haploidentical blood and marrow transplantation is closely correlated with early disease status,[19,26] higher numbers of CD56^{bright} cells reconstituted on day 14 posttransplant,[41] lower CD4/CD8 in G-BM,[26] a short time from diagnosis to transplant (≤450 days) for CML patients,[19] and higher absolute counts of lymphocytes (more than 300/μl) on day 30 posttransplant. Peking university researchers[5] reported that the 2-year probability of LFS was 68% for standard-risk patients and 42% for high-risk patients, in 171 patients who underwent unmanipulated HLA-mismatched/haploidentical transplantation.

For 42 pediatric patients, 27 survived with a 3-year probability of LFS, 57.3 ± 8%; 18 of them were in the high-risk group.[17] With respect to CML patients, Huang *et al.*[19] demonstrated that the probability of 1-year and 4-year LFS was 76.5% and 74.5% for CP1 patients, 85.7% and 85.7% for CP2/CR2 patients, 80% and 66.7% for AP patients, and 53.8% and 53.8% for BC patients. In a large cohort of AL patients,[13] the 3-year probability of LFS for AML was 70.7% and 55.9% and for ALL 59.7% and 24.8% in the standard- and high-risk groups, respectively. Eighteen of the 25 patients were classified as high-risk candidates before transplantation, with a 52.2 ± 9.5% probability of LFS. Seven of 9 patients in the standard-risk group survived free of leukemia. The 3-year probability of LFS for all patients was 57.3 ± 8%.[13] Similar LFS was achieved using the GIAC protocol compared with HLA-matched sibling transplantation or unrelated donor transplantation.

Posttransplant immune reconstitution

In unmanipulated haploidentical blood and marrow transplant settings, the immune reconstitution (IR) of NK cells in 43 patients was first investigated.[41] Our results showed that only 16 of 43 patients survived without leukemia and were exempt from grade II–IV aGvHD; the reconstitution kinetics of NK cells were analyzed in all 43 patients, as well as in those 16 who never developed GvHD. The absolute number of CD56^{bright} NK subsets in white blood cells (WBCs) and the number of CD56^{bright} NK subsets had recovered to the donor's level by day 14, and continuously increased up to their highest levels by day 60 in those 16 who never developed GvHD or by day 120 in all 43 patients, which were higher than those of healthy controls. The ratio of CD56^{dim}/CD56^{bright} NK subsets in patients eventually reached a level similar to that of healthy controls by day 120 in those 16 who never developed GvHD, or by day 180 in all 43 patients. The dose of CD56^{dim} NK cells in the allograft was positively associated with the day 14 CD56^{bright} NK cells and inversely correlated with the day 14 ratio of CD56^{dim}/CD56^{bright} cells. Patients with more CD56^{bright} NK cells in the recovery stage had a higher survival rate, and patients with a higher ratio of T/NK had a higher chance of getting aGvHD and chronic GvHD.

Ruggeri *et al.*[33,34] found that donor-versus-recipient NK cell alloreactivity could eliminate leukemia relapse and graft rejection and protect patients against GvHD after haploidentical transplantation with T cell depletion. In contrast to Ruggeri's results,[33,34] our findings showed that KIR ligand mismatch is associated with higher aGvHD, a greater relapse rate and inferior survival. The cumulative incidence of 3-year DFS, overall survival (OS) and TRM were best predicted by the number of KIR ligands carried by patients (P = 0.002 for DFS; P = 0.014 for OS; P = 0.030 for TRM). We also found that the KIR ligand–ligand mismatch model is a good predictor of acute GvHD (P = 0.002). Meanwhile, the presence of donor-activating KIR2DS3 also contributed significantly to acute and chronic GvHD. These data suggest that prognosis after transplantation is associated with the numbers of KIR ligands in recipients, and that T cell alloreaction may play a predominant role in the GIAC model.[42,43] Zhao *et al.*[42] also demonstrated that high levels of CD94 expression in donors or in recipients by day 60 after transplantation might be a good predictor of poor prognosis. Taken together, our results suggest that the role of NK cell alloreactivity could be covered by a large numbers of T cells in the GIAC protocol.[41–43]

Chang *et al.*[44] retrospectively compared the IR of patients who underwent HLA-matched transplantation and of those after unmanipulated HLA-mismatched/haploidentical transplantation. They found that $CD3^+$ cells approached normal levels between 2 and 4 months, primarily due to an increase in $CD8^+$ T cell numbers in both group A (haploidentical transplant) and group B (HLA-identical transplant); the counts of $CD3^+$ cells were significantly higher in group B than in group A at 1 month. During the first 12 months posttransplant, CD4 cell counts were lower in group A than in group B, whereas there was no difference at 6 and 9 months. The number of $CD4^+CD45RA^+$ cells was very low throughout the study in both groups, being lower in group A than in group B, especially during the first 6 months posttransplant. Normal levels of $CD4^+CD45RA^+$ cells were not achieved 12 months posttransplant in both groups. Normal levels of

CD8[+] cells were reached by 1 month and 2 months posttransplant in group B and group A, respectively. B lymphocytes (CD19[+]) showed low or undetectable counts throughout the first 4 months in both groups, achieving the normal range at 12 months. The results suggest that the IR, especially CD4[+] cells, and CD4[+]CD45RA[+] cells, during the first 6 months following HLA-mismatched/haploidentical transplantation without *in vitro* T cell depletion, was somewhat delayed compared with those after HLA-matched sibling transplantation. Currently, a prospective study is being carried out at our center to investigate the kinetics of T cells dendritic cells and regulatory T cells after unmanipulated HLA-mismatched/haploidentical transplantation.

Immune Tolerance Basis for Unmanipulated HLA-Mismatched Blood and Marrow HSCT

Simultaneous Induction of T Cell Tolerance in Bone Marrow and Peripheral Blood Grafts by Treating Healthy Donors with G-CSF

Initial studies showed that G-CSF leads to T cell hyporesponsiveness and modulates the balance between Th1 and Th2 immune responses by skewing T cell differentiation toward a Th2 type with an increase of interleukin-4 (IL-4) and a decrease of interferon-γ (IFN-γ) production. The immune modulatory effect of G-CSF on T cells was originally believed to be mediated exclusively through other effector cells, such as monocytes, CD40[+] GM cells and type 2 dendritic cells (DC2, plasmacytoid DCs).[28,29,45] However, Franzke *et al.*[46] provided evidence and suggested that G-CSF acts as a strong immune regulator in T cells and directly modulates T cell immune responses via G-CSFR on T cells. Morris *et al.*[47] suggested that three key immunomodulatory effects after the treatment of healthy donors with G-CSF may lead to the attenuation of GvHD. First, donor T cells upregulate GATA-3 expression and are biased toward TH2 differentiation, limiting TH1-dependent monocyte activation after SCT. Second, G-CSF induces the generation of Tr1 regulatory cells through IL-10 production. Third, G-CSF expands regulatory APCs within the donor (immature myeloid precursors and plasmacytoid DCs), which, after transplantation, promote the generation of classical $CD4^+CD25^+$ IL-10-producing T_{reg}. The generation of IL-10 and TGF-β from Tr1 and T_{reg} serves to further inhibit the inflammatory effector phase of GvHD, limiting target tissue damage.[47]

In human studies, the immunoregulatory effects of G-CSF on immune characteristics of bone marrow grafts were demonstrated by Shiers and by us.[29,48] Our data suggest that *in vivo* administration of G-CSF might alter the composition of bone marrow grafts, polarize Th1 to Th2, and induce hyporesponsiveness of T cells. Downregulation of CD28/B7 costimulatory signals and the preferential increase of monocytes and DC2 may contribute to the hyporesponsiveness of T cells. Our studies suggest that treating healthy donors with G-CSF could induce T cell hyporesponsiveness and polarize T cells from Th1 to Th2 simultaneously.[29] More recently, we found that G-CSF administration significantly decreased the expression of VLA-4, ICAM-1, L-selectin and LFA-1 on naïve $CD4^+$ and $CD8^+$ T cells in bone marrow grafts. G-CSF also polarized bone marrow naïve $CD4^+$ and $CD8^+$ T cells from Th1 to Th2 phenotype.[48] Therefore, the clinical significance of these alterations warrants further study.

Maintaining the Hyporesponsiveness of T Cells After in vitro Mixture of G-PB and G-BM in Different Proportions

Further evidence showed that the quantities of nucleated cells and monocytes in G-PB were, respectively, 4- and 43-fold higher than in G-BM harvests; all lymphocyte subsets exhibited 26- to 46-fold higher cell counts. The quantities of IFN-γ and IL-4 secreted per microliter of G-PB mononuclear cells were, respectively, 8.5- and 4.5-fold higher than those of G-BM mononuclear cells. The lymphocyte proliferation ability in G-PB was significantly higher than in G-BM. These findings suggest that quantitative and qualitative differences in immune cells and type 1 and type 2 cytokines exist between G-BM and G-PB.[49]

To clarify the mechanism of clinical application of G-BM and G-PB, these were mixed *in vitro* according to the proportions of G-PB:G-BM equal to 2:1, 1:1 and 1:2, respectively. This matches the clinical data, in which the median ratio of G-PB:G-BM was 1.16 (range 0.15–5.73). Our studies showed that the quantities of IFN-γ and IL-4 secreted by lymphocytes per microliter in the three mixture grafts were 2–4-fold lower than in G-PB and 1–3-fold higher than in SS-BM and G-BM, while the IL-4/IFN-γ ratio was higher than SS-BM and G-PB and lower than G-BM, although no significant difference was confirmed. Lymphocyte proliferation ability in the three mixture grafts was comparable to G-BM and significantly lower than SS-BM and G-PB. These results suggest that T cell hyporesponsiveness and polarization of the T cell from Th1 to Th2 could be maintained after *in vitro* mixture of G-PB and G-BM in different proportions. Although the relevance of this highly simplified *in vitro* system with PHA to the complex situation of *in vivo* alloreactivity cannot be completely established, we think that our data might partly explain the fact that the incidence of GvHD could be comparable after HLA-mismatched/haploidentical transplantation using G-PB plus G-BM, as compared with HLA-identical sibling transplantation.[50]

Combination of Immunologic Suppressive Agents

ATG present a broad spectrum of immunoregulatory effects, such as T cell depletion, IL-2 pathway suppression, and triggering of Fas (CD95)–mediated T cell apoptosis. Using a mouse model, Ruzek *et al.*[51] found that culture of mice splenocytes with mATG resulted in expansion of $CD4^+CD25^+$ T cells; these cells can suppress immune responses of normal splenocytes *in vitro* and protect against acute GvHD *in vivo*. A randomized clinical trial from Gruppo Italiano Trapianti Midollo Osseo (GITMO) suggests that 15 mg/kg ATG before BMT significantly reduces the risk of grade III–IV acute GvHD and that extensive chronic GvHD is significantly reduced in patients receiving ATG.[52] Finke *et al.*[53] found that a certain degree of one-antigen mismatching might not compromise the outcome after unrelated donor HSCT when rabbit ATG, in addition to the standard GvHD prophylaxis regimen, was used.

CsA is a neutral hydrophobic cyclic peptide composed of 11 amino acids, whose mechanisms of action dissect the pathways of T cell activation by the blockade of the calcium-dependent signal transduction pathways distal to engagement of the TCR. So far, it has been the most commonly used agent for GvHD prophylaxis after allogeneic BMT and, alone or in combination with methotrexate, it is included in the GvHD prophylaxis schedule of more than 70% of transplant recipients. MMF, an interesting agent for GvHD prophylaxis and therapy, can act at a late stage of T and B lymphocyte proliferation and promote $CD4^+CD25^+FoxP3^+$ regulatory T cell–mediated suppression of alloreactivity. A prospective randomized trial in a matched sibling allo-BMT setting which compared CsA and MTX with CsA and MMF showed that the incidences of grades II–IV aGvHD were 48% in the MMF group and 37% in the MTX group ($P = 0.49$).[54]

Recently, Lai *et al.*[55] suggested that a combination of CsA, MTX, low dose and short course of MMF in related HLA-matched and single-antigen-mismatched allo-PBSCT can effectively decrease the risk of acute GvHD without adversely impacting other outcomes, such as survival and disease relapse in standard-risk patients. In the GIAC protocol, the use of CSA and MMF was shifted from the conventional day −1 to day −9; this may contribute to immune tolerance. Together with ATG, G-BM/G-PB and the application of G-CSF on day +5 posttransplant, successful engraftment and an acceptable incidence of GvHD were achieved at Peking University.[5,13,17,19]

Conclusions

For patients requiring an allograft but without an HLA-identical sibling donor, how to choose an ideal alternative stem cell source remains difficult and controversial. Because of a lack of randomized comparisons, when one is selecting the best alternative donor and type of regimen, many aspects should be considered, including age, disease status, performance status, HLA typing, financial status, urgency of transplant, and donor availability. Of course, the experience of the transplant center is also an important aspect. Matched unrelated donor (MUD) has been accepted worldwide and has increased fast during the past two decades; however, high TRM and severe GvHD, which lead to morbidity and mortality, remain the problem. The long time of processing is another disadvantage, especially for patients who are in urgent need of a transplant. Unrelated cord blood has the advantage of easy procedure and immediate availability. A low cell dose which is related to poor engraftment is always the obstacle for adult patients with high body weight before multiunit cord blood transplantation. Haploidentical transplantation is a relatively new style which offers a high cell dose, almost unlimited donor availability, no time restriction for transplant, and the potential of graft engineering.

Based on the previous studies, if an allograft is crucial for disease treatment, a partially matched family donor could be an option for patients without perfectly matched unrelated donors. Sometimes, haploidentical HSCT is an even better choice at an experienced transplant center and in the following special circumstances: (1) urgency for early transplant, such as acute leukemia, but without an available HLA-matched donor; (2) posttransplant DLI is highly recommended due to the high risk of leukemia relapse; (3) an ethnic minority, in whom the chances of finding an available matched unrelated donor are very low.

Haploidentical HSCT provides an opportunity for patients to benefit from HSCT when an HLA-matched donor is not available. The final goal of haploidentical transplant is to successfully overcome the HLA barrier and capture an optimal GvL effect without GvHD. There are several novel approaches which may be promising in the future: (1) selective but effective allodepletion which facilitates successful donor engraftment, improves posttransplant immune reconstitution, and maximally reduces the indidence of GvHD; (2) improvement of DLI, in order to acquire GvL effect without or limiting GvHD; (3) adoptive cellular immunotherapy, such as $T_{reg}s$, $NK/T_{reg}s$, MSCs and donor-derived NK cell as well as the third-party cell infusion; (4) pathogen- or leukemia-specific donor-derived T cell infusion could be an additional approach to preventing opportunistic infection and reducing the leukemia relapse rate after haploidentical transplantation.

References

1. Friedrich W, Goldmann SF, Vetter U *et al.* (1984) Immunoreconstitution in severe combined immunodeficiency after transplantation of HLA-haploidentical, T cell-depleted bone marrow. *Lancet* **1**: 761–764.
2. Aversa F. (2008) Haploidentical haematopoietic stem cell transplantation for acute leukaemia in adults: Experience in Europe and the United States. *Bone Marrow Transplant* **41**: 473–481.
3. Huang XJ. (2008) Current status of haploidentical stem cell transplantation for leukemia. *J Hematol Oncol* **1**: 27.
4. Kang Y, Chao NJ, Aversa F. (2008) Unmanipulated or CD34 selected haplotype mismatched transplants. *Curr Opin Hematol* **15**: 561–567.
5. Huang XJ, Liu DH, Liu KY *et al.* (2006) Haploidentical hematopoietic stem cell transplantation without *in vitro* T cell depletion for the treatment of hematological malignancies. *Bone Marrow Transplant* **38**: 291–297.
6. Lu DP, Dong L, Wu T *et al.* (2006) Conditioning including antithymocyte globulin followed by unmanipulated HLA-mismatched/haploidentical blood and marrow transplantation can achieve comparable outcomes with HLA-identical sibling transplantation. *Blood* **107**: 3065–3073.
7. Aversa F, Terenzi A, Carotti A *et al.* (1999) Improved outcome with T cell-depleted bone marrow transplantation for acute leukemia. *J Clin Oncol* **17**: 1545–1550.
8. Aversa F, Terenzi A, Tabilio A *et al.* (2005) Full haplotype-mismatched hematopoietic stem-cell transplantation: A phase II study in patients with acute leukemia at high risk of relapse. *J Clin Oncol* **23**: 3447–3454.

9. Beatty PG, Clift RA, Mickelson EM *et al.* (1985) Marrow transplantation from related donors other than HLA-identical siblings. *N Engl J Med* **313**: 765–771.

10. Aversa F, Tabilio A, Velardi A *et al.* (2007) Hematopoietic stem cell transplantation from alternative donors for high-risk acute leukemia: The haploidentical option. *Curr Stem Cell Res Ther* **2**: 105–112.

11. Luznik L, O'Donnell PV, Symons HJ *et al.* (2008) HLA-haploidentical bone marrow transplantation for hematologic malignancies using nonmyeloablative conditioning and high-dose, posttransplantation cyclophosphamide. *Biol Blood Marrow Transplant* **14**: 641–650.

12. Brodsky RA, Luznik L, Bolanos-Meade J *et al.* (2008) Reduced intensity HLA-haploidentical BMT with post-transplantation cyclophosphamide in nonmalignant hematologic diseases. *Bone Marrow Transplant* **42**: 523–527.

13. Huang XJ, Liu DH, Liu KY *et al.* (2009) Treatment of acute leukemia with unmanipulated HLA-mismatched/haploidentical blood and bone marrow transplantation. *Biol Blood Marrow Transplant* **15**: 257–265.

14. Ogawa H, Ikegame K, Kaida K *et al.* (2008) Unmanipulated HLA 2–3 antigen-mismatched (haploidentical) bone marrow transplantation using only pharmacological GvHD prophylaxis. *Exp Hematol* **36**: 1–8.

15. Ichinohe T, Uchiyama T, Shimazaki C *et al.* (2004) Feasibility of HLA-haploidentical hematopoietic stem cell transplantation between noninherited maternal antigen (NIMA)–mismatched family members linked with long-term fetomaternal microchimerism. *Blood* **104**: 3821–3828.

16. van Rood JJ, Loberiza FR, Jr, Zhang MJ *et al.* (2002) Effect of tolerance to noninherited maternal antigens on the occurrence of graft-versus-host disease after bone marrow transplantation from a parent or an HLA-haploidentical sibling. *Blood* **99**: 1572–1577.

17. Liu D, Huang X, Liu K *et al.* (2008) Haploidentical hematopoietic stem cell transplantation without *in vitro* T cell depletion for treatment of hematological malignancies in children. *Biol Blood Marrow Transplant* **14**: 469–477.

18. Huang YJ, Sun QY, Liu LH *et al.* (2006) Kinetic study of various cytokine mRNA expressions in rhesus treated with haploidentical peripheral blood stem cell transplantation. *Zhongguo Shi Yan Xue Ye Xue Za Zhi* **14**: 571–576.

19. Xiao-Jun H, Lan-Ping X, Kai-Yan L *et al.* (2008) HLA-mismatched/ haploidentical hematopoietic stem cell transplantation without *in vitro* T cell depletion for chronic myeloid leukemia: Improved outcomes in patients in accelerated phase and blast crisis phase. *Ann Med* **40**: 444–455.

20. Aversa F, Terenzi A, Felicini R *et al.* (1998) Mismatched T cell-depleted hematopoietic stem cell transplantation for children with high-risk acute leukemia. *Bone Marrow Transplant* **22**(Suppl. 5): S29–S32.

21. Chang YJ, Xu LP, Liu DH *et al.* (2009) Platelet engraftment in patients with hematologic malignancies following unmanipulated haploidentical blood and marrow transplantation: Effects of CD34$^+$ cell dose and disease status. *Biol Blood Marrow Transplant* **15**: 632–638.

22. Sartor MM, Garvin F, Antonenas V *et al.* (2007) Failure to achieve a threshold dose of CD34$^+$ CD110$^+$ progenitor cells in the graft predicts delayed platelet engraftment after autologous stem cell transplantation. *Bone Marrow Transplant* **40**: 851–857.

23. Kim DH, Won DI, Lee NY *et al.* (2006) Non-CD34$^+$ cells, especially CD8$^+$ cytotoxic T cells and CD56$^+$ natural killer cells, rather than CD34 cells, predict early engraftment and better transplantation outcomes in patients with hematologic malignancies after allogeneic peripheral stem cell transplantation. *Biol Blood Marrow Transplant* **12**: 719–728.

24. Jansen EM, Hanks SG, Terry C *et al.* (2007) Prediction of engraftment after autologous peripheral blood progenitor cell transplantation: CD34, colony-forming unit-granulocyte-macrophage, or both? *Transfusion* **47**: 817–823.

25. Chang YJ, Xu LP, Liu DH *et al.* (in press) The impact of CD34$^+$ cell dose on platelet engraftment in pediatric patients following

unmanipulated haploidentical blood and marrow transplantation. *Pediatr Blood Cancer.*

26. Luo XH, Chang YJ, Xu LP *et al.* (2009) The impact of graft composition on clinical outcomes in unmanipulated HLA-mismatched/ haploidentical hematopoietic SCT. *Bone Marrow Transplant* **43**: 29–36.

27. Huang XJ, Xu LP, Liu KY *et al.* (in press) Partially matched related donor transplantation can achieve outcomes comparable to unrelated donor transplantation for patients with hematologic malignancies. *Clin Cancer Res.*

28. Chen SH, Li X, Huang XJ. (2004) Effect of recombinant human granulocyte colony-stimulating factor on T-lymphocyte function and the mechanism of this effect. *Int J Hematol* **79**: 178–184.

29. Jun HX, Jun CY, Yu ZX. (2004) *In vivo* induction of T cell hyporesponsiveness and alteration of immunological cells of bone marrow grafts using granulocyte colony-stimulating factor. *Haematologica* **89**: 1517–1524.

30. Koh LP, Rizzieri DA, Chao NJ. (2007) Allogeneic hematopoietic stem cell transplant using mismatched/haploidentical donors. *Biol Blood Marrow Transplant* **13**: 1249–1267.

31. Zhao XY, Chang YJ, Xu LP *et al.* Association of natural killer cells in allografts with transplant outcomes in patients receiving G-CSF-mobilized PBSC grafts and G-CSF-primed BM grafts from HLA-haploidentical donors. *Bone Marrow Transplant* [doi:10.1038/ bmt.2009.73].

32. Chang YJ, Zhao XY, Huo MR *et al.* Expression of CD62L on donor CD4$^+$ T cells in allografts: correlation with graft-versus-host disease after unmanipulated allogeneic blood and marrow transplantation. *J Clin Immunol*, [doi:10.1007/s10875-009-9293-9].

33. Ruggeri L, Capanni M, Casucci M *et al.* (1999) Role of natural killer cell alloreactivity in HLA-mismatched hematopoietic stem cell transplantation. *Blood* **94**: 333–339.

34. Ruggeri L, Capanni M, Urbani E *et al.* (2002) Effectiveness of donor natural killer cell alloreactivity in mismatched hematopoietic transplants. *Science* **295**: 2097–2100.

35. Huang XJ, Liu DH, Liu KY *et al.* (2008) Modified donor lymphocyte infusion after HLA-mismatched/haploidentical T cell-replete hematopoietic stem cell transplantation for prophylaxis of relapse of leukemia in patients with advanced leukemia. *J Clin Immunol* **28**: 276–283.

36. Maury S, Cordonnier C, Kuentz M *et al.* (2008) Searching for factors to improve the antileukemic effect of donor lymphocyte infusion. *Blood* **111**: 5256; author's reply 5256–5257.

37. Huang XJ, Liu DH, Liu KY *et al.* (2007) Donor lymphocyte infusion for the treatment of leukemia relapse after HLA-mismatched/haploidentical T cell-replete hematopoietic stem cell transplantation. *Haematologica* **92**: 414–417.

38. Huang XJ, Liu DH, Xu LP *et al.* (2006) Prophylactic infusion of donor granulocyte colony stimulating factor mobilized peripheral blood progenitor cells after allogeneic hematological stem cell transplantation in patients with high-risk leukemia. *Leukemia* **20**: 365–368.

39. Huang XJ, Wang Y, Liu DH *et al.* (2008) Modified donor lymphocyte infusion (DLI) for the prophylaxis of leukemia relapse after hematopoietic stem cell transplantation in patients with advanced leukemia — feasibility and safety study. *J Clin Immunol* **28**: 390–397.

40. Liu KY, Chen YH, Liu DH *et al.* (2008) A pilot study of low-dose recombinant interleukin-2 for acute lymphoblastic malignancy after unmanipulated allogeneic blood and marrow transplantation. *Bone Marrow Transplant* **42**: 535–539.

41. Chang YJ, Zhao XY, Huang XJ. (2008) Effects of the NK cell recovery on outcomes of unmanipulated haploidentical blood and marrow transplantation for patients with hematologic malignancies. *Biol Blood Marrow Transplant* **14**: 323–334.

42. Zhao XY, Huang XJ, Liu KY *et al.* (2007) Reconstitution of natural killer cell receptor repertoires after unmanipulated HLA-mismatched/haploidentical blood and marrow transplantation: Analyses of CD94:NKG2A and killer immunoglobulin-like receptor expression and their associations with clinical outcome. *Biol Blood Marrow Transplant* **13**: 734–744.

43. Zhao XY, Huang XJ, Liu KY *et al.* (2007) Prognosis after unmanipulated HLA-haploidentical blood and marrow transplantation is correlated to the numbers of KIR ligands in recipients. *Eur J Haematol* **78**: 338–346.

44. Chang YJ, Zhao XY, Huo MR *et al.* (2008) Comparison of immune reconstitution after unmanipulated HLA-mismatched/haploidentical blood and marrow transplantation and unmanipulated HLA-matched sibling transplantation in patients with hematological malignancies. *Blood* **112**: abstract 2221.

45. Rutella S, Zavala F, Danese S *et al.* (2005) Granulocyte colony-stimulating factor: A novel mediator of T cell tolerance. *J Immunol* **175**: 7085–7091.

46. Franzke A, Piao W, Lauber J *et al.* (2003) G-CSF as immune regulator in T cells expressing the G-CSF receptor: Implications for transplantation and autoimmune diseases. *Blood* **102**: 734–739.

47. Morris ES, MacDonald KP, Hill GR. (2006) Stem cell mobilization with G-CSF analogs: A rational approach to separate GvHD and GVL? *Blood* **107**: 3430–3435.

48. Chang YJ, Zhao XY, Huo MR, Huang XJ. (2009) Expression profiles of adhesion molecules on naive T cells in bone marrow grafts of healthy donors treated with granulocyte colony-stimulating factor. *Transpl Immunol.*

49. Jun HX, Jun CY, Yu ZX. (2005) A direct comparison of immunological characteristics of granulocyte colony-stimulating factor (G-CSF)–primed bone marrow grafts and G-CSF-mobilized peripheral blood grafts. *Haematologica* **90**: 715–716.

50. Huang XJ, Chang YJ, Zhao XY. (2007) Maintaining hyporesponsiveness and polarization potential of T cells after *in vitro* mixture of G-CSF mobilized peripheral blood grafts and G-CSF primed bone marrow grafts in different proportions. *Transpl Immunol* **17**: 193–197.

51. Ruzek MC, Waire JS, Hopkins D *et al.* (2008) Characterization of *in vitro* antimurine thymocyte globulin-induced regulatory T cells that inhibit graft-versus-host disease *in vivo*. *Blood* **111**: 1726–1734.

52. Bacigalupo A, Lamparelli T, Bruzzi P *et al.* (2001) Antithymocyte globulin for graft-versus-host disease prophylaxis in transplants from unrelated donors: 2 randomized studies from Gruppo Italiano Trapianti Midollo Osseo (GITMO). *Blood* **98**: 2942–2947.

53. Finke J, Schmoor C, Lang H *et al.* (2003) Matched and mismatched allogeneic stem-cell transplantation from unrelated donors using combined graft-versus-host disease prophylaxis including rabbit anti-T lymphocyte globulin. *J Clin Oncol* **21**: 506–513.

54. Hu KX, Zhao SF, Sun QY *et al.* (2007) Effect of bone marrow mesenchymal stem cells on immunoregulation in H-2 haploidentical bone marrow transplantation mice. *Zhonghua Xue Ye Xue Za Zhi* **28**: 505–509.

55. Latini P, Aristei C, Aversa F *et al.* (1992) Interstitial pneumonitis after hyperfractionated total body irradiation in HLA-matched T-depleted bone marrow transplantation. *Int J Radiat Oncol Biol Phys* **23**: 401–405.

Chapter 5

Alloanergization in Haploidentical Hematopoietic Stem Cell Transplantation

Jeff K. Davies[†,¶]*, Lee M. Nadler*[†,¶] *and Eva C. Guinan*[*,‡,§]

Introduction

Allogeneic hematopoietic stem cell transplantation (HSCT) offers the best chance of curing a variety of diseases. Unfortunately, most patients lack fully HLA-matched related donors and many also lack available HLA-matched unrelated donors, particularly patients from minority populations. Although umbilical cord blood (UCB) registries have increased donor availability to some such patients, its use currently remains limited by lack of UCB units from ethnically diverse populations, inadequate stem cell doses for ensuring engraftment in adult recipients and poor immune reconstitution after HSCT.[1–3] In contrast, almost all patients will have available haploidentical family donors, the use of whom would significantly increase the availability of HSCT as a treatment modality.[4] However, haploidentical HSCT leads to increased frequency and severity of acute graft-versus-host disease (GvHD), mediated by alloreactive donor T cells.[5] Although profound nonselective T cell depletion of haploidentical donor grafts effectively prevents severe acute GvHD, this

*Corresponding author. E-mail: Eva_Guinan@dfci.harvard.edu.
Departments of [†]Medical Oncology and [‡]Pediatric Oncology, Dana-Farber Cancer Institute, Boston, MA, [¶]Department of Medicine, Brigham and Women's Hospital and [§]Division of Hematology/Oncology, Children's Hospital, Boston, MA.

process also removes pathogen- and tumor-antigen-specific T cells, delays immune reconstitution and increases both infectious complications and relapse rates, limiting the overall success of nonselective T cell depletion in haploidentical HSCT.[6–10]

Several strategies have therefore been developed to selectively remove or destroy alloreactive T cells within the donor hematopoietic stem cell graft or donor lymphocyte populations to either prevent or limit acute GvHD while preserving beneficial pathogen- and tumor-specific T cells within the remaining nonalloreactive donor T cell pool.[11–17] Most of these "allodepletion" approaches utilize a common mechanistic platform of *ex vivo* donor T cell stimulation by recipient alloantigens and subsequent removal or destruction of alloreactive T cells, identified by activation marker expression, metabolic activity or proliferation. One alternative to selective allodepletion is the strategy of induction of alloantigen-specific hyporesponsiveness in donor T cells by recipient alloantigen presentation with concurrent costimulatory blockade (CSB).[18] This "alloanergization" strategy has been successfully employed in two clinical pilot studies in which very large doses of haploidentical alloanergized donor T cells were infused *en masse* with donor bone marrow, resulting in less severe acute GvHD than for historical control recipients of non-T cell-depleted haploidentical bone marrow transplantation.[19–21]

This chapter will summarize the immunological basis underlying the strategy of alloanergization and the previous clinical experience of alloanergization strategies in the setting of haploidentical HSCT. The experimental evidence that pathogen- and tumor-specific T cell responses are selectively retained by the strategy of alloanergization will also be reviewed. Finally, the design of our current multicenter phase 1 clinical study of delayed infusion of alloanergized donor T cells after haploidentical HSCT will be discussed.

The Immunological Basis of Alloanergization

T cells require at least two signals to become activated: cognate antigen/MHC binding to the T cell receptor (signal 1) and positive costimulation

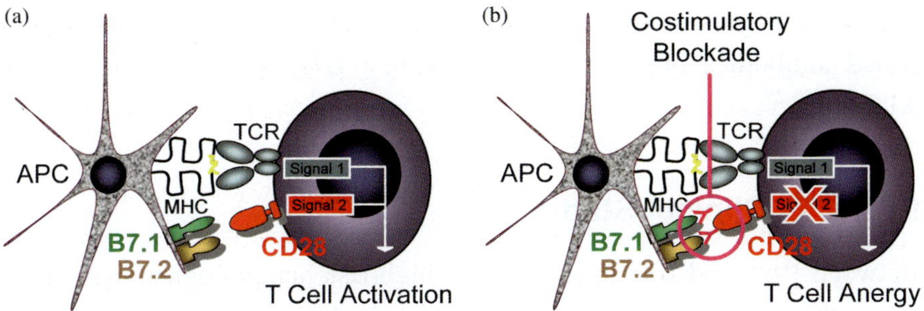

Fig. 1. (a) The delivery of both signal 1 (cognate antigen) and signal 2 (postive costimulation) from APCs to human T cells results in T cell activation. (b) When signal 1 is present but signal 2 is blocked by monoclonal antibodies (costimulatory blockade. shown in pink), the T cell enters a state of persistent antigen-specific hyporesponsiveness, or anergy. APC — antigen-presenting cell; TCR — T cell receptor; MHC — major histocompatibility complex.

by antigen-presenting cells (APCs, signal 2).[22] The predominant positive costimulatory signal to human CD4[+] T cells is delivered via the CD28 receptor (constitutively expressed on the surface of 95% of human CD4[+] cells) via the ligands B7.1 and B7.2 on APCs. When both signal 1 and signal 2 are present, the net result is T cell activation. T cells stimulated only with signal 1 when signal 2 is blocked undergo a cascade of intracellular signaling events resulting in a state of antigen-specific hyporesponsiveness (anergy), defined by absent proliferation upon restimulation with the same antigen, even if signal 2 is present; see Fig. 1.[23]

Thus, recipient-allospecific donor T cells can be rendered anergic by *ex vivo* stimulation with recipient alloantigens in the presence of CSB with molecules which block signals delivered by APCs to the CD28 receptor on the T cell. *In vitro* studies on human peripheral blood mononuclear cells (PBMCs) demonstrated that a complete blockade of both B7.1 and B7.2 during allostimulation was required for effective induction of alloanergy, and that this could be achieved either with the use of CTLA4-Ig, a bioengineered fusion molecule containing the extracellular portion of the CTLA4 receptor (which binds to both the B7.1 and B7.2

ligands, thus preventing their ligation of CD28), or with separate mono-clonal antibodies binding to the individual B7.1 and B7.2 ligands on APCs.[18,24,25]

Previous Clinical Studies

Between 1996 and 2001, patients with high-risk hematological malignan-cies or bone marrow failure underwent haploidentical alloanergized bone marrow transplantation after full intensity conditioning.[19,20]

Patients, Donors and Preparative Regimen

A total of 24 patients enrolled in two pilot studies. The median age of adult patients was 26 years (range 19–50; $n = 7$), while that of those aged <18 was 6.5 years (range 0.5–16; $n = 17$). The haploidentical family donors consisted of parents ($n = 16$), full siblings ($n = 5$), half-siblings ($n = 2$) and children ($n = 1$). The patients received 1400 cGy total body irradiation (175 cGy BID D-6-D-3) and cyclophosphamide 1800 mg/m^2 on D-2 and D-1. Cytosine arabinoside 3g/m^2 q12h for 6 doses was included in the regimen of the first 8 patients. All patients also received methylprednisolone q12h for 4 doses ending no later than 2 h prior to bone marrow transplantation.

Ex Vivo Alloanergization of Bone Marrow

Prior to conditioning, patient PBMCs obtained by leukapheresis were cryopreserved for subsequent use as APCs during *ex vivo* coculture. These cells were subsequently thawed, irradiated and cocultured for 36 h *ex vivo* with donor bone marrow in the presence of CSB, as shown in Fig. 2.

Ex vivo CSB was with CTLA4-Ig (Repligen, Waltham, Massachusetts, USA) for the initial 19 patients, following which a sec-ond pilot study with identical parameters was conducted in which humanized monoclonal anti-B7.1 and -B7.2 antibodies (Wyeth, Madison,

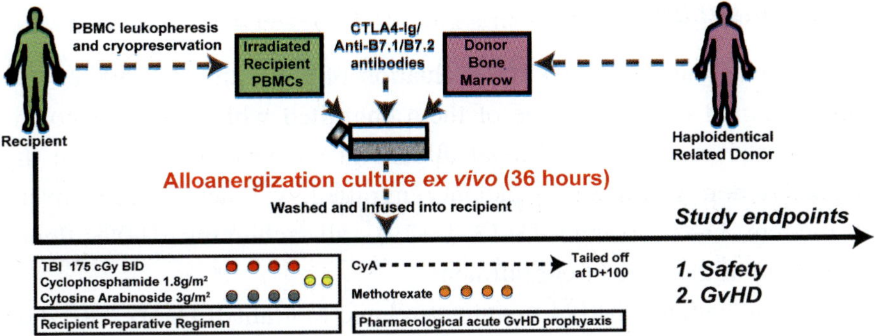

Fig. 2. Schematic design of previous clinical studies of haploidentical alloanergized bone marrow transplantation. PBMC — peripheral blood mononuclear cells; TBI — total body irradiation; CyA — cyclosporin A.

New Jersey, USA) replaced CTLA4-Ig for 5 patients. Patients received alloanergized bone marrow containing median doses of 3.5×10^6/kg $CD34^+$, 29×10^6/kg $CD3^+$, 16×10^6/kg $CD4^+$ and 11×10^6/kg $CD8^+$ cells.

Pharmacological GvHD Prophylaxis and Supportive Care

Conventional GvHD prophylaxis (with short-course methotrexate and cyclosporine) was used. Patients received oral, nonabsorbable antibiotics from admission until neutrophil engraftment, fluconazole for fungal prophylaxis and *Pneumocystis carinii* prophylaxis with trimethoprim-sulfamethoxazole or pentamidine during conditioning and after D+30 or discharge. They received acyclovir prophylaxis at 100 mg/m² q12h if they were seropositive for HSV or at 250 mg/m² q8h if the donor or recipient was CMV-seropositive. Intravenous immunoglobulin (IVIg) was given weekly (400–500 mg/kg) until levels of IgG > 500 mg/dL were sustained without intervention. Patients were monitored for CMV-reactivation at weekly intervals by detection of CMV antigenemia. Those who became CMV-antigenemic received intravenous ganciclovir therapy.

Engraftment and TRM

Two patients died too early for evaluation of engraftment. Another two patients failed to engraft; one of them engrafted without further conditioning after receiving additional alloanergized bone marrow from the original donor. All remaining patients engrafted, with neutrophil recovery at median D+21 (range D+13–D+29), all achieving 100% donor chimerism at the time of engraftment.

Twelve patients died of treatment-related mortality (TRM). Two died of fungal and three of bacterial infection; four of these infection-related deaths occurred in patients with progressive disease at the time of transplant. Five patients died from noninfectious toxicity; four from regimen-related end-organ failure and one, for whom acute GvHD was considered the primary cause of death, died with presumptive fungal infection while receiving immunosuppressive therapy. One patient was found dead at home, cause undetermined. Three-quarters of TRM occurred before D+100 and all before D+200. The overall cumulative incidence of TRM was 50%, with recipient age above 18 years the only factor significantly associated with the overall TRM.

GvHD

Eight of 21 evaluable patients (38%) had clinical findings consistent with acute GvHD, clinically graded B ($n = 3$), C ($n = 4$) and D ($n = 1$). In addition, one patient developed diarrhea immediately prior to death from VOD, with postmortem GI biopsies consistent with acute GvHD. Seven patients had acute GvHD involving the GI tract, and disease was limited to the GI tract in six of these patients. In contrast, only three patients had acute GvHD affecting the skin and/or liver. Eight patients received treatment with systemic corticosteroids, with only two requiring additional treatment. All patients responded with improvement of symptoms. The only death attributable to acute GvHD occurred in a patient who developed a presumed fungal infection on immunosuppressive treatment. There was no significant difference in median infused cell doses of CD34$^+$,

CD3$^+$, CD4$^+$ or CD8$^+$ cells or helper T lymphocyte precursor frequency (or dose) in patients who developed acute GvHD and those who did not. Only one of 12 evaluable patients developed *de novo* chronic GvHD (with GI tract and skin involvement), which resolved after receiving slowly tapering immunosuppression. The cumulative incidence of chronic GvHD (at 8 years) was only 8%.

Viral Reactivation and Infection

Of 11 at-risk patients (donor and/or recipient seropositive for CMV), 5 experienced a total of 7 episodes of CMV reactivation (45%). Only one patient, who had a history of severe CMV disease immediately prior to transplantation had recurrent CMV reactivation. This resolved after prolonged antiviral therapy. No CMV disease and no other clinically significant viral infection or posttransplant lymphoproliferative disorder (PTLD) occurred.

Immune Reconstitution

Eight of nine evaluable patients surviving without relapse beyond D+100 were assessed for T cell subset reconstitution. CD4$^+$ T cell reconstitution was rapid with a median CD4$^+$ count of 90/µL at 1 month and almost 500/µL at 3 months. CD4$^+$ T cell counts above 200/µL were achieved by 3/8, 5/8 and all patients by 2, 4 and 9 months, respectively. CD8$^+$ T cell reconstitution was also rapid; CD8$^+$ counts greater than 200/µL were achieved by 5/8, 7/8 and all patients by 2, 4 and 12 months, respectively. B cell reconstitution was less rapid, although the median CD19 count was greater than 200/µL by 4 months. Reconstituting CD4$^+$ T cells were predominantly memory cells. Naive CD4$^+$ T cells emerged after 6 months. In patients who had CD8 memory cell subsets measured, the majority of reconstituting memory CD8 cells had a CD45RA$^-$ CD62L$^-$ effector memory phenotype. Endogenous immunoglobulin production also recovered rapidly and IVIg replacement was discontinued at a median of 4 months posttransplantation. Quantitative immune reconstitution is depicted in Fig. 3.

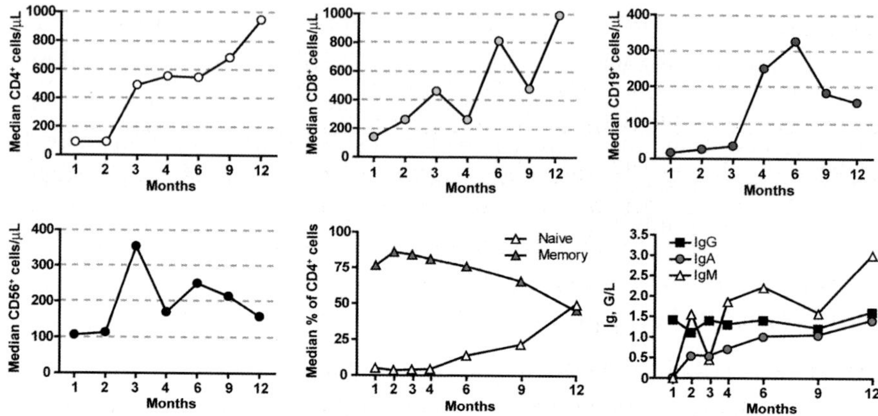

Fig. 3. Reconstitution of T, B and NK cell subsets, naive and memory CD4 T cells and immunoglobulin (Ig) levels after alloanergized haploidentical bone marrow transplantation. Median values are shown for nine assessable patients who survived without disease relapse to D+100. Figure adapted from: Davies *et al.* (2008) *Blood* **112**.

To evaluate factors in the kinetics of T cell reconstitution after haploidentical alloanergized bone marrow transplantation, we performed an area under curve (AUC) analysis. The only factor that was associated with significantly greater CD4[+] T cell reconstitution was patient age (below versus above median). Disease status at time of transplantation, infused cell doses and acute GvHD did not significantly affect CD4[+] T cell subset reconstitution. However, significantly greater CD8[+] T cell reconstitution was observed in patients who reactivated CMV compared to those who did not — consistent with antigen-driven expansion. These early studies were not primarily designed to evaluate reconstitution of antigen-specific immunity, and the data are therefore limited. However, the three patients in whom serial frequencies of CMV-specific pentamer[+] CD8[+] T cells were determined recovered and sustained absolute levels of CMV-specific pentamer[+] CD8[+] T cells above 10 cells/μL (the level identified as protective against CMV infection in early studies of CMV-specific T cell reconstitution after HSCT)[26] as early as D+50. A rapid and sustained expansion of EBV-specific pentamer[+] CD8[+] T cells was also observed in all four evaluated patients.

Outcome

Overall actuarial event-free survival (EFS) was 33% at 10 years, with increased early TRM in adult patients limiting EFS in those aged >18 years. No other factors significantly affected EFS. All three patients transplanted for bone marrow failure are long-term disease-free survivors. The cumulative incidence of relapse/progression (competing risk death in CR/without progression) was 17%. One third of the total cohort has survived to date with a median followup of over 7 years. The survivors have normal performance scores and, specifically, are all disease-free, with normal peripheral blood counts. All have normal immunoglobulin levels and have demonstrated humoral responses to posttransplant vaccinations. None are on immunosuppressive or anti-infectious medications.

Summary

In these two phase 1 clinical studies, myeloablative haploidentical bone marrow transplantation containing very large doses of alloanergized donor T cells resulted in acceptable engraftment and a lower incidence of severe acute GvHD than expected based on that reported after unmanipulated haploidentical bone marrow transplantation. Moreover, alloanergized bone marrow transplantation was associated with rapid T cell reconstitution, *in vivo* expansion of pathogen-specific CD8[+] T cells and early recovery of immunoglobulin production. While substantial early TRM was observed, particularly in adult patients, no TRM was related to viral infection, suggesting that alloanergized T cells were able to confer functional protection against pathogens. Long-term disease-free survival uncomplicated by chronic GvHD or infection was seen in one third of the patients.

In Vitro Studies of Efficacy and Specificity of Alloanergization of Human Peripheral Blood Mononuclear Cells

Our previous clinical studies demonstrated that severe acute GvHD was limited but not prevented after haploidentical alloanergized bone marrow transplantation whilst reconstitution of T cell subsets was very rapid and morbidity due to viral infection was very low. This suggested that donor T cells contained within alloanergized bone marrow may have conferred functional pathogen-specific immunity. We therefore hypothesized that infusion of alloanergized donor T cells might be used to augment immune reconstitution after T cell-depleted HSCT and adapted our *ex vivo* strategy accordingly. We used an *in vitro* HLA-mismatched PBMC model to examine the reduction of alloresponses in both CD4[+] and CD8[+] T cells and the retention of beneficial immune responses prior to implementation of this strategy in a new clinical study.

Alloanergization Reduced Alloproliferative Responses in both CD4[+] and CD8[+] Donor T Cells

Healthy volunteer donor PBMCs were allostimulated for 72 h with irradiated HLA-mismatched PBMCs in the presence of humanized anti-B7.1 and anti-B7.2. Residual proliferation was measured by ^{3}H-thymidine incorporation after allogeneic or mitogenic (soluble CD3 and CD28) stimulation. Alloanergization significantly and consistently reduced subsequent alloproliferation. Median residual alloproliferation was 1.2%, a median 85-fold reduction. In contrast, alloanergized responders retained proliferation after mitogenic stimulation. We also used CFSE labeling of responder PBMCs to measure the reduction in subsets of alloproliferative cells after allorestimulation. First-party-specific alloanergization resulted in a median 30-fold and 8-fold reduction in the percentage of first-party-alloproliferative CD4[+] and CD8[+] cells respectively, when compared to untreated responders, whereas third-party-alloproliferative responses were retained after first-party alloanergization, as shown in Fig. 4.

Importantly, these data demonstrated for the first time that the strategy of alloanergization reduces alloproliferation in both CD4[+] and CD8[+] T cells.[25] Alloresponses were more efficiently reduced in CD4[+] than in CD8[+] cells, probably reflecting the higher frequency of human

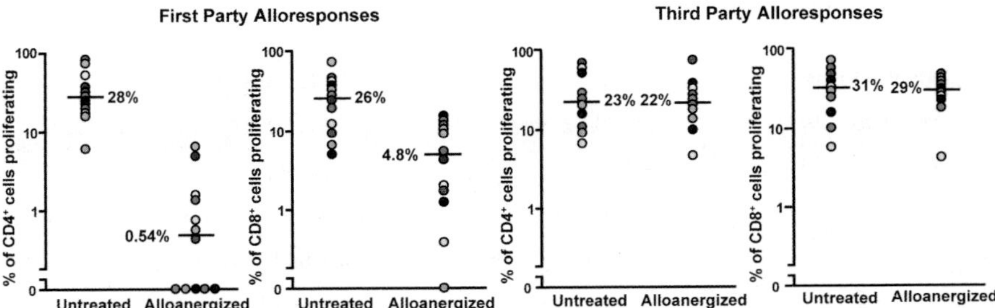

Fig. 4.   Alloanergization of healthy volunteer donor PBMCs resulted in a median 30-fold and 8-fold reduction in first-party-specific CD4 and CD8 alloproliferative responses, respectively (left hand panels). Third-party-specific alloresponses were maintained (right hand panels). Horizontal bars and adjacent numbers represent medians. Adapted from: Davies *et al.* (2008) Transplantation **86**.

CD28⁻CD8⁺ (30%) compared with CD28⁻CD4⁺ cells (5%) found in normal healthy donors.

Functional CD4⁺ and CD8⁺ T Cell Responses to Human Herpes Viruses Were Retained after Alloanergization

Intracellular cytokine secretion and CD107a flow cytometry assays have been developed for assessment of functional low-frequency CD4⁺ and CD8⁺ T cell responses specific to viral pathogens.[27,28] These assays were therefore used to assess the degree of retention of beneficial pathogen-specific immune responses after *in vitro* alloanergization of HLA-mismatched PBMCs from healthy volunteer donors. The frequencies of virus-specific Th1-type cytokine⁺ CD4⁺ and CD8⁺ cells were retained after alloanergization. The ability of CD8⁺ cells to upregulate CD107a (a lysosomal protein associated with degranulation of cytotoxic T cells) was also maintained (Fig. 5). CMV-specific proliferative responses were assessed by measuring CFSE dye dilution in CD4⁺ cells cultured with mock- or CMV-infected lysate for seven days. CMV-specific proliferation was retained after alloanergization in all donors tested.

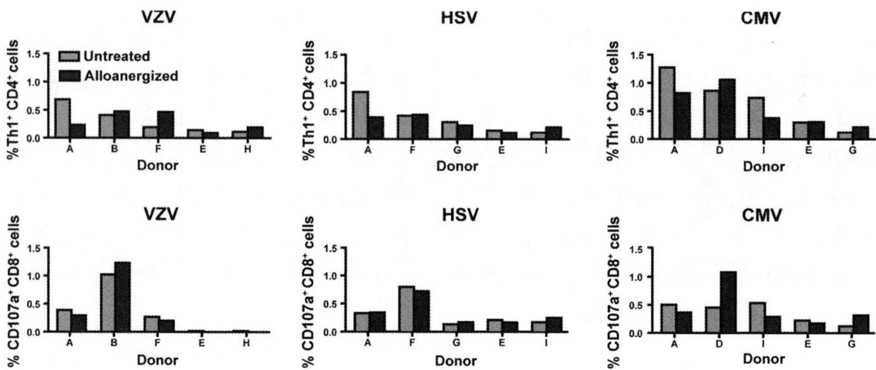

Fig. 5. Functonal viral-pathogen-specific CD4+and CD8+ T cell responses are maintained after alloanergization of healthy volunteer donor PBMCs. Viral-specific Th1 cytokine+ CD4+ cell frequencies are shown specific to VZV, HSV and CMV before and after alloanergization (top row). Similarly, viral-specific CD107a+ CD8+ cell frequencies before and after alloanergization are shown (bottom row).

Tumor-associated Antigen-specific CD8+ and CD4+ T Cell Responses Were Also Retained after Alloanergization

CD8+ T cells specific to the tumor-associated antigen Wilms tumor 1 (WT1) have been identified by IFN-γ secretion.[29,30] We used this approach, measuring IFN-γ secretion by intracellular cytokine secretion flow cytometry after stimulation with a peptide pool derived from the WT1 antigen, in order to assess retention of potential graft–vs-leukemia (GvL) activity in alloanergized PBMCs. WT1-specific IFN-γ+ CD8+ cells were retained after alloanergization in four of five donors and WT1-specific CD107a+ CD8+ cells were retained after alloanergization in all donors. Importantly, four of five alloanergized responders retained WT1-specific IFN-γ+ CD4+ cells.[25]

Summary

The reduction in alloresponses we observed *in vitro* after alloanergization was similar to that reported after many alternate strategies to selectively reduce alloreactivity of human donor T cells. The potential advantages of this approach include: (1) the ability to use PBMC sensitizers rather than specialized allostimulator APCs;[12,13,31] (2) retention of functional viral-pathogen-specific CD4[+] and CD8[+] T cells in similar frequencies to untreated PBMCs and (3) retention of functional WT1-specific T cells, which are detectable at low frequency in up to 50% of healthy donors.[32] This latter observation suggests that alloanergization of PBMCs does not obviate this potential GvL mechanism.[30,33]

New Clinical Study

Encouraged by the rapid immune reconstitution seen in the first two pilot studies of alloanergized haploidentical bone marrow transplantation but mindful of the high early TRM, we chose to design a new multicenter study utilizing delayed infusion of alloanergized donor T cells to improve immune reconstitution after haploidentical T cell-depleted HSCT. The new trial strategy attempts to minimize TRM by utilizing key advances in both our alloanergization strategy and other aspects of transplantation medicine, and is depicted in Fig. 6.

Stem Cell Source and Conditioning Regimen

The use of large numbers of CD34-selected donor cells after myeloablative and immunosuppressive conditioning regimens was first reported by the Perugia group.[34] Since 1999 they have successfully employed a one-step CD34 selection procedure using the CliniMACS device, resulting in a >90% pure CD34[+] product with very low levels of contaminating T cells ($<5 \times 10^4$ CD3[+] cells/kg). While producing markedly delayed immune reconstitution and considerable infectious morbidity and mortality, the use of very-high-dose CD34[+] cells with profound T cell depletion and no pharmacological GvHD prophylaxis resulted in marked improvement in both engraftment rates and prevention of severe acute GvHD after haploidentical HSCT.[7,35,36] We therefore selected a TBI/Fludarabine/ Thiotepa/antithymocyte globulin regimen piloted in Perugia, with

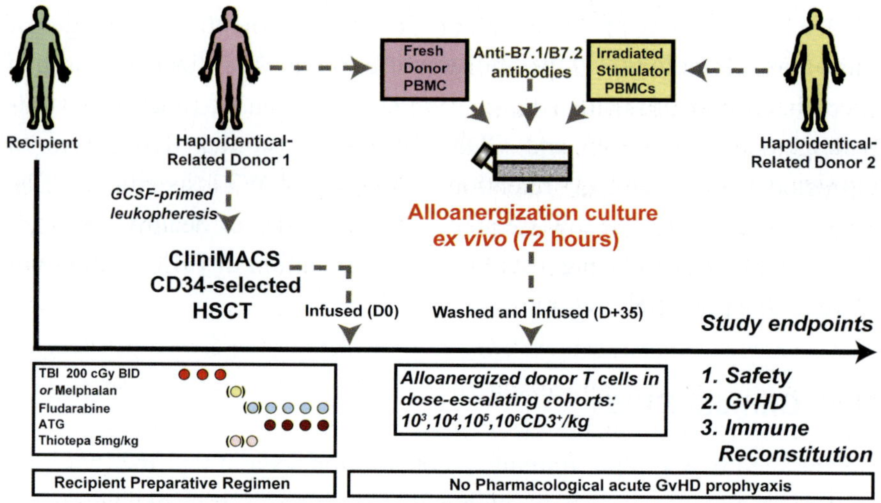

Fig. 6. Schematic design of the new clinical study of delayed infusion of escalating doses of alloanergized donor PBMCs after haploidentical CD34-selected HSCT (cryopreserved recipient PBMCs are used as allostimulators if haploidentical-related donor 2 is unavailable). PBMCs — peripheral blood mononuclear cells; TBI — total body irradiation; ATG — antithymocyte globulin.

modified TBI fractionation shown to be effective by the Emory group.[37] For patients not suitable for TBI we selected a reduced intensity conditioning regimen consisting of Melphalan, Fludarabine and Thiotepa, which has a demonstrated track record in the setting of haploidentical HSCT at the MD Anderson Cancer Center, Texas (personal communication). The median day of neutrophil engraftment in our prior clinical studies of alloanergized bone marrow transplantation was D+21 (range 13–29), with a substantial incidence of early bacterial infection. It is hoped that the use of large doses of CD34-selected peripheral blood stem cells as our HSC source will expedite neutrophil engraftment and therefore reduce early TRM associated with bacterial infection. In addition, cryopreservation of donor HSCs prior to administration of myeloablative conditioning provides an extra measure of patient safety by ensuring an adequate number of donor HSCs and obviating the difficulties of intercurrent donor illness.

Donor T Cell and Allostimulator Sources

Our previous studies used patient PBMCs as allostimulators, raising theoretical concerns both that tumor cells contaminating recipient PBMCs might induce anergy to tumor-associated antigens, and that frozen-thawed PBMCs would not present antigen optimally. Also, cell collection from patients with treatment- or disease-related cytopenia proved difficult. These problems have been addressed by using PBMC allostimulators from a family member with the recipient haplotype disparate in donor and recipient, a strategy successfully implemented by other groups.[38] Patients lacking a family member suitable to act as the donor of stimulator cells for alloanergy induction may donate autologous cells for this purpose.

Timing of Infusion of Alloanergized Donor T Cells

The new protocol temporally separates infusion of CD34-selected (and T cell-depleted) HSCs and infusion of alloanergized T cells. This trial design allows us to address past concerns about the *in vivo* exposure of alloanergized donor T cells to high levels of cytokines. Such high cytokine concentrations have been shown to result in temporary reversal of clonal alloanergy *in vitro*.[39,40] By delaying alloanergized T cell infusion until D+35 after HSCT, chemo-radiotherapy-induced cytokine levels can subside.[41] Delaying administration of the manipulated cells until much of the toxicity from conditioning and neutropenia has resolved also serves to clarify issues of attribution regarding adverse events. We recognize, however, that the substantial infection rates noted at this time in reports from Perugia may weaken both these theoretical advantages.

Dose Escalation of Alloanergized Donor
T Cell Infusion

In order to ascertain the optimal dose of alloanergized donor T cells conferring beneficial cellular immunity while maintaining control of acute GvHD, we have elected to use a Bayesian adaptive dose-escalating trial design provided by Peter Thall, Ph.D. (M.D. Anderson Cancer Center, Houston, Texas). Using a "learn as you proceed" approach characteristic of outcome-adaptive statistical methods, Bayesian models and methods will be used to monitor serious adverse events prior to the patient receiving alloanergized cells and to choose alloanergized cell doses for individual patients, based on efficacy and toxicity seen in previous patients from D+35–100. The dose-finding portion of the design will stop the trial if the D+35–100 toxicity rate at the lower cell doses is unacceptably high, providing an extra measure of safety. The method chooses a cell dose level for each cohort, with the constraint that no untried level may be skipped. The algorithm can escalate, de-escalate, or repeat a dose. In practice, the method treats a substantial number of patients at each dose, provided that it is acceptably safe, with the sample most concentrated on the dose(s) giving the best efficacy–toxicity tradeoff. Covariate-adjusted Bayesian regression analyses of the final data (appropriate to the small sample size and unequal distribution of patients among doses, which characteristically result from any outcome-adaptive dose-finding method) will be employed.

Measurement of Functional Antigen-specific Immune Reconstitution

Recent evidence has shown that the effective provision of pathogen-specific immunity post-HSCT requires antigen-specific memory $CD4^+$ T cells as well as $CD8^+$ effector T cells.[42–44] In addition, the significance of qualitative as well as quantitative impairment of antigen-specific immunity after allogeneic HSCT has become increasingly clear, emphasizing the need for functional rather than just quantitative assays to provide surrogate end points.[45] MHC class I– and II–restricted peptide multimers limit analysis to a single MHC locus/antigen and do not give any measurement of functionality. Therefore, in addition to the use of $CD8^+$ MHC class I–restricted multimers, we are employing non-HLA-restricted approaches described earlier to measure functional $CD4^+$ and $CD8^+$ T cell responses to multiple immunogenic epitopes after stimulation with human herpes virus–infected cell lysates and multiple peptide pools derived from viral pathogens, and to the tumor–associated WT1 antigens. In addition to broader applicability in terms of HLA restriction, this approach stimulates immune responses to multiple antigenic epitopes. Therefore, responses detected are quantitatively larger (and therefore easier to detect) and also likely to more closely represent *in vivo* antigen presentation of important pathogens and tumor-associated antigens.

Final Summary

The clinical pilot studies described have demonstrated the proof of principle that an immunological strategy of *ex vivo* alloanergization can be successfully applied at a clinical scale. After infusion of large doses of haploidentical donor T cells contained within a marrow graft, T cell subsets reconstituted rapidly with relatively low frequencies of severe acute and chronic GvHD and no mortality related to viral infections. This suggested that the infused donor T pool had a diminished response to specific alloantigens and yet retained functional pathogen-specific T cells. However, these studies were limited by a high early TRM, particularly in adult patients, and were not designed to examine optimal efficacy-versus-toxicity tradeoffs.

Recent advances in conditioning regimens and HSC sources have resulted in reliable engraftment after T cell-depleted haploidentical HSCT, suggesting that a new platform of delayed infusion of alloanergized donor PBMCs after T cell-depleted haploidentical HSCT may be one feasible and productive approach to improving immune reconstitution. There are considerable practical advantages to generating alloanergized donor T cells for adoptive use after allogeneic HSCT. More than 10^8 alloanergized donor T cells can routinely be generated from 200 mL of blood, sufficient for an adoptive T cell dose of 10^6/kg for a 70 kg recipient — tenfold more than the dose of selectively allodepleted T cells reported to improve immune reconstitution without significant acute GvHD after haploidentical HSCT in recent key clinical studies.[46,47] PBMCs for use as allostimulator APCs are obtained easily and require no *ex vivo* culture prior to use. We have therefore embarked on a new multicenter clinical trial to assess the use of delayed infusion of escalating doses of alloanergized donor PBMCs after haploidentical T cell-depleted HSCT.

References

1. Ballen KK, Hicks J, Dharan B *et al.* (2002) Racial and ethnic composition of volunteer cord blood donors: Comparison with volunteer unrelated marrow donors. *Transfusion* **42**: 1279.
2. Samuel GN, Kerridge IH, Vowels M *et al.* (2007) Ethnicity, equity and public benefit: A critical evaluation of public umbilical cord blood banking in Australia. *Bone Marrow Transplant* **40**: 729.
3. Brunstein CG, Wagner JE. (2006) Cord blood transplantation for adults. *Vox Sang* **91**: 195.
4. Spitzer TR. (2005) Haploidentical stem cell transplantation: The always present but overlooked donor. *Hematol Am Soc Hematol Educ Program* 390.
5. Szydlo R, Goldman JM, Klein JP *et al.* (1997) Results of allogeneic bone marrow transplants for leukemia using donors other than HLA-identical siblings. *J Clin Oncol* **15**: 1767.
6. Munn RK, Henslee-Downey PJ, Romond EH *et al.* (1997) Treatment of leukemia with partially matched related bone marrow transplantation. *Bone Marrow Transplant* **19**: 421.
7. Aversa F, Tabilio A, Velardi A *et al.* (1998) Treatment of high-risk acute leukemia with T-cell-depleted stem cells from related donors with one fully mismatched HLA haplotype. *N Engl J Med* **339**: 1186.
8. Keever CA, Small TN, Flomenberg N *et al.* (1989) Immune reconstitution following bone marrow transplantation: Comparison of recipients of T-cell-depleted marrow with recipients of conventional marrow grafts. *Blood* **73**: 1340.
9. Horowitz MM, Gale RP, Sondel PM *et al.* (1990) Graft-versus-leukemia reactions after bone marrow transplantation. *Blood* **75**: 555.
10. Henslee PJ, Thompson JS, Romond EH *et al.* (1987) T cell depletion of HLA and haploidentical marrow reduces graft-versus-host disease

but it may impair a graft-versus-leukemia effect. *Transplant Proc* **19**: 2701.

11. Cavazzana-Calvo M, Fromont C, Le Deist F *et al.* (1990) Specific elimination of alloreactive T cells by an anti-interleukin-2 receptor B chain-specific immunotoxin. *Transplantation* **50**: 1.

12. Davies JK, Koh MB, Lowdell MW *et al.* (2004) Antiviral immunity and T-regulatory cell function are retained after selective alloreactive T-cell depletion in both the HLA-identical and HLA-mismatched settings. *Biol Blood Marrow Transplant* **10**: 259.

13. Amrolia PJ, Muccioli-Casadei G, Yvon E *et al.* (2003) Selective depletion of donor alloreactive T cells without loss of antiviral or antileukemic responses. *Blood* **102**: 2292.

14. Mielke S, Nunes R, Rezvani K *et al.* (2007) A clinical scale selective allodepletion approach for the treatment of HLA-mismatched and matched donor–recipient pairs using expanded T lymphocytes as antigen-presenting cells and a TH9402-based photodepletion technique. *Blood.*

15. Wehler TC, Nonn M, Brandt B *et al.* (2007) Targeting the activation-induced antigen CD137 can selectively deplete alloreactive T cells from antileukemic and antitumor donor T-cell lines. *Blood* **109**: 365.

16. Chen BJ, Cui X, Liu C, Chao NJ *et al.* (2002) Prevention of graft-versus-host disease while preserving graft-versus-leukemia effect after selective depletion of host-reactive T cells by photodynamic cell purging process. *Blood* **99**: 3083.

17. Martins SL, St. John LS, Champlin RE *et al.* (2004) Functional assessment and specific depletion of alloreactive human T cells using flow cytometry. *Blood* **104**: 3429.

18. Gribben JG, Guinan EC, Boussiotis VA *et al.* (1996) Complete blockade of B7 family-mediated costimulation is necessary to induce human alloantigen-specific anergy: A method to ameliorate graft-versus-host disease and extend the donor pool. *Blood* **87**: 4887.

19. Guinan EC, Boussiotis VA, Neuberg D *et al.* (1999) Transplantation of anergic histoincompatible bone marrow allografts. *N Engl J Med* **340**: 1704.

20. Davies JK, Gribben JG, Brennan LL *et al.* (2008) Outcome of alloanergized haploidentical bone marrow transplantation after *ex vivo* costimulatory blockade: Results of 2 phase 1 studies. *Blood* **112**: 2232.

21. Powles RL, Kay HEM, Clink HM *et al.* (1983) Mismatched family donors for bone-marrow transplantation as treatment for acute leukaemia. *Lancet* **1**: 612.

22. Bretscher P, Cohn M. (1970) A theory of self–nonself discrimination. *Science* **169**: 1042.

23. Gimmi CD, Freeman GJ, Gribben JG *et al.* (1993) Human T-cell clonal anergy is induced by antigen presentation in the absence of B7 costimulation. *Proc Natl Acad Sci USA* **90**: 6586.

24. Tan P, Anasetti C, Hansen JA *et al.* (1993) Induction of alloantigen-specific hyporesponsiveness in human T lymphocytes by blocking interaction of CD28 with its natural ligand B7/BB1. *J Exp Med* **177**: 165.

25. Davies JK, Yuk D, Nadler LM, Guinan EC. (2008) Induction of alloanergy in human donor T cells without loss of pathogen or tumor immunity. *Transplantation* **86**: 854.

26. Cwynarski K, Ainsworth J, Cobbold M *et al.* (2001) Direct visualization of cytomegalovirus-specific T-cell reconstitution after allogeneic stem cell transplantation. *Blood* **97**: 1232.

27. Jung T, Schauer U, Heusser C *et al.* (1993) Detection of intracellular cytokines by flow cytometry. *J Immunol Methods* **159**: 197.

28. Betts MR, Brenchley JM, Price DA *et al.* (2003) Sensitive and viable identification of antigen-specific CD8$^+$ T cells by a flow cytometric assay for degranulation. *J Immunol Methods* **281**: 65.

29. Oka Y, Tsuboi A, Taguchi T *et al.* (2004) Induction of WT1 (Wilms' tumor gene)–specific cytotoxic T lymphocytes by WT1 peptide vaccine and the resultant cancer regression. *Proc Natl Acad Sci USA* **101**: 13885.

30. Rezvani K, Yong AS, Savani BN *et al.* (2007) Graft-versus-leukemia effects associated with detectable Wilms tumor-1 specific T lymphocytes following allogeneic stem cell transplantation for acute lymphoblastic leukemia (ALL). *Blood* **110**: 1924.

31. Comoli P, Locatelli F, Moretta A *et al.* (2001) Human alloantigen-specific anergic cells induced by a combination of CTLA4-Ig and CsA maintain anti-leukemia and anti-viral cytotoxic responses. *Bone Marrow Transplant* **27**: 1263.

32. Rezvani K, Brenchley JM, Price DA *et al.* (2005) T-cell responses directed against multiple HLA-A*0201-restricted epitopes derived from Wilms' tumor 1 protein in patients with leukemia and healthy donors: Identification, quantification, and characterization. *Clin Cancer Res* **11**: 8799.

33. Rezvani K, Grube M, Brenchley JM *et al.* (2003) Functional leukemia-associated antigen-specific memory CD8[+] T cells exist in healthy individuals and in patients with chronic myelogenous leukemia before and after stem cell transplantation. *Blood* **102**: 2892.

34. Aversa F, Tabilio A, Terenzi A *et al.* (1994) Successful engraftment of T-cell-depleted haploidentical "three-loci" incompatible transplants in leukemia patients by addition of recombinant human granulocyte colony-stimulating factor-mobilized peripheral blood progenitor cells to bone marrow inoculum. *Blood* **84**: 3948.

35. Aversa F, Terenzi A, Carotti A *et al.* (1999) Improved outcome with T-cell-depleted bone marrow transplantation for acute leukemia. *J Clin Oncol* **17**: 1545.

36. Aversa F, Terenzi A, Tabilio A *et al.* (2005) Full haplotype-mismatched hematopoietic stem-cell transplantation: A phase II study in patients with acute leukemia at high risk of relapse. *J Clin Oncol* **23**: 3447.

37. Redei I, Langston AA, Lonial S *et al.* (2002) Rapid hematopoietic engraftment following fractionated TBI conditioning and transplantation with CD34(+) enriched hematopoietic progenitor cells from partially mismatched related donors. *Bone Marrow Transplant* **30**: 335.

38. Andre-Schmutz I, Le Deist F, Hacein-Bey-Abina S *et al.* (2002) Immune reconstitution without graft-versus-host disease after haemopoietic stem-cell transplantation: A phase 1/2 study. *Lancet* **360**: 130.

39. Essery G, Feldmann M, Lamb JR. (1988) Interleukin-2 can prevent and reverse antigen-induced unresponsiveness in cloned human T lymphocytes. *Immunology* **64**: 413.

40. Beverly B, Kang SM, Lenardo MJ, Schwartz RH. (1992) Reversal of *in vitro* T cell clonal anergy by IL-2 stimulation. *Int Immunol* **4**: 661.

41. Ferrara JL, Levy R, Chao NJ. (1999) Pathophysiologic mechanisms of acute graft-vs.-host disease. *Biol Blood Marrow Transplant* **5**: 347.

42. Walter EA, Greenberg PD, Gilbert MJ *et al.* (1995) Reconstitution of cellular immunity against cytomegalovirus in recipients of allogeneic bone marrow by transfer of T-cell clones from the donor. *N Engl J Med* **333**: 1038.

43. Hebart H, Einsele H. (2004) Clinical aspects of CMV infection after stem cell transplantation. *Hum Immunol* **65**: 432.

44. Lacey SF, Diamond DJ, Zaia JA. (2004) Assessment of cellular immunity to human cytomegalovirus in recipients of allogeneic stem cell transplants. *Biol Blood Marrow Transplant* **10**: 433.

45. Ozdemir E, St. John LS, Gillespie G *et al.* (2002) Cytomegalovirus reactivation following allogeneic stem cell transplantation is associated with the presence of dysfunctional antigen-specific CD8$^+$ T cells. *Blood* **100**: 3690.

46. Roy DC, Cohen S, Busque L *et al.* (2006) Phase 1 clinical study of donor lymphocyte infusion depleted of alloreactive T cells after haplotype mismatched myeloablative stem cell transplantation to limit infections and malignant relapse without causing GVHD. *Blood* **108**: 309.

47. Amrolia PJ, Muccioli-Casadei G, Huls H *et al.* (2006) Adoptive immunotherapy with allodepleted donor T-cells improves immune reconstitution after haploidentical stem cell transplantation. *Blood* **108**: 1797.

Chapter 6

Hematopoietic Stem Cell Transplantation Across Genetic Barriers Using a Nonmyeloablative Conditioning Regimen

Liang-Piu Koh[*,†]*, David A. Rizzieri*[*] *and Nelson J. Chao*[*]

Introduction

Allogeneic hematopoietic stem cell transplantation (HSCT) has been successfully used to treat many high risk hematologic malignancies and marrow failure syndromes. The best results with allogeneic HSCT have been obtained in patients receiving an allograft from a human leukocyte antigen (HLA)–matched sibling. As the chance of finding an HLA-genotypically-identical sibling donor is only 25%, much attention has been focused on the use of alternative donors — either unrelated volunteer adult donors, umbilical cord blood or partially matched related donors. Despite the expansion of worldwide unrelated donor registries that have markedly improved the chances of finding a donor for many patients,[1] the application of transplantation using unrelated volunteer adult donors remains limited by some major obstacles,[2] including: (i) the variable chance of finding a suitably genotypically matched unrelated donor, from 60–70% for Caucasians to under 10% for ethnic minorities;

*Adult Bone Marrow and Stem Cell Transplantation Program, Duke University Medical Center, Durham, North Carolina, USA.
[†]Adult Stem Cell Transplant Program, Department of Hematology–Oncology, National University Cancer Institute, National University Health System, Singapore.

(ii) the cumbersome process of identifying, typing, and harvesting an unrelated donor translating to the median time interval between the initiation of a search and the donation of marrow of about four months, rendering this option less viable for patients who urgently need transplantation. Many such patients do not maintain a remission or survive the long waiting period until a donation is available. Moreover, ablative allogeneic transplantation using a matched unrelated donor is still associated with a high transplant-related mortality (TRM) (30–40%) and high long-term morbidity. Umbilical cord blood donations, on the other hand, overcome some of these limitations due to easy procurement, the absence of risk for donors, the potential reduced risk of GvHD, and less stringent criteria for HLA matching for donor–recipient selection. However, engraftment remains a significant concern, in part due to the low number of progenitor cells contained in a single umbilical cord blood unit. Delayed neutrophil recovery and TRM remain the chief obstacles to successful UCB transplantation, particularly in patients receiving a myeloablative preparative regimen.[3]

The use of hematopoietic stem cells from relatives who are only partially HLA-matched provides some advantages for patients lacking fully HLA-matched sibling or unrelated donors. Virtually all patients have at least one HLA-partially-matched parent, sibling, or child, who is immediately available to serve as a donor. Further, the immediate availability of this mismatched family member could have important treatment implications as patients will not be lost to early relapse, and financial implications as the considerable expenditure of additional typing and procurement of unrelated donor grafts, can be avoided.

This review will focus on the recent development of T cell depletion strategies and available data on the transplantation from haploidentical/mismatched donors using nonmyeloablative conditioning.

Evolving Strategies to Overcome HLA Barriers

It becomes clear from these early clinical reports that haploidentical or partially matched HSCT with T cell-replete marrow grafts following myeloablative conditioning was associated with high TRM from GvHD, graft failure, delayed immune reconstitution, vulnerability to life-threatening infections, and relapse.[4–11] Thus, haploidentical transplant could not be widely adopted as a routine procedure, leading to subsequent efforts focusing on strategies to overcome these barriers, which include: (i) reducing the intensity of conditioning and hence ameliorating the regimen-related toxicity; (ii) promoting the engraftment capacity of the graft by means of GCSF-mobilized PBSCs, and the use of megadoses of stem cells; (iii) effective T cell depletion methods for decreasing both graft rejection and GvHD by different *in vivo* ± *ex vivo* T cell depletion procedures; (iv) exploiting the concept of alloreactive NK cells, which may play a vital role in facilitating engraftment and in preventing relapse.[12]

The initial attempts at overcoming the HLA barrier focused on strategies for effective host and graft T cell depletion. However, the benefit of a decrease in GvHD from donor T cell depletion was offset by a higher incidence of graft rejection, relapse, and infections.[13,14] Another major step toward induction of tolerance was achieved following the pioneering work by Reisner[15] and the clinical results of Aversa *et al.* using "megadoses" of hematopoietic stem cells mobilized into the peripheral blood by growth-factor use as a supplement to the heavily T cell-depleted mismatched bone marrow stem cells. A remarkably high 95% engraftment rate was seen in patients receiving an allograft from haploidentical 3/6 HLA-matched family members in the absence of severe GvHD despite there being no postgrafting immunosuppression.[16] The encouraging results of their subsequent study using strategies involving large doses of T cell-depleted blood-derived stem cells spurred further interest in exploring the option of using haploidentical/mismatched related donors for patients who may benefit from a transplant but do not have a readily available matched donor.

Effective T Cell Depletion: A Pivotal Platform in the Development of Haploidentical/Mismatched Transplantation

Despite the problems associated with T cell depletion (TCD), great interest remains in developing this technology due to the negative effects of severe GvHD, particularly for recipients of HLA-mismatched or haploidentical allografts. The past decade has witnessed the development of different graft manipulation strategies (see Table 1), moving from E-rosetting and soybean agglutination, through a combination of negative and positive selection of HSCs, to the current method of one-step positive selection using immunoadsorption columns and monoclonal antibody for *ex vivo* or *in vivo* purging. The rapid progress in this area has resulted in effective prophylaxis of GvHD and provides a pivotal platform in the development of haploidentical transplant.[2] It also leads to the enthusiastic application of TCD in allogeneic HSCT, with the general anticipation that pharmacological immunosuppression in this setting is not adequate. While large bodies of clinical evidence attest to the efficacy of TCD strategies in crossing the immunological barrier and GvHD suppression, they have also revealed new and important limitations associated with TCD HSCT. These include potentially a higher incidence of graft failure, relapse, and complications associated with delayed immune reconstitution with resultant risk of infection and EBV-PTLD.

Table 1. Methods of T Cell Depletion

---

1. *Ex vivo* TCD
1.1. *Negative selection*

    Physical — DACS (density-adjusted cell sorting)
         — Counterflow centrifugal elutriation

    Immunological — soybean lectin and erythrocyte rosette
         Monoclonal antibody + rabbit/human complement
         Monoclonal antibody formulated as immunotoxin
         Monoclonal antibody bound to magnetic beads

    Photodynamic cell purging

1.2. *Positive selection*
    CD34$^+$ immunoadsorption column (e.g. CliniMACS)

2. *In vivo* TCD
    Monoclonal antibody (e.g. alemtuzumab/campath)
    Antithymocyte globulin (e.g. thymoglobulin)

Early Development in T Cell Depletion

Early efforts at TCD were thus intended to maximally purge lymphocytes without compromising hematopoietic precursors. Positive and/or negative selection of the hematopoietic stem cells are the most commonly used techniques in graft manipulation today. In the negative selection, unwanted T cells are eliminated from the allogeneic grafts. The early techniques of negative selection developed were based on combining E-rosetting and soybean lectin aggutination, which removes cells producing graft-vs-host reactions by differential agglutination with the galactose binding lectin soybean agglutinin.[17] This approach had first been attempted in animal models,[17] then applied in transplantation for patients with severe combined immunodeficiency and leukemia.[18,19] Investigators in Perugia made further advances in successful TCD in pioneering the megadose $CD34^+$ stem cell dosage. This approach utilizes G-CSF-mobilized peripheral blood stem cells and bone marrow cells, both *ex vivo*-depleted of T cells by soybean agglutination and E-rosetting, following an intensive total body irradiation (TBI)–based conditioning regimen. Clinical studies showed convincingly that prompt engraftment was achieved with a low occurrence of GvHD.[16,20]

Since the 1990s, several investigators have started evaluating haploidentical transplant by using partial TCD combined with intensive immunosuppression. Henslee Downey *et al.*[21] were among the pioneers in exploiting a novel sequential immunomodulation strategy pre- and posttransplant using *ex vivo* TCD with the $T_{10}B_9$ monoclonal antibody and *in vivo* T cell lysis with immunotoxin H65-RTA, following an intensive TBI-based myeloablative conditioning. Seventy-two patients received partially mismatched related donor grafts from haploidentical family members using this treatment protocol. The engraftment rate of 88%, the 16% probability of acute GvHD grades II–IV, and the 51% probability of extensive chronic GvHD were encouraging. At a median follow up of 21.5 months, the 2-year disease-free survival (DFS) was 31%, with a 53% probability of DFS seen among the low risk patients.

Drobyski *et al.*[22] in a single institution analysis, compared the outcome of patients who received transplant from a matched unrelated donor, mismatched unrelated donor, or haploidentical donor. All patients had received a T cell-depleted marrow graft, using either $T_{10}B_9$ or OKT3. There was a decrease in relapse and increase in survival in matched unrelated donor recipients compared with the other two groups, but the degree of TCD might not have been sufficient for the haploidentical setting. The higher TRM after transplantation from a mismatched unrelated or haploidentical related donor transplant compared to matched unrelated donor transplant demonstrated a clear effect of HLA disparity.

These studies highlighted the feasibility of partial TCD in preventing GvHD in mismatched hematopoietic transplant and the importance of postgrafting immunosuppression in lowering the risk of graft failure, significantly broadening the array of patients who may now be offered immunotherapy from those with matched donors to those with at least a partially matched family member.

Recent Advances in T Cell Depletion

While a wide range of T cell-depleting techniques (Table 1) have been employed, three different strategies of TCD have emerged to show promising results: (1) positive $CD34^+$ selection; (2) *ex vivo* $CD3^+/CD19^+$ TCD (negative selection); (3) *in vivo* TCD using alemtuzumab or ATG. Although it is impossible to make a definite conclusion with regard to the best option available in the absence of propective comparative studies, some of the merits and limitations of each technique will be compared and discussed.

A wide array of monoclonal antibodies, either used alone.[23–25] or in conjunction with homologous or heterologous complement,[26–28] have been employed, with successful 2–4-log T cell reduction. Alemtuzumab (Campath), an anti-CD52 monoclonal antibody, has been widely used for both *in vitro* and *ex vivo* TCD. It has been incorporated into many myeloablative and nonmyeloablative conditioning regimens, with encouraging outcomes in terms of GvHD management, and has also broadened the applicability of transplant using both matched and mismatched donors.[29–31]

Positive CD34 Selection

Using CD34[+] hematopoietic stem cell selection for elimination of T cells represents an important breakthrough in the field of HSCT, especially haploidentical transplantation. Introduced by investigators from Tuebingen, CD34[+] selection was primarily developed to enrich hematopoietic progenitor cells and passive depletion of tumor or lymphoma cell contamination in the autologous apheresis product.[32–34] The first system available for large, clinical scale CD34[+] selection was based on an immunoaffinity device using an avidin-coated column and biotinylated anti-CD34 antibody (Ceprate SC).[35] During subsequent years new methodologies based on immunomagnetic enrichment with ferromagnetic particles (Isolex 300) have been developed, which allowed better recovery of CD34[+] cells and purities $\geq 95\%$.[34,36] The technology of immunomagnetic CD34[+] selection has now been optimized toward a closed system which allows each site to adhere to the principles of good manufacturing practice, leading to approval for clinical use in Europe and the United States. Importantly, the availability of the CD34[+] enrichment technique using the CliniMACS system (Miltenyi Biotec Gmbh, Bergish Gladbach, Germany) has provided a reproducible TCD of >4.5 logs in several studies.[34] This technology, initially intended to prepare stem cell grafts for autologous transplantation, was later extended to allogeneic transplantation settings. Moreover, positive stem cell selection techniques can be followed by antibody-based negative selection to further deplete specific T cell populations. Several studies have shown the feasibility of transplanting allogeneic CD34[+]-selected PBSCs from matched related donors,[37] haploidentical related donors[16,38] and unrelated donors.[39] In contrast to the time-consuming and "difficult-to-standardize" TCD techniques by the older physical separation methods discussed above, the availability of CD34[+] selection has allowed effective, reproducible TCD to be performed in a relatively simple and automated manner.

CD3$^+$/CD19$^+$ Depletion

The delayed immune reconstitution in CD34$^+$-selected cells is partly attributed to the absence of NK cells, monocytes or granulocytes. A negative T and B cell depletion strategy was thus developed to overcome this limitation. Using anti-CD3$^-$ and anti-CD19-coated microbeads on a CliniMACS device, this negative T and B cell (CD3/CD19) depletion strategy resulted in grafts with up to a four-log reduction in T cells. The CD34$^+$ dose was approximately half of that collected from the CD34$^+$ selection strategies reported above.[40] This approach preserves a high content of NK cells and other non-CD34$^+$ cells in the graft, which may contribute to the important engraftment-facilitating function and graft-versus-tumor effects after transplantation, especially in the setting of killer inhibitory receptor (KIR) mismatch situations. Further, the cellular preparations depleted of B cells minimize development of Epstein–Barr-virus-associated lymphoproliferative diseases. This CD3/CD19 depletion approach has been tested in a pilot study of 10 patients with advanced hematological malignancies receiving transplant from mismatched donors. Using a reduced intensity conditioning regimen, the study showed that stable engraftment could be achieved in all patients with a low incidence of GvHD.[40] Treatment-related mortality was still 30%, though, and overall survival was 50%, with 4 patients alive and in complete remission at a median followup of >1 year. Importantly, favorable immune reconstitution with fast reconstitution of NK cells was noted with this approach, resulting in fewer infectious complications. In their most recently published, updated report, which included 19 more patients, engraftment occurred in all except 1 patient. Grade ≥2 acute GvHD occurred in 48% of the patients. However, the first 100-day TRM was 20% and the event-free and overall survival at 12 months were both 35%.[41] The fast engraftment seen in this CD3/CD19 group with CD34 doses as low as 5.2×10^6 CD34$^+$ cells/kg demonstrates that successful haploidentical transplant may be feasible even without megadoses of CD34$^+$ stem cells. This may have logistic implications, as mobilization and/or harvesting and processing of megadoses of CD34$^+$ cells can be labor-intensive, expensive, and can place considerable demands on both the donors and the pheresis service.

In vivo T cell Depletion Using Alemtuzumab or ATG

Another method of immunosuppression commonly used to reduce graft failure and GvHD in unrelated or mismatched/haploidentical transplant is the simultaneous depletion of host and donor immune cells using ATG or alemtuzumab at the time of transplant. Significant *in vivo* depletion of donor T cells from the graft can be achieved with alemtuzumab and ATG persisting in the patient's circulation for weeks after the allograft, thereby allowing a prolonged donor TCD and reduction in the risk of GvHD. Several investigators have incorporated antithymocyte globulin (ATG), with some confirming that the addition to ATG pretransplant reducing the risk of severe aGvHD, the incidence of extensive cGvHD, and of non-relapse mortality (NRM).[42–44] This has led to the results of matched unrelated donor transplant approaching those of matched sibling donor transplant in some series.[45–47] However, there are also disadvantages to this approach, because there is evidence for delayed immune reconstitution and a higher risk of infectious complications and of disease relapse.[48] At least one phase III study is underway in the MUD population to assess the outcomes with and without ATG in the preparative regimen.

Alemtuzumab (Campath-1H), a humanized rat monoclonal anti-CD52 antibody, targets the CD52 antigen, which is expressed by all lymphocytes, monocytes, and dendritic cells, but not by adult hematopoietic stem cells.[49] The long half-life of alemtuzumab also results in the depletion of donor $CD52^+$ cells, including circulating antigen-presenting dendritic cells.[50,51] This humanized antibody is uniquely suited to managing both graft rejection and GvHD because of its ability to deplete T cells as well as B cells from both host and recipient.[52] Furthermore, recent evidence has suggested that alemtuzumab may be selective in the T cells that it targets for elimination, thus allowing it to limit GvHD while promoting engraftment and maintaining the allogeneic antitumor effect. The preferential targeting of CD52 expressing monocyte-derived dendritic cells, and sparing of Langerhans cells and dermal-interstitial dendritic cells, has been speculated to facilitate immune reconstitution and mediation of the GvL effect.[53]

Alemtuzumab has been used over the last two decades in stem cell transplantation for depletion of donor and recipient T cells to prevent graft-vs-host disease and graft rejection.[30,31] Several clinical trials evaluated its ability to prevent GvHD following conventional or reduced-intensity conditioning allografts, in the settings of either matched related, unrelated, or mismatched/haploidentical donor transplants.[54–58] By depleting T cells in both the donor and the recipient, alemtuzumab has been shown to prevent development of both acute and chronic GvHD, without impairing engraftment or inhibiting the benefits associated with the graft-versus-leukemia effect.[55]

In the context of haploidentical transplant, the use of alemtuzumab or ATG for *in vitro* TCD without any *ex vivo* graft manipulation has resulted in a low incidence of grade II–IV and III–IV acute GvHD ranging between 16–40% and 8–16%, respectively, in several series.[57–59]

This approach, while allowing the omission of *ex vivo* graft manipulation without compromising its efficacy in risk of GvHD reduction and facilitating engraftment, also confers the advantage of simplifying the transplant procedure and lowering costs. Moreover, this technique provides the additional advantage of allowing TCD to be performed in the absence of a cell-processing facility.[2]

The Rationale of Haploidentical/Mismatched Transplantation Using Nonmyeloablative Conditioning

Several studies have been published on the use of T cell-depleted grafts from haploidentical/mismatched donors following myeloablative conditioning.[20,59–63] While the highly immunosuppressive and myeloablative conditioning regimen and a megadose of extensively T cell-depleted GCSF-mobilized PBSCs has demonstrated encouraging survival results, it is not without limitations. Firstly, the procedure is associated with significant regimen-related toxicity and high treatment-related mortality (35–40%)[60,61] due primarily to infections. Secondly, a megadose of purified CD34$^+$ cells is crucial in overcoming the barrier of residual antidonor cytotoxic T lymphocyte precursors in T-depleted mismatched transplant. There is continuing concern with regard to the slow engraftment or graft failure in patients receiving a lower cell dose. Previous studies from Tuebingen have shown delayed engraftment at CD34 doses less than 8×10^6/kg body weight.[64] As such, most physicians would usually target for a megadose of stem cells (>10×10^6 CD34$^+$ cells/kg body weight) from the donor while planning for haploidentical transplants. This can place considerable demands on both the donors and the pheresis service, for the following reasons: (i) the high graft content is an obstacle in large adults; (ii) the long hours of multiple days of pheresis can be exhausting, with a slight increase in pheresis-related adverse effects on donors; (iii) for the pheresis and stem-cell-processing laboratory staff, the procedures involved can be time-consuming and labor-intensive. Also, the remarkable results achieved by the Perugia group using the haploidentical megadose PBSC approach did not seem to be reproducible by other investigators in the United States. Even with high cell doses, graft failure in the range of 5–14% has been reported by some.[65–67] Communications from investigators and reports given at conferences on haploidentical transplantation have indicated that both graft failure and GvHD remained a problem and there were few survivors.[68] Developing new strategies of T depletion or graft manipulation in mismatched HSCT, with the aim of improving engraftment with better-tolerated, less toxic conditioning has become an important area of research.

Although the number of mismatched allogeneic HSCTs has increased steadily over the past few decades, this high risk ablative procedure can be offered only to a minority of patients, since most subjects are beyond the age when myeloablative preparative regimens can be delivered with a reasonable degree of safety. GvHD and high transplant-related mortality in the range of 35–40%, contributed mainly by posttransplant infectious complications and other toxicities, remain significant deterrents and have limited use in otherwise healthy, younger patients as well. To extend allogeneic HSCT to older patients with comorbidities, reduced-intensity or nonmyeloablative conditioning lacking significant regimen-related toxicities has been developed.

Recent Studies Using T Cell-depleted Hematopoietic Cell Grafts Involving Nonmyeloablative Conditioning (Table 2)

Results from Tuebingen/Dresden

Based on the promising experience gained at St. Jude Children's Research Hospital (SJCRH), Memphis, USA, from the pediatric population,[69,70] investigators from Tuebingen explored a new TCD strategy in adult patients following dose-reduced conditioning.[40] Using this new approach, T and B cells (CD3/CD19) are negatively depleted from PBSCs with 3.5–4-log T depletion using anti-CD3- and anti-CD19-coated microbeads on a CliniMACS device. In contrast to the CD34$^+$ selection strategy pioneered by the Perugia group, CD3/CD19-depleted grafts harvested using this strategy not only contain CD34$^+$ stem cells but also CD34$^-$ progenitors and natural killer, dendritic, and graft-facilitating cells. Dose-reduced conditioning made up of fludarabine (150–200 mg/m^2), thiotepa (10 mg/kg), melphalan (120 mg/m^2), and OKT-3 (5 mg/day, day -5 to $+14$) was used. Ten adult patients with a median age of 43 and advanced hematological malignancies received mismatched transplant using this approach. Rapid engraftment with full donor chimerism was seen after two weeks in all patients. Six patients developed grade II GvHD and one developed lethal grade IV GvHD. Treatment-related mortality was 30% and overall survival was 50%, with four patients in complete remission with a median followup of >1 year. The fast engraftment seen in this CD3/CD19 group with CD34 doses as low as 5.2×10^6 CD34$^+$ cells/kg demonstrates that successful haploidentical transplant may be feasible even without megadoses of CD34$^+$ stem cells. Importantly, the favorable immune reconstitution with fast reconstitution of NK cells was noted with this approach, resulting in few infectious complications.

Table 2. Summary of Outcome of Nonmyeloablative Mismatched/Haploidentical Stem Cell Transplantation

Institutions (Authors, Year)	Number of Patients	Preparative Regimens	GvHD Prophylaxis	Median Cell Dose ($\times 10^6$/kg) CD34/CD3	Method of T Cell Depletion	Primary Graft Failure	GvHD	NRM	Outcome/ Survival
Duke University (Rizzieri, 2007)[57]	49	Flu/Cy/Campath	MMF ± CSP	13.5/460[†]	*In vivo* ± *ex vivo* TCD with Campath	6%	Gd III–IV: 16% Gd III–IV: 8%	10.2%	OS: 31% @ 1 year
Tuebingen/ Dresden (Bethge, 2006)[40]	10	Flu/TT/Melphalan/ OKT3	TCD	7.8/0.02	*Ex vivo* CD3/ CD19% negative depletion with anti-CD3 and CD19 Mab	0%	Gd II: 6/10 Gd IV: 1/10	30%	OS: 50% @ >1 year
Tuebingen (Hand-gretinger, 2007)[71]	38	Flu/TT/Melphalan	TCD	16/0.049	*Ex vivo* CD3/CD19 negative depletion with anti-CD3 and CD19 Mab	17%	Gd II–IV: 27%	2.6%	EFS: 70% in good risk patients EFS: 20% in poor risk patients

(*Continued*)

Table 4.2. (*Continued*)

Institutions (Authors, Year)	Number of Patients	Preparative Regimens	GvHD Prophylaxis	Median Cell Dose ($\times 10^6$/kg) CD34/CD3	Method of T Cell Depletion	Primary Graft Failure	GvHD	NRM	Outcome/ Survival
MGH (Spitzer, 2003)[73–75]	12	Cy/Anti-CD2 Mab/Thymic RT	CsP ± *ex vivo* TCD PBSC	10.6*/8.9*	*Ex vivo* CD 34 selection+ *in vivo* TCD using anti-CD 2 Mab	0%	Gd II–IV: 2/12	25%	17% DFS, 25% OS @ 15–34 months
JHU/FHCRC (Luznik, 2008)[77]	68	TBI/Cy/Flu/ Post BMT Cy	FK506/MMF	4.8/42	Not done	13%	Gd II–IV: 34%	15%	26% EFS, 36% OS @ 2 years
Osaka University (Ogawa, 2006)[78]	26	Flu/Bu/ATG	FK506/MP	6.55/254[†]	*In vitro* TCD with ATG	4%	Gd II: 20%	15%	EFS 55% @ 3 years OS 58% at median FU 664 days

(*Continued*)

Table 4.2. (*Continued*)

Institutions (Authors, Year)	Number of Patients	Preparative Regimens	GvHD Prophylaxis	Median Cell Dose ($\times 10^6$/kg) CD34/CD3	Method of T Cell Depletion	Primary Graft Failure	GvHD	NRM	Outcome/ Survival
Tokyo University (Kanda, 2005)[58]	12	Myeloablative ($N = 6$): TBI/ Cy/Campath Reduced intensity ($N = 6$): Flu/Bu/ Campath ± TBI 4 Gy	CsP/MTX	5.1/260[†]	*In vivo* TCD with Campath	0%	Gd III–IV: 9%	17%	≈35% OS @ 1 year

GvHD: graft-vs-host disease; NRM: nonrelapse mortality; MPD: myeloproliferative disease; Flu: fludarabine; Cy: cyclophosphamide; MMF: mycophenolate mofetil; CSP: cyclosporin A; OS: overall survival; TT: Thiotepa; HM: hematological malignancies; AA: aplastic anemia; CR: complete remission; MGH: Massachusetts General Hospital; JHU: Johns Hopkins University; FHCRC: Fred Hutchinson Cancer Research Center; RT: irradiation; FK506: tacrolimus; Mab: monoclonal antibody; MP: methylprednisolone; TCD: T cell depletion; DFS: disease-free survival; EFS: event-free survival TBI: total body irradiation; Bu: busulphan; FU: followup; ATG: antithymocyte globulin; Campath: alemtuzumab.

*Cell dose for a subgroup of patients.

[†]Cell dose before T cell depletion.

In another recent study from Tuebingen,[71] Handgretinger *et al.* reported the outcome of 38 pediatric patients with high risk hematological malignancies and severe aplastic anemia who received haploidentical transplant using this approach. The dose-reduced conditioning was modified to a lower dose of fludarabine (to reduce neurotoxicity), and OKT3 was omitted. Primary sustained engraftment occurred in 83% of the patients and final engraftment was 98% when the remaining patients with graft failure had a repeat transplant. Grade II–IV acute GvHD occurred in only 27% of the patients. Overall TRM was low at 2.6%. The favorable event-free survival of 70% seen only in patients with nonmalignant disease and those in remission at the time of transplant, suggests that disease relapse is a major obstacle among patients with refractory malignancies who undergo haploidentical transplant.

Results from Massachusetts General Hospital

Based on murine models established by Sykes and colleagues,[72] a series of haploidentical stem cell transplantations have been conducted at Massachusetts General Hospital. To address the problems of graft failure and GvHD, the initial regimen has been modified to its current form, which includes cyclophosphamide, fludarabine, MEDI-507 (a monoclonal anti-CD2 antibody), and thymic irradiation. Mixed "split lineage" lymphohematopoietic chimerism has been achieved in most cases with this strategy, with a predominance of donor myeloid chimerism and a much lower percentage of donor T cell chimerism. In addition, mixed chimerism, including the low percentage of donor T cell chimerism, can be successfully converted to full or nearly full donor chimerism with either no GvHD or manageable, primarily cutaneous GvHD. Recurrent malignancy and late infections have been the chief reasons for treatment failure with this approach. Efforts are underway to optimize the *ex vivo* TCD of the product and to explore different doses of delayed DLI.[73–75]

Results from Johns Hopkins University/ Fred Hutchinson Cancer Research Center

O'Donnell *et al.* from Johns Hopkins University have performed non-myeloablative haploidentical transplant on 13 patients with hematological malignancies using low-dose TBI 2 Gy and fludarabine (with or without cyclophosphamide) as conditioning. High-dose posttransplant cyclophosphamide, given at 50 mg/kg on day 3, was added to tacrolimus/mycophenolate mofetil to improve GvHD prophylaxis.[76] The median time to absolute neutrophil count >500/μL in 8 patients with engraftment was 15 days (range 13–16 days). Acute GvHD developed in 6 of the 13 patients. Six of the 13 patients were alive, and 5 were in a complete remission at a median of 191 days posttransplant, including 2 patients with graft rejection. The results suggest possible benefits of pre- and post-transplant cyclophosphamide in promoting engraftment and prevention of GvHD. In the recent publication which involved collaboration with investigators from Fred Hutchinson Cancer Research Center in Seattle, USA, Luznik *et al.*[77] presented the updated series involving 67 patients with a variety of advanced hematological malignancies treated with fludarabine, cyclophosphamide, and TBI 2 Gy as conditioning, with tacrolimus, MMF, and cyclophosphamide (either 1 or 2 doses) given as prophylaxis for GvHD. Graft rejection occurred in only 13% of the evaluable patients. Acute grade II–IV and II–IV GvHD occurred in 34% and 6% of the patients, respectively, with no statistically significant difference for patients receiving 1 versus 2 doses of cyclophosphamide. At a median followup among survivors of 745 days, the actuarial overall and event-free survival at 2 years were 36% and 26%, respectively.

Results from Osaka University

Ogawa *et al.*[78] from Osaka University Hospital in Japan investigated the use of an ATG-based nonmyeloablative conditioning regimen as previously reported by Slavin *et al.*[79] in the haploidentical transplant of 26 patients who had hematologic malignancies in an advanced stage or with a poor prognosis. Using a conditioning made up of fludarabine, busulfan, and anti–T-lymphocyte globulin and GvHD prophylaxis consisting of tacrolimus and methylprednisolone (1mg/kg/day), 26 patients underwent transplantation using peripheral blood stem cells from 2–3 antigen HLA-mismatched donors. All patients except for 1 achieved donor-type engraftment. Full donor chimerism was achieved by day 14. Only 5 (25%) of the 20 evaluable patients developed grade II GvHD. Sixteen of the 26 patients are alive, in complete remission. Four died of transplantation-related causes and 6 died of progressive disease. The event-free survival at 3 years was 55%.

Results from Tokyo University

Kanda *et al.*[58] evaluated the feasibility of haploidentical unmanipulated PBSC transplantation from 2 or 3 locus-mismatched family members using *in vivo* alemtuzumab in 12 patients (median age 49.5 years) with high-risk hematological malignancies. Six patients received a TBI-based myeloablative regimen, whereas the remaining 6 patients older than 50 years received less intensive or nonmyeloablative fludarabine-based conditioning. Alemtuzumab was added on days −8 to −3 and CsP+MTX was used as GvHD prophylaxis. There was no graft rejection, and the incidence of grade III–IV acute GvHD was only 9%. The nonrelapse mortality was observed in only 2/12 patients. None of the patients died of infectious causes despite impaired T cell immune reconstitution during the first 2 months after transplantation.

Results from Duke University

Rizzieri *et al.*[57] from Duke University recently reported one of the largest series of adult patients with nonmyeloablative transplant using 3–5/6 HLA-matched family donors. Forty-nine patients with hematological malignancies or marrow failure were accrued. The patients in this group were, on average, older (median age 48) than those in most other reported series haploidentical transplants. Using a nonmyeloablative preparative regimen consisting of fludarabine and cyclophosphamide in combination with alemtuzumab for *in vivo* and *in vitro* TCD, the group reported successful engraftment in 94% of the patients, low treatment-related mortality rates of 10.2%, and severe GvHD of 8%. With more than half of the patients not in the first CR at transplantation, the high CR rate of 75% was encouraging. With 4.25 years of median followup, 1-year overall survival in this high-risk group was 31%. Subgroup analysis of 19 standard-risk patients showed 63% 1-year overall survival and 3-year median survival, which compared favorably to reports using alternative matched unrelated donors or cord blood. Despite the use of a T cell-depleting regimen, immune reconstitution analysis demonstrated encouraging evidence of quantitative lymphocyte recovery through expansion of transplanted T cells by 3–6 months.

Most of the studies discussed above included patients of a poor prognostic group with either relapsed chemoresistant or primary refractory hematological diseases. The results showed that this reduced intensity conditioning regimen is associated with less immediate regimen-related toxicities. Importantly, despite the less ablative conditioning regimen and the use of mismatched donors, the graft failure rate is low, ranging between 0% and 17%. This is attributed to a combination of factors, including the use of immunosuppressive regimens and the effective *ex vivo* ± *in vivo* TCD strategies employed. The incidence of grade III–IV acute GvHD is lower than 20% and the nonrelapse mortality is in the range of 10–30%. While these reduced-intensity preparative regimens have decreased immediate procedural mortality and GvHD, cardinal problems related to delayed immune reconstitution causing posttransplant infectious complications and relapse still exist. It remains to be seen if these barriers can all be safely overcome to gain long-term improvements in survival. As will be discussed in the following section, new directions in the use of adoptive cellular immunity appear promising.[80] Preliminary data have demonstrated the great potential of selective allodepletion in rapidly reconstituting immunity without GvHD.[81,82] It appears that in some T cell-depleted haploidentical transplants, the benefit of NK alloreactivity is expected to encourage the greater use of haploidentical transplants for a larger number of leukemia patients without matched donors.[83] In addition, there are emerging data to suggest the use of NIMA-mismatched donors in providing an especially attractive strategy for patients to further minimize the risk of GvHD.[84–87]

Strategies to Improve the Outcome of Patients with Haploidentical Transplantation Using TCD Allografts

Harnessing the Beneficial Effects of the Natural Killer Cell/KIR Ligand

The translation of NK cell recognition of "missing self" into clinical practice of haploidentical transplantation has opened innovative perspectives in the cure of leukemia. Donor-derived NK cells have the potential to promote engraftment, suppress GvHD, and promote GVT, whereas host-derived NK cells can mediate graft rejection and affect GvHD by eliminating donor hematopoietic stem cells (HSCs) and activated T cells, respectively. NK cells are negatively regulated by major histocompatibility complex (MHC) class-I-specific alleles.[88] Lack of expression of self-MHC molecules on mismatched allogeneic targets results in susceptibility to NK cell-mediated lysis (missing self recognition). In humans, inhibitory cell killer immunoglobulin (Ig) receptors (KIRs) recognize groups of HLA-C and HLA-B molecules (KIR ligands). Consequently, when faced with KIR-ligand-mismatched allogeneic targets, KIR-bearing NK cells sense the missing expression of self-class-I alleles and mediate cell killing.

The important role of alloreactive NK cells in the setting of haploidentical transplantation has previously been demonstrated. Extensive TCD to prevent GvHD in the setting of haploidentical transplantation allows rapid regeneration of NK cells in the graft. Ruggeri *et al.* have shown that NK alloreactivity reduced the risk of leukemia relapse in 57 AML patients receiving haploidentical transplantation, while improving engraftment and protecting against GvHD.[89] In a recent updated analysis of 112 adult high-risk AML patients who had received haploidentical transplantation from 1993 to 2006,[90] the Perugia investigators demonstrated that transplantation from NK alloreactive donors does not cause GvHD and helps to control leukemia relapse in patients who are transplanted in remission. The marked graft-vs-leukemia effect has translated into a marked survival advantage (65% event-free survival in patients in any CR). While such a positive effect of KIR-ligand-mismatched haploidentical transplantation is seen only in acute myeloid leukemia for adults in the Perugia study, similar benefit with a lower risk of relapse was observed in a study at St. Jude's Children Research Hospital among pediatric patients with acute lymphocytic leukemia who had received transplantation from haploidentical NK-alloreactive donors.[91,92] Several groups of investigators subsequently tested the KIR ligand incompatibility model in patients given grafts from HLA-mismatched unrelated donors.[93–96] Two studies found lower risks of relapse in patients with KIR ligand incompatibility in the graft-versus-host direction,[93,96] though two others did not find such associations.[94,95] The heterogeneous results are likely attributable to other factors, such as the extent of donor TCD,[97] the speed at which NK cells recover, and/or the use of posttransplant immune modulation. These data point to the need for further study under different transplant procedures and conditions. Nevertheless, the recently demonstrated benefits of NK alloreactivity are expected to encourage greater use of haploidentical transplantation in the future.

In patients with advanced or refractory malignancies, the alloreactivity of NK cells has been exploited as a form of adoptive immunotherapy, providing a potential role as an adjunct to HSCT. Miller *et al.*[98] recently demonstrated the safety and potential benefit of adoptive haploidentically related NK cell therapy without HSCT following high-dose intensity conditioning. All NK cell donors were haploidentical family members; few were KIR-ligand-mismatched in the GVH direction. Twenty-six percent of a small cohort of poor prognosis patients with acute myelogenous leukemia achieved complete hematological remission of their leukemia. Intriguingly, a significantly higher complete remission rate was observed when KIR-mismatched donors were used. The study also demonstrated *in vivo* expansion of donor-derived NK cells in the majority of the treated patients, in association with increased levels of endogenous IL-15. More importantly, donor NK cell infusions were well tolerated, without evidence for induction of GvHD. These findings suggest that haploidentical NK cells can persist and expand *in vivo* and may have a role in the treatment of selected malignancies when used alone or in association with HSCT. Additional studies are needed to determine how best to exploit the potential benefit of NK cells in allogeneic HSCT by promoting their recovery with cytokines such as IL-15 or by selection of specific subsets.

Harnessing the Beneficial Effects of the Nonfetal Maternal Antigen

The potential benefit of fetomaternal immunologic tolerance in allogeneic HSCT was recently demonstrated[87,99–101] and may serve as a new parameter in selection of donors. Based on the results of a nationwide HSCT survey conducted in Japan[87] and a large IBMTR analysis,[99] maternal stem cell donation was found to be better for HSCT than paternal donation in mismatched transplantation. Van Rood *et al.*,[99] in their large IBMTR analysis, have shown that the recipients of non-T cell-depleted maternal transplants had a significantly lower incidence of chronic GvHD than the recipients of paternal transplants in haploidentical one- or two-antigen-mismatched transplantation. They have also demonstrated a lower rate of acute GvHD and transplant-related mortality in sibling transplants mismatched for noninherited maternal antigens (NIMAs) compared with those mismatched for noninherited paternal antigens (NIPAs). Separate studies from Japan have confirmed the tolerizing effect of NIMAs after myeloablative[84,87] and reduced-intensity[85,86] conditioning. Although no differences in risk of clinically significant acute GvHD were noted in one study,[87] five-year overall survival was significantly higher and TRM was lower among recipients of maternal grafts compared to paternal grafts. In other studies, significantly lower risks of GvHD were observed among

NIMA-mismatched transplant recipients.[84] NIMA-mismatched sibling donor and recipient share the inherited paternal antigens (IPAs) and are mismatched at the maternal antigens, but there are microchimeric cells expressing the NIMAs. These observations support the hypothesis that offspring may be tolerant to haploidentical relatives expressing NIMAs (mother or NIMA-mismatched siblings), and the microchimeric mother may be hyporesponsive to IPAs of the offspring. These encouraging results reported so far provide the rationale to assessing the feasibility of haploidentical SCT using either a myeloablative or nonmyeloablative conditioning regimen, from mother to offspring and vice versa, or from NIMA-mismatched siblings. The approach may provide a more appropriate donor selection in HLA-haploidentical HSCT, resulting in both less toxicity and better antitumor effect.

Selective T Cell Depletion of Allografts

In an effort to diminish the problems of engraftment failure and relapse probability risk of *ex vivo* TCD, recent investigations have focused on the depletion of selective T cell subsets. One of the promising approaches is to selectively remove the T cells responsible for mediating GvHD, while conserving GvL and antimicrobial immune responses. This can be accomplished by deleting T cells that become activated in response to recipient APCs. This approach has the advantage that alloreactive T cells are permanently eliminated and cannot influence the function of the remaining T cells. In several murine transplant models, GvHD can be reduced or prevented by removal or inactivation of alloreactive donor T cells using anti-CD25,[102,103] anti-CD69,[104] anti-CD95,[105] or photodepletion.[106] This promising approach has been tested by a number of clinical trials involving both HLA-matched sibling donor and haploidentical donor transplants, and the results suggest that the concept is feasible.[81,82,102,107] In a recently published report, Solomon *et al.*[81] performed transplants on 16 older patients (median age 65 years) with selective allodepletion allografts following reduced-intensity conditioning and compared their results with a historical cohort of older transplant recipients receiving unmanipulated allografts. The results demonstrate that *ex vivo* selective depletion of alloreactive T cells from PBSC allografts, using an anti-CD25 immunotoxin, is feasible and safe, and that GvHD severity may be diminished in patients treated by this approach. Furthermore, the severity of GvHD was found to be related to the efficiency of selective allodepletion, as measured by the helper T lymphocyte precursor (HTLp) frequency assay. Finally, unlike other methods of TCD, engraftment, GvL, and immune recovery were not adversely affected in these patients. More recently, Amrolia *et al.*[82] reported the results from a dose escalation study using allodepleted T cells following haploidentical transplantation in 16 patients with a median age of 9 years (range 2–58), treated mostly for high-risk hematologic malignancies. Each patient was scheduled to receive three infusions of allodepleted donor T cells on days 30, 60, and 90 after HSCT. Eight patients received dose level 1 (10^4 cells/kg/dose) and another eight patients received dose levels 10^5 cells/kg/dose. Only two patients developed significant acute GvHD, followed by extensive, chronic GvHD, with death in one of them from liver failure associated with GvHD and adenovirus. Patients at dose level 1 had T cell reconstitution consistent with other patients undergoing haploidentical HSCT without allodepleted T cell addback. However, patients at dose level 2 (10^5 cells/kg/dose) showed significantly improved T cell recovery time, particularly at 3–5 months after HSCT, which is most often the time period in which patients die of infection following haploidentical HSCT.

Cotransplantation of Mesenchymal Stem Cells

In addition to HSCs, bone marrow contains a second type of stem cells — mesenchymal stem cells (MSCs), capable of giving rise to multiple mesenchymal lineages.[108,109] Convincing evidence shows that MSCs possess immunomodulatory properties, which may play a role in the maintenance of peripheral tolerance, the induction of transplantation tolerance, and the control of autoimmunity.[110] In allogeneic stem cell transplant, MSCs may be used to enhance engraftment of white blood cells and platelets, modulate the immune system, as prophylaxis to prevent GvHD, and treatment of established GvHD. The first experience with the use of MSCs was reported in two patients for the prevention and treatment of acute GvHD after HLA-matched or mismatched HCT.[111,112] Following the encouraging results of these anecdotal case reports, the immunosuppressive capacities of MSCs to prevent GvHD have been evaluated in several clinical studies. In an open-label multicenter clinical trial involving adult patients undergoing transplantation from an HLA-identical sibling, MSC infusion has been shown by Lazarus *et al.* to be safe and possibly to accelerate hematopoietic recovery, as well as to reduce the incidence of both acute and chronic GvHD.[113] Ball *et al.* recently reported the results of a phase I–II study on children undergoing haploidentical HSC transplantation. The cotransplantation of MSCs from the same HSC donor was associated with a significant reduction of the graft failure rate as compared to historic controls.[114] Although very encouraging, the long-term outcome of both anecdotal and full series is not yet available. More recently, Ning *et al.* from Beijing published the results of the first randomized trial addressing benefits and disadvantages of MSC infusions in the context of HSC allografting.[115] The study showed that while cotransplantation successfully prevents GvHD, it is not without its drawbacks as the prevention of GvHD is associated with a higher incidence of leukemia relapse. Further large-scale randomized studies are needed to evaluate the potential benefits and hazards of MSC cotransplantation in malignant hematopoietic diseases.

Prophylatic/Pre-emptive Donor Lymphocyte Infusion

Although there has been a modest trend to reduce transplantation-related mortality in the past few years, there has been no clear reduction in disease relapse, which still surpasses 50% in high-risk patients.[21,60] The risk of day-100 TRM has been reduced to below 20% in several recent series of haploidentical transplants using reduced-intensity conditioning protocols[21,57,60,71,78] The high relapse rate observed in most series, apart from the inclusion of a large proportion of high-risk patients or patients with refractory diseases at the time of transplant, is attributable to the delayed immune recovery and abrogated GvL effect with the use of T cell-depleted grafts. Intensification of conditioning regimens is unlikely to compensate for the loss of T cell-related GvL effect, as the benefit usually is offset by the increase in the regimen-related toxicity. Additional posttransplant strategies such as donor lymphocyte infusion are potential therapeutic options for relapse prevention.

Donor lymphocyte infusion (DLI) provides direct and potent GvL activity to treat relapse in patients who have undergone HLA-matched, related, or unrelated HSCT.[116,117] Reports on the use of unmanipulated DLI in haploidentical transplant, both prophylactically and therapeutically, remain scanty.[118–125] The diverse results reported in terms of efficacy, adverse events, and survival outcome are more a reflection of the heterogeneity of patients being treated using this therapeutic strategy. In addition, given the limited number of patients in most of these reports, it is difficult to draw definite conclusions about the relationship between the cell dose given, GvHD and GvL effects. Nevertheless, several important observations were made: (1) GvHD remains an important risk after DLI, which can be a severe complication leading to death; (2) DLI is significantly more effective when it is given during an early stage of relapse, when the disease burden is minimal.[124,125]

To minimize the risk of GvHD, modified strategies have been developed, such as partially T cell-depleted DLI.[126] In haploidentical SCT, studies have been initiated in which purified donor NK cells have been used in DLI with the aim of facilitating engraftment and inducing GvL effects.[127,128] Although no firm conclusions can be made regarding the clinical efficacy of NK cell-based DLI at this stage, the available data indicate that NK cell infusions are safe and can generate antitumor responses and long-term remission in some patients after leukemia relapse. The development of NK-cell-based DLI presents new possibilities of treating patients with tumor relapse after haploidentical or cord blood SCT in which T cell-based DLIs are not feasible.

Adoptive Immunotherapy and Vaccination

Dendritic cells (DCs), NK cells, and cytotoxic lymphocytes have been shown to mediate antitumor response in HSCT.[129–133] Specifically, these cells have been incorporated into vaccines or expanded and directed against tumor cells. In patients with leukemia such as AML, ALL, or CLL, malignant cells can be induced to differentiate and mature into relatively mature malignant DCs capable of generating an alloimmune response. Vaccination of patients in a state of minimum residual disease after allogeneic HSCT may evoke an appropriate immune response to control the disease. The malignant DCs can be used to induce a leukemia reactive T cell response from donor cells *in vitro*, resulting in the production of large numbers of activated T cells that may be capable of controlling the disease after allogeneic HSCT.[133] Although the feasibility of this approach has been demonstrated, the logistics of generation of these T cell responses is still complex. Further clinical and preclinical investigations are needed to improve the specificity and efficacy of these *in vitro* immune responses.

A promising method for restoring specific immunity against infections after transplants, albeit highly specialized and cumbersome, relies upon adoptive transfer of specific T cell clones. Adoptive transfer of donor-derived virus-specific CD8$^+$ T cells has been shown to be safe and effective in prophylaxis and treatment of cytomegalovirus (CMV) and Epstein–Barr virus (EBV) infection following stem cell transplantation from an HLA-identical related and unrelated donor.[134–136] Due to the high degree of mismatching between donor and patient in haploidentical transplantation, transfer of donor T cells to improve immune reconstitution in these patients is associated with a high risk of severe acute GvHD. But immunotherapy with highly enriched polyclonal virus-specific CD4$^+$ T cells has been reported to be safe and effective in a small cohort of patients, including one recipient of a haploidentical transplant.[137] The most recent and exciting data have come from investigators in Perugia, who have generated large numbers of donor pathogen-specific T cell clones, screened them individually for alloreactivity against recipient cells, identified and deleted those cross-reacting against recipient alloantigens, and infused them into 35 high-risk adults with diverse advanced-stage, heavily pretreated hematologic malignancies who had undergone haploidentical hematopoietic transplantation.[80] This study has demonstrated that transfer of immunity to *Aspergillus* and CMV to recipients of a haploidentical transplant can be performed without triggering GvHD. Interestingly, despite the small number of pathogen-specific T cells administered, specific T cell responses could be detected in all patients in the study. All the patients showed a surprisingly prompt increase in CD4[+] as well as CD8[+] T cell responses to CMV as soon as three weeks after transfer, suggesting that even extensively *in-vitro*-cultured T cells were able to rapidly expand *in vivo* when administered to lymphopenic patients not receiving immunosuppressive medication for GvHD prophylaxis. When compared with a control group, patients receiving CMV-directed immunotherapy had a lower risk of CMV reactivation and disease. Importantly, this is the first study to describe adoptive T cell therapy not only for viral but also for invasive fungal infection. *Aspergillus*-directed CD4[+] T_h1 responses were detected in all recipients as soon as three weeks after the transfer, and nine out of ten treated patients showed a decrease in their galactomannan antigenemia and resolution of pulmonary infiltrates. Although not a routine laboratory procedure, the development of such adoptive therapy clearly offers promise for improving the overall outcome following haploidentical SCT by reducing infectious complications without worsening GvHD.

Conclusions

Haploidentical HSCT provides an opportunity for patients to benefit from HSCT when a 6/6 HLA-genotypically-matched sibling is not available. It presents an easier logistic and practical alternative to matched unrelated donor transplantation as well. This may be especially important when one is dealing with a patient suffering from a disease with a rapid tempo and also for non-Caucasian patients, in whom the chances of finding an available matched unrelated match are still low. Recent advances with effective T cell depletion and reduced-intensity conditioning have significantly decreased the early transplant-related mortality and risk of severe GvHD, while enabling reliable engraftment, and hence enhancing the therapeutic benefits of haploidentical transplantation. However, posttransplant infectious complications and relapse remain important barriers to overcome. New directions in the use of adoptive cellular immunity, mesenchymal stem cell and selective allodepletion in rapidly reconstituting immunity without GvHD appear promising. Preliminary data have demonstrated the great potential of selective allodepletion in rapidly reconstituting immunity without GvHD. It appears that in some T cell-depleted haploidentical transplants, the benefit of NK alloreactivity is expected to encourage the greater use of haploidentical transplants for a larger number of leukemia patients without matched donors. In addition, there are emerging data to suggest the use of NIMA-mismatched donors in providing an especially attractive strategy for patients to further minimize the risk of GvHD. There are many issues that remain unresolved, including the role in certain diseases and the timing of haploidentical HSCT. The relative merits of a haploidentical family donor versus a mismatched unrelated or umbilical cord blood donor remain to be defined. The data presented to date provide an important framework for future improvements via more appropriate patient selection, better donor selection, development of conditioning regimens that are safer yet result in reliable engraftment, and more effective strategies that eliminate the high risk of severe GvHD while preserving antitumor and antimicrobial immunocompetence.

References

1. Confer DL. (1997) Unrelated marrow donor registries. *Curr Opin Hematol* **4**: 408–412.
2. Koh LP, Rizzieri DA, Chao NJ. (2007) Allogeneic hematopoietic stem cell transplant using mismatched/haploidentical donors. *Biol Blood Marrow Transplant* **13**: 1249–1267.
3. Koh LP, Chao NJ. (2004) Umbilical cord blood transplantation in adults using myeloablative and nonmyeloablative preparative regimens. *Biol Blood Marrow Transplant* **10**: 1–22.

4. Anasetti C, Beatty PG, Storb R *et al.* (1990) Effect of HLA incompatibility on graft-versus-host disease, relapse, and survival after marrow transplantation for patients with leukemia or lymphoma. *Hum Immunol* **29**: 79–91.

5. Kernan NA, Flomenberg N, Dupont B, O'Reilly RJ. (1987) Graft rejection in recipients of T-cell-depleted HLA-nonidentical marrow transplants for leukemia. Identification of host-derived antidonor allocytotoxic T lymphocytes. *Transplantation* **43**: 842–847.

6. Buckley RH, Schiff SE, Schiff RI *et al.* (1999) Hematopoietic stem-cell transplantation for the treatment of severe combined immunodeficiency. *N Engl J Med* **340**: 508–516.

7. Beatty PG, Clift RA, Mickelson EM *et al.* (1985) Marrow transplantation from related donors other than HLA-identical siblings. *N Engl J Med.* **313**: 765–771.

8. Anasetti C, Amos D, Beatty PG *et al.* (1989) Effect of HLA compatibility on engraftment of bone marrow transplants in patients with leukemia or lymphoma. *N Engl J Med* **320**: 197–204.

9. Powles RL, Morgenstern GR, Kay HE *et al.* (1983) Mismatched family donors for bone-marrow transplantation as treatment for acute leukaemia. *Lancet* **1**: 612–615.

10. Szydlo R, Goldman JM, Klein JP *et al.* (1997) Results of allogeneic bone marrow transplants for leukemia using donors other than HLA-identical siblings. *J Clin Oncol.* **15**: 1767–1777.

11. Kanda Y, Chiba S, Hirai H *et al.* (2003) Allogeneic hematopoietic stem cell transplantation from family members other than HLA-identical siblings over the last decade (1991–2000). *Blood* **102**: 1541–1547.

12. Ruggeri L, Capanni M, Casucci M *et al.* (1999) Role of natural killer cell alloreactivity in HLA-mismatched hematopoietic stem cell transplantation. *Blood* **94**: 333–339.

13. Soiffer RJ, Mauch P, Tarbell NJ *et al.* (1991) Total lymphoid irradiation to prevent graft rejection in recipients of HLA non-identical T cell-depleted allogeneic marrow. *Bone Marrow Transplant* **7**: 23–33.

14. Kernan NA, Flomenberg N, Dupont B *et al.* (1987) Graft rejection in recipients of T-cell-depleted HLA-nonidentical marrow transplants for leukaemia: identification of host-derived antidonor allocytotoxic T lymphocytes. *Transplantation* **43**: 842–847.
15. Reisner Y, Martelli MF. (1995) Bone marrow transplantation across HLA barriers by increasing the number of transplanted cells. *Immunol Today* **16**: 437–440.
16. Aversa F, Tabilio A, Terenzi A *et al.* (1994) Successful engraftment of T-cell-depleted haploidentical "three-loci" incompatible transplants in leukemia patients by addition of recombinant human granulocyte colony-stimulating factor-mobilized peripheral blood progenitor cells to bone marrow inoculum. *Blood* **84**: 3948–3955.
17. Reisner Y, Itzicovitch L, Meshorer A, Sharon N. (1978) Hemopoietic stem cell transplantation using mouse bone marrow and spleen cells fractionated by lectins. *Proc Natl Acad Sci USA* **75**: 2933–2936.
18. Reisner Y, Kapoor N, Kirkpatrick D *et al.* (1981) Transplantation for acute leukemia with HLA-A and B nonidentical parental marrow cells fractionated with soybean agglutinin and sheep red blood cells. *Lancet* **2**: 327–331.
19. Reisner Y, Kapoor N, Kirkpatrick D *et al.* (1983) Transplantation for severe combined immunodeficiency with HLA-A, B, D, DR incompatibility parental marrow cells fractionated by soybean agglutinin and sheep red blood cells. *Blood* **61**: 341–348.
20. Aversa F, Tabilio A, Velardi A *et al.* (1998) Treatment of high-risk acute leukemia with T-cell-depleted stem cells from related donors with one fully mismatched HLA haplotype. *N Engl J Med* **339**: 1186–1193.
21. Henslee-Downey PJ, Abhyankar SH, Parrish RS *et al.* (1997) Use of partially mismatched related donors extends access to allogeneic marrow transplant. *Blood* **89**: 3864–3872.
22. Drobyski WR, Klein J, Flomenberg N *et al.* (2002) Superior survival associated with transplantation of matched unrelated versus one-antigen-mismatched unrelated or highly human leukocyte antigen-disparate haploidentical family donor marrow grafts for

the treatment of hematologic malignancies: Establishing a treatment algorithm for recipients of alternative donor grafts. *Blood* **99**: 806–814.

23. Prentice HG, Blacklock HA, Janossy G *et al.* (1982) Use of anti-T-cell monoclonal antibody OKT3 to prevent acute graft versus host disease in allogeneic bone marrow transplantation for acute leukemia. *Lancet* **1**: 700–703.

24. Filipovich AH, McGlave PB, Ramsay NKC *et al.* (1982) Pretreatment of donor bone marrow with monoclonal antibody OKT3 for prevention of acute graft versus host disease in allogeneic histocompatible bone marrow transplantation. *Lancet* **1**: 1266–1269.

25. Martin PJ, Hansen JA, Thomas ED. (1984) Preincubation of donor bone marrow cells with a combination of murine monoclonal anti-T-cell antibodies without complement does not prevent graft-versus-host disease after allogeneic marrow transplantation. *J Clin Immunol* **4**: 18–22.

26. Waldmann HG, Hale G, Cividalli G *et al.* (1984) Elimination of graft-versus-host disease by *in vitro* depletion of alloreactive lymphocytes with a monoclonal rat anti-human lymphocyte antibody (Campath-1). *Lancet* **2**: 483–486.

27. Mitsuyasu RT, Champlin RE, Gale RP *et al.* (1986) Treatment of donor bone marrow with monoclonal anti-T-cell antibody and complement for the prevention of graft versus host disease. *Ann Intern Med* **105**: 20–26.

28. Soiffer RJ, Murray C, Mauch P *et al.* (1992) Prevention of graft-versus-host disease by selective depletion of CD6-positive T lymphocytes from donor bone marrow. *J Clin Oncol* **10**: 1191–2000.

29. Hale G, Slavin S, Goldman JM. (2002) Alemtuzumab (Campath-1H) for treatment of lymphoid malignancies in the age of nonmyeloablative conditioning? *Bone Marrow Transplant* **30**: 797–804.

30. Chakrabarti S, Hale G, Waldmann H. (2004) Alemtuzumab (Campath-1H) in allogeneic stem cell transplantation: Where do we go from here? *Transplant Proc* **36**: 1225–1227.

31. Hale G. (2002) Alemtuzumab in stem cell transplantation. *Med Oncol* **19**(Suppl): S33–S47.

32. Handgretinger R, Lang P, Ihm K *et al.* (2002) Isolation and transplantation of highly purified autologous peripheral CD34(+) progenitor cells: Purging efficacy, hematopoietic reconstitution and long-term outcome in children with high-risk neuroblastoma. *Bone Marrow Transplant* **29**: 731–736.

33. Lang P, Schumm M, Taylor G *et al.* (1999) Clinical scale isolation of highly purified peripheral CD34$^+$ progenitors for autologous and allogeneic transplantation in children. *Bone Marrow Transplant* **24:** 583–589.

34. Schumm P, Lang P, Taylor G *et al.* (1999) Isolation of highly purified autologous and allogeneic peripheral CD34$^+$ cells using the CliniMACS device. *J Hematother* **8**: 209–218.

35. Heimfeld S, Fogarty B, McGuire K *et al.* (1992) Peripheral blood stem cell mobilization after stem cell factor or G-CSF treatment: Rapid enrichment for stem and progenitor cells using the CEPRATE immunoaffinity separation system. *Transplant Proc* **24**: 2818.

36. Rowley SD, Loken M, Radich J *et al.* (1998) Isolation of CD34$^+$ cells from blood stem cell components using the Baxter Isolex system. *Bone Marrow Transplant* **21**: 1253–1262.

37. Elmaagacli AH, Peceny R, Steckel N *et al.* (2003) Outcome of transplantation of highly purified peripheral blood CD34$^+$ cells with T-cell add-back compared with unmanipulated bone marrow or peripheral blood stem cells from HLA-identical sibling donors in patients with first chronic phase chronic myeloid leukemia. *Blood* **101**: 446–453.

38. Lang P, Greil J, Bader P *et al.* (2004) Long-term outcome after haploidentical stem cell transplantation in children. *Blood Cells Mol Dis* **33**: 281–287.

39. Lang P, Handgretinger R, Niethammer D *et al.* (2003) Transplantation of highly purified CD34$^+$ progenitor cells from unrelated donors in pediatric leukemia. *Blood* **101**: 1630–1636.

40. Bethge WA, Haegele M, Faul C *et al.* (2006) Haploidentical allogeneic hematopoietic cell transplantation in adults with

reduced-intensity conditioning and CD3/CD19 depletion: Fast engraftment and low toxicity. *Exp Hematol* **34**: 1746–1752.

41. Bethge WA, Faul C, Bornhäuser M *et al.* (2008) Haploidentical allogeneic hematopoietic cell transplantation in adults using CD3/CD19 depletion and reduced intensity conditioning: An update. *Blood Cells Mol Dis* **40**: 13–19.

42. Bacigalupo A, Lamparelli T, Bruzzi P *et al.* (2001) Antithymocyte globulin for graft-versus-host disease prophylaxis in transplants from unrelated donors: 2 randomized studies from Gruppo Italiano Trapianti Midollo Osseo (GITMO). *Blood* **98**: 2942–2947.

43. Basara N, Baurmann H, Kolbe K *et al.* (2005) Antithymocyte globulin for the prevention of graft-versus-host disease after unrelated hematopoietic stem cell transplantation for acute myeloid leukemia: Results from the multicenter German cooperative study group. *Bone Marrow Transplant* **35**: 1011–1018.

44. Remberger M, Storer B, Ringden O *et al.* (2002) Association between pretransplant thymoglobulin and reduced non-relapse mortality rate after marrow transplantation from unrelated donors. *Bone Marrow Transplant* **29**: 391–397.

45. Kalhs P, Brugger S, Reiter E *et al.* (1999) Low transplant-related mortality in patients receiving unrelated donor marrow grafts for leukemia. *Bone Marrow Transplant* **23**: 753–758.

46. Duggan P, Booth K, Chaudhry A *et al.* (2002) Unrelated donor BMT recipients given pretransplant low-dose antithymocyte globulin have outcomes equivalent to matched sibling BMT: A matched pair analysis. *Bone Marrow Transplant* **30**: 681–686.

47. Finke J, Bertz H, Schmoor C *et al.* (2000) Allogeneic bone marrow transplantation from unrelated donors using *in vivo* anti-T-cell globulin. *Br J Haematol* **111**: 303–313.

48. Bacigalupo A. (2005) Antilymphocyte/thymocyte globulin for graft versus host disease prophylaxis: efficacy and side effects. *Bone Marrow Transplant* **35**: 225–231.

49. Hale G, Rebello P, Brettman LR. (2004) Blood concentrations of alemtuzumab and antiglobulin responses in patients with chronic

lymphocytic leukemia following intravenous or subcutaneous routes of administration. *Blood* **104**: 948–955.

50. Klangsinsirikul P, Carter GI, Byrne JL *et al.* (2002) Campath-1G causes rapid depletion of circulating host dendritic cells (DCs) before allogeneic transplantation but does not delay donor DC reconstitution. *Blood* **99**: 2586–2591.

51. Buggins AGS, Mufti GJ, Salisbury J *et al.* (2002) Peripheral blood but not tissue dendritic cells express CD52 and are depleted by treatment with alemtuzumab. *Blood* **100**: 1715–1720.

52. Hale G, Slavin S, Goldman JM. (2002) Alemtuzumab (Campath-1H) for treatment of lymphoid malignancies in the age of nonmyeloablative conditioning? *Bone Marrow Transplant* **30**: 797–804.

53. Ratzinger G, Reagan JL, Heller G. (2003) Differential CD52 expression by distinct myeloid dendritic cell subsets: Implications for alemtuzumab activity at the level of antigen presentation in allogeneic graft–host interactions in transplantation. *Blood* **101**: 1422–1429.

54. von dem Borne PA, Beaumont F, Starrenburg CW *et al.* (2006) Outcomes after myeloablative unrelated donor stem cell transplantation using both *in vitro* and *in vivo* T-cell depletion with alemtuzumab. *Haematologica* **91**: 1559–1562.

55. Perez-Simon JA, Kottaridis PD, Martino R. (2002) Nonmyeloablative transplantation with or without alemtuzumab: Comparison between 2 prospective studies in patients with lymphoproliferative disorders. *Blood* **100**: 3121–3127.

56. Chakraverty R, Peggs K, Chopra R *et al.* (2002) Limiting transplantation-related mortality following unrelated donor stem cell transplantation by using a nonmyeloablative conditioning regimen. *Blood* **99**: 1071–1078.

57. Rizzieri DA, Koh LP, Long GD *et al.* (2007) Partially matched, non-myeloablative allogeneic transplantation: Clinical outcomes and immune reconstitution. *J Clin Oncol* **25**: 690–697.

58. Kanda Y, Oshima K, Asano-Mori Y *et al.* (2005) *In vivo* alemtuzumab enables haploidentical human leukocyte antigen-mismatched

hematopoietic stem-cell transplantation without *ex vivo* graft manipulation. *Transplantation* **79**: 1351–1357.

59. Lu DP, Dong L, Wu T *et al.* (2006) Conditioning including antithymocyte globulin followed by unmanipulated HLA-mismatched/haploidentical blood and marrow transplantation can achieve comparable outcomes with HLA-identical sibling transplantation. *Blood* **107**: 3065–3073.

60. Aversa F, Terenzi A, Tabilio A *et al.* (2005) Full haplotype-mismatched hematopoietic stem-cell transplantation: A phase II study in patients with acute leukemia at high risk of relapse. *J Clin Oncol* **23**: 3447–3454.

61. Lang P, Greil J, Bader P *et al.* (2004) Long-term outcome after haploidentical stem cell transplantation in children. *Blood Cells Mol Dis* **33**: 281–287.

62. Kato S, Yabe H, Yasui M *et al.* (2000) Allogeneic hematopoietic transplantation of CD34$^+$ selected cells from an HLA haplo-identical related donor: A long-term follow-up of 135 patients and a comparison of stem cell source between the bone marrow and the peripheral blood. *Bone Marrow Transplant* **26**: 1281–1290.

63. Walker I, Shehata N, Cantin G *et al.* (2004) Canadian multicenter pilot trial of haploidentical donor transplantation. *Blood Cells Mol Dis* **33**: 222–226.

64. Lang P, Bader P, Schumm M *et al.* (2004) Transplantation of a combination of CD133$^+$ and CD34$^+$ selected progenitor cells from alternative donors. *Br J Haematol* **124**: 72–79.

65. Kawano Y, Takaue Y, Watanabe A *et al.* (1998) Partially mismatched pediatric transplants with allogeneic CD34($^+$) blood cells from a related donor. *Blood* **92**: 3123–3130.

66. Peters C, Matthes-Martin S, Fritsch G *et al.* (1999) Transplantation of highly purified peripheral blood CD34$^+$ cells from HLA-mismatched parental donors in 14 children: Evaluation of early monitoring of engraftment. *Leukemia* **13**: 2070–2078.

67. Passweg, Jr., Kuhne T, Gregor M *et al.* (2000) Increased stem cell dose, as obtained using currently available technology, may not be

sufficient for engraftment of haploidentical stem cell transplants. *Bone Marrow Transplant* **26**: 1033–1036.

68. Henslee-Downey PJ. (2001) Allogeneic transplantation across major HLA barriers. *Best Pract Res Clin Haematol* **14**: 741–754.

69. Barfield RC, Otto M, Houston J *et al.* (2004) A one-step large-scale method for T- and B-cell depletion of mobilized PBSC for allogeneic transplantation. *Cytotherapy* **6**: 1–6.

70. Hale G, Kimberly K, Lovins R *et al.* (2005) CD3 depleted hematopoietic peripheral blood stem cell grafts in children with refractory hematologic malignancies undergoing transplantation from mismatched related donors [*abstract*]. *Blood* **106**: 451b.

71. Handgretinger R, Chen X, Pfeiffer M *et al.* (2007) Feasability and outcome of reduced intensity conditioning in haploidentical transplantation. *Ann N Y Acad Sci* **1106**: 279–289.

72. Pelot MR, Pearson DA, Swenson K *et al.* (1999) Lympho-hematopoietic graft-vs.-host reactions can be induced without graft-vs.-host disease in murine mixed chimeras established with a cyclophosphamide-based nonmyeloablative conditioning regimen. *Biol Blood Marrow Transplant* **5**: 133–143.

73. Spitzer TR, McAfee SL, Dey BR *et al.* (2003) Nonmyeloablative haploidentical stem-cell transplantation using anti-CD2 monoclonal antibody (MEDI-507)-based conditioning for refractory hematologic malignancies. *Transplantation* **75**: 1448–1751.

74. Dey BR, Spitzer TR. (2006) Current status of haploidentical stem cell transplantation. *Br J Haematol* **135**: 423–437.

75. Spitzer TR. (2005) Haploidentical stem cell transplantation: The always present but overlooked donor. *Hematol Am Soc Hematol Educ Program* 390–395.

76. O'Donnell PV, Luznik L, Jones RJ *et al.* (2002) Nonmyeloablative bone marrow transplantation from partially HLA-mismatched related donors using posttransplantation cyclophosphamide. *Biol Blood Marrow Transplant* **8**: 377–386.

77. Luznik L, O'Donnell PV, Symons HJ *et al.* (2008) HLA-haploidentical bone marrow transplantation for hematologic malignancies

using nonmyeloablative conditioning and high-dose, posttransplantation cyclophosphamide. *Biol Blood Marrow Transplant* **14**: 641–650.

78. Ogawa H, Ikegame K, Yoshihara S *et al.* (2006) Unmanipulated HLA 2–3 antigen-mismatched (haploidentical) stem cell transplantation using nonmyeloablative conditioning. *Biol Blood Marrow Transplant* **12**: 1073–1084.

79. Slavin S, Nagler A, Naparstek E *et al.* (1998) Nonmyeloablative stem cell transplantation and cell therapy as an alternative to conventional bone marrow transplantation with lethal cytoreduction for the treatment of malignant and nonmalignant hematologic diseases. *Blood* **91**: 756–763.

80. Perruccio K, Tosti A, Burchielli E *et al.* (2005) Transferring functional immune responses to pathogens after haploidentical hematopoietic transplantation. *Blood* **106**: 4397–4406.

81. Solomon SR, Mielke S, Savani BN *et al.* (2005) Selective depletion of alloreactive donor lymphocytes: A novel method to reduce the severity of graft-versus-host disease in older patients undergoing matched sibling donor stem cell transplantation. *Blood* **106**: 1123–1129.

82. Amrolia PJ, Muccioli-Casadei G, Huls H *et al.* (2006) Adoptive immunotherapy with allodepleted donor T-cells improves immune reconstitution after haploidentical stem cell transplantation. *Blood* **108**: 1797–1808.

83. Ruggeri L, Mancusi A, Burchielli E *et al.* (2007) Natural killer cell alloreactivity in allogeneic hematopoietic transplantation. *Curr Opin Oncol* **19**: 142–147.

84. Shimazaki C, Ochiai N, Uchida R *et al.* (2003) Non-T-cell-depleted HLA haploidentical stem cell transplantation in advanced hematologic malignancies based on the feto-maternal microchimerism. *Blood* **101**: 3334–3336.

85. Obama K, Utsunomiya A, Takatsuka Y *et al.* (2004) Reduced-intensity non-T-cell-depleted HLA-haploidentical stem cell

transplantation for older patients based on the concept of feto-maternal tolerance. *Bone Marrow Transplant* **34**: 897–899.

86. Shimazaki C, Fuchida S, Ochiai N *et al.* (2004) Non-T-cell-depleted HLA-haploidentical stem cell transplantation after reduced-intensity conditioning in advanced haematological malignancies based on feto-maternal microchimerism, *Br J Haematol* **127**: 474–475.

87. Tamaki S, Ichinohe T, Matsuo K *et al.* (2001) Superior survival of blood and marrow stem cell transplants given maternal grafts over recipients given paternal grafts. *Bone Marrow Transplant* **28**: 375–380.

88. Ljunggren HG, Karre K. (1990) In search of the "missing self": MHC molecules and NK cell recognition. *Immunol Today* **11**: 237–244.

89. Ruggeri L, Capanni M, Urbani E *et al.* (2002) Effectiveness of donor natural killer cell alloreactivity in mismatched hematopoietic transplants. *Science* **295**: 2097–2100.

90. Ruggeri L, Mancusi A, Capanni M *et al.* (2007) Donor natural killer cell allorecognition of missing self in haploidentical hematopoietic transplantation for acute myeloid leukemia: Challenging its predictive value. *Blood* **110**: 433–440.

91. Leung W, Iyengar R, Turner V *et al.* (2004) Determinants of antileukemia effects of allogeneic NK cells. *J Immunol* **172**: 644–650.

92. Leung W, Iyengar R, Triplett B *et al.* (2005) Comparison of killer Ig-like receptor genotyping and phenotyping for selection of allogeneic blood stem cell donors. *J Immunol* **174**: 6540–6545.

93. Giebel S, Locatelli F, Lamparelli T *et al.* (2003) Survival advantage with KIR ligand incompatibility in hematopoietic stem cell transplantation from unrelated donors, *Blood* **102**: 814–819.

94. Davies SM, Ruggieri L, DeFor T *et al.* (2002) Evaluation of KIR ligand incompatibility in mismatched unrelated donor hematopoietic transplants: Killer immunoglobulin-like receptor. *Blood* **100**: 3825–3827.

95. Bornhauser M, Schwerdtfeger R, Martin H *et al.* (2004) Role of KIR ligand incompatibility in hematopoietic stem cell transplantation using unrelated donors. *Blood* **103**: 2860–2861.

96. Beelen DW, Ottinger HD, Ferencik S *et al.* (2005) Genotypic inhibitory killer immunoglobulin-like receptor ligand incompatibility enhances the long-term antileukemic effect of unmodified allogeneic hematopoietic stem cell transplantation in patients with myeloid leukemias. *Blood* **105**: 2594–2600.

97. Bishara A, De Santis D, Witt CC *et al.* (2004) The beneficial role of inhibitory KIR genes of HLA class I NK epitopes in haploidentically mismatched stem cell allografts may be masked by residual donor-alloreactive T cells causing GVHD. *Tissue Antigens* **63**: 204–211.

98. Miller JS, Soignier Y, Panoskaltsis-Mortari A *et al.* (2005) Successful adoptive transfer and *in vivo* expansion of human haploidentical NK cells in patients with cancer. *Blood* **105**: 3051–3057.

99. van Rood JJ, Loberiza FR, Zhang MJ *et al.* (2002) Effect of tolerance to noninherited maternal antigens on the occurrence of graft-versus-host disease after bone marrow transplantation from a parent or an HLA-haploidentical sibling. *Blood* **96**: 1572–1577.

100. Ichinohe T, Uchiyama T, Shimazaki C *et al.* (2004) Feasibility of HLA-haploidentical hematopoietic stem cell transplantation between noninherited maternal antigen (NIMA)–mismatched family members linked with long-term fetomaternal microchimerism. *Blood* **104**: 3821–3828.

101. Ochiai N, Shimazaki C, Fuchida S *et al.* (2002) Successful non-T-cell-depleted HLA haplo-identical 3-loci mismatched hematopoietic stem cell transplantation from mother to son based on the fetomaternal microchimerism in chronic myelogenous leukemia. *Bone Marrow Transplant* **30**: 793–796.

102. Cavazzana-Calvo M., Fromont C, Le DF *et al.* (1990) Specific elimination of alloreactive T cells by an anti-interleukin-2 receptor B chain-specific immunotoxin. *Transplantation* **50**: 1–7.

103. Harris DT, Sakiestewa D, Lyons C *et al.* (1999) Prevention of graft-versus-host disease (GvHD) by elimination of recipient-reactive

donor T cells with recombinant toxins that target the interleukin 2 (IL-2) receptor. *Bone Marrow Transplant* **23**: 137–144.

104. Koh MB, Prentice HG, Corbo M *et al.* (2002) Alloantigen-specific T-cell depletion in a major histocompatibility complex fully mismatched murine model provides effective graft-versus-host disease prophylaxis in the presence of lymphoid engraftment. *Br J Haematol* **118**: 108–116.

105. Hartwig UF, Robbers M, Wickenhauser C *et al.* (2002) Murine acute graft-versus-host disease can be prevented by depletion of alloreactive T lymphocytes using activation-induced cell death. *Blood* **99**: 3041–3049.

106. Chen BJ, Cui X, Liu C, Chao NJ. (2002) Prevention of graft-versus-host disease while preserving graft-versus-leukemia effect after selective depletion of host-reactive T cells by photodynamic cell purging process. *Blood* **99**: 3083–3088.

107. Andre-Schmutz I, Le DF, Hacein-Bey-Abina S *et al.* (2002) Immune reconstitution without graft-versus-host disease after haemotopoietic stem-cell transplantation: A phase 1/2 study. *Lancet* **360**: 130–137.

108. Pittenger MF, Mackay AM, Beck SC *et al.* (1999) Multilineage potential of adult human mesenchymal stem cells. *Science* **284**: 143–147.

109. Horwitz EM, Le Blanc K, Dominici M *et al.* (2005) Clarification of the nomenclature for MSC: The International Society for Cellular Therapy position statement. *Cytotherapy* **7**: 393–395.

110. Le Blanc K, Ringdén O. (2005) Immunobiology of human mesenchymal stem cells and future use in hematopoietic stem cell transplantation. *Biol Blood Marrow Transplant* **11**: 321–334.

111. Lee ST, Jang JH, Cheong JW *et al.* (2002) Treatment of high-risk acute myelogenous leukaemia by myeloablative chemoradiotherapy followed by co-infusion of T-cell-depleted haematopoietic stem cells and culture-expanded marrow mesenchymal stem cells from a related donor with one fully mismatched human leucocyte antigen haplotype. *Br J Haematol* **118**: 1128–1131.

112. Le Blanc K, Rasmusson I, Sundberg B *et al.* (2004) Treatment of severe acute graft-versus-host disease with third party haploidentical mesenchymal stem cells. *Lancet* **363**: 1439–1441.

113. Lazarus HM, Koc ON, Devine SM *et al.* (2005) Co-transplantation of HLA-identical sibling culture-expanded mesenchymal stem cells and hematopoietic stem cells in hematologic malignancy patients. *Biol Blood Marrow Transplant* **11**: 389–398.

114. Ball LM, Bernardo ME, Roelofs H *et al.* (2007) Cotransplantation of *ex vivo* expanded mesenchymal stem cells accelerates lymphocyte recovery and may reduce the risk of graft failure in haploidentical hematopoietic stem-cell transplantation. *Blood* **110**: 2764–2767.

115. Ning H, Yang F, Jiang M *et al.* (2008) The correlation between cotransplantation of mesenchymal stem cells and higher recurrence rate in hematologic Malignancy patients: Outcome of a pilot clinical study. *Leukemia* **22**: 593–599.

116. Dazzi F, Szydlo RM, Cross NC *et al.* (2000) Durability of responses following donor lymphocytes infusions for patients who relapse after allogeneic stem cell transplantation for chronic myeloid leukemia. *Blood* **96**: 2712–2716.

117. Porter DL, Collins RH, Hardy C *et al.* (2000) Treatment of relapsed leukemia after unrelated donor marrow transplantation with unrelated donor leukocyte infusions. *Blood* **95**: 1214–1221.

118. Mehta J, Singhal S, Gee AP *et al.* (2004) Bone marrow transplantation from partially HLA-mismatched family donors for acute leukemia: Single-center experience of 201 patients. *Bone Marrow Transplant* **33**: 389–396.

119. Handgretinger R, Klingebiel K, Lang P *et al.* (2001) Megadose transplantation of purified peripheral blood CD34(+) progenitor cells from HLA-mismatched parental donors in children. *Bone Marrow Transplant* **27**: 777–783.

120. Klingebiel T, Handgretinger R, Lang P *et al.* (2004) Haploidentical transplantation for acute lymphoblastic leukemia in childhood. *Blood Rev* **18**: 181–192.

121. Wu BY, Guo KY, Song CY *et al.* (2000) Mixed chimera converted into full donor chimera with powerful graft-versus-leukemia effects but no graft-versus-host disease after non-T-cell-depleted HLA-mismatched peripheral blood stem cell transplantation. *Bone Marrow Transplant* **26:** 691–693.

122. Lewalle P, Triffet A, Delforge A *et al.* (2003) Donor lymphocyte infusions in adult haploidentical transplant: A dose finding study. *Bone Marrow Transplant* **31**: 39–44.

123. Pati AR, Godder K, Lamb L *et al.* (1995) Immunotherapy with donor leukocyte infusions for patients with relapsed acute myeloid leukemia following partially mismatched related donor bone marrow transplantation. *Bone Marrow Transplant* **15**: 979–981.

124. Or R, Hadar E, Bitan M *et al.* (2006) Safety and efficacy of donor lymphocyte infusions following mismatched stem cell transplantation. *Biol Blood Marrow Transplant* **12**: 1295–1301.

125. Huang XJ, Liu DH, Liu KY *et al.* (2007) Donor lymphocyte infusion for the treatment of leukemia relapse after HLA-mismatched/haploidentical T-cell-replete hematopoietic stem cell transplantation. *Haematologica* **92**: 414–417.

126. Soiffer RJ, Alyea EP, Hochberg E *et al.* (2002) Randomized trial of CD8$^+$ T-cell depletion in the prevention of graft-versus-host disease associated with donor lymphocyte infusion. *Biol Blood Marrow Transplant* **8**: 625–632.

127. Passweg JR, Tichelli A, Meyer-Monard S *et al.* (2004) Purified donor NK-lymphocyte infusion to consolidate engraftment after haploidentical stem cell transplantation. *Leukemia* **18**: 1835–1838.

128. Passweg JR, Stern M, Koehl U *et al.* (2005) Use of natural killer cells in hematopoetic stem cell transplantation. *Bone Marrow Transplant* **35**: 637–643.

129. Ruggeri L, Mancusi A, Burchielli E *et al.* (2007) Natural killer cell alloreactivity in allogeneic hematopoietic transplantation. *Curr Opin Oncol* **19**: 142–147.

130. Dazzi F, Szydlo RM, Cross NC *et al.* (2000) Durability of responses following donor lymphocytes infusions for patients who relapse after

allogeneic stem cell transplantation for chronic myeloid leukemia. *Blood* **96**: 2712–2716.

131. Fong L, Engleman EG. (2000) Dendritic cells in cancer immunotherapy. *Annu Rev Immunol* **18**: 245–273.

132. O'Neill DW, Adams S, Bhardwaj N. (2004) Manipulating dendritic cell biology for the active immunotherapy of cancer. *Blood* **104**: 2235–2246.

133. Falkenburg JH, Wafelman AR, Joosten P *et al.* (1999) Complete remission of accelerated phase chronic myeloid leukemia by treatment with leukemia-reactive cytotoxic T lymphocytes. *Blood* **94**: 1201–1208.

134. Riddell SR, Watanabe KS, Goodrich JM *et al.* (1992) Restoration of viral immunity in immunodeficient humans by the adoptive transfer of T cell clones. *Science* **257**: 238–241.

135. Peggs KS, Verfuerth S, Pizzey A *et al.* (2003) Adoptive cellular therapy for early cytomegalovirus infection after allogeneic stem-cell transplantation with virus-specific T-cell lines. *Lancet* **362**: 1375–1377.

136. Rooney CM, Smith CA, Ng CY *et al.* (1995) Use of gene-modified virus-specific T lymphocytes to control Epstein–Barr-virus-related lymphoproliferation. *Lancet* **345**: 9–13.

137. Einsele H, Roosnek E, Rufer N *et al.* (2002) Infusion of cytomegalovirus (CMV)–specific T cells for the treatment of CMV infection not responding to antiviral chemotherapy. *Blood* **99**: 3916–3922.

Chapter 7

Deploying Natural Killer Cell Allotherapy in the Setting of HLA-Haplotype-Mismatched Hematopoietic Stem Cell Transplantation

Andrea Velardi, Loredana Ruggeri, Antonella Mancusi, Franco Aversa and Massimo F. Martelli*

Introduction

For almost all leukemia patients who do not have a matched sibling donor, transplantation from family donors who are matched for one HLA haplotype but fully mismatched at the HLA class I and II loci of the unshared haplotype (haploidentical) is an option. Unlike unrelated donors or unrelated cord blood units, haploidentical donors are immediately available, circumventing the delays and limitations of the other alternative transplants. Their use offers a chance of cure for those patients who urgently need a transplant.

All haploidentical transplant recipients are at high risk of T cell-mediated alloreactions in the GvH direction, as well as in the host-versus-graft (rejection) direction. These are largely controlled by appropriate immunosuppressive intensity of the conditioning regimen followed by transplantation of a large dose of hematopoietic stem cells to

*Corresponding author. Division of Hematology and Clinical Immunology, Department of Clinical and Experimental Medicine, University of Perugia, Perugia, Italy.
*E-mail: velardi@unipg.net

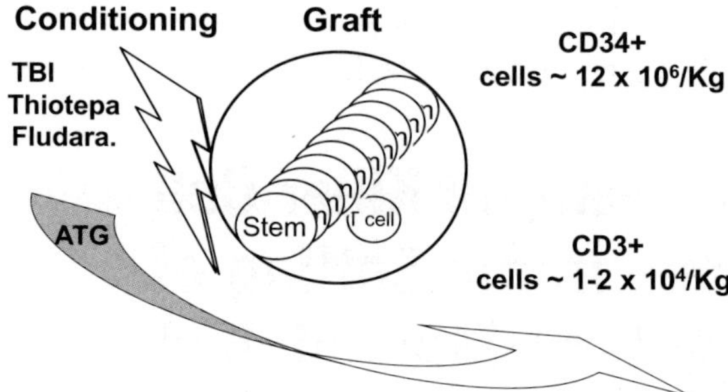

Fig. 1. The protocol for HLA haploidentical transplantation for acute leukemia as designed by Aversa *et al.*[4] Conditioning consists of 8 Gy total-body irradiation on day −9 before transplant in a single fraction at an instantaneous dose rate of 0.16 Gy per minute; lungs shielded to receive 0.04 Gy; thiotepa (5 mg/kg daily) on days −8 and −7; fludarabine (40 mg/m^2 daily) from day −7 to day −3; rabbit antithymocyte globulin (ATG) at 5 mg/kg daily from days −5 to −2. The graft contains ~12 × 10^6 CD34$^+$ cells and ~1–2 × 10^4 CD3$^+$ cells/kg body weight. *Ex vivo* T cell depletion of the graft combined with *in vivo* T depletion exerted by ATG prevents GvHD, without the need for posttransplant pharmacological immune suppression. The stem cell "megadose" ensures engraftment across HLA barriers.

prevent graft rejection, and extensive T cell depletion of the graft to prevent GvHD (Fig. 1).

The need for extensive T cell depletion might be expected to result in a weak or no GvL effect, as it is conventionally achieved through T cell-mediated alloreactions directed against the recipient's histocompatibility antigens. However, another cell of the immune system influences the outcome of hematopoietic cell transplantation in a surprisingly favorable way. In haploidentical hematopoietic stem cell transplantation, NK cells of donor origin were recently shown to bypass the obstacles inherent in T cell alloreactivity. They prevent leukemia relapse, while not increasing the risk of GvHD.

In recent years, intensive research on mice and humans has unraveled the biology of NK cells. Dramatic progress has been made in our understanding of how they function and their exploitation in therapy for leukemia.

This review focuses on recent research demonstrating the role NK cells play in adoptive immunotherapy of leukemia in mismatched hematopoietic transplantation. It also covers studies investigating other possible NK cell-related effector mechanisms in transplantation.

NK Cell Alloreactivity in Allogeneic Hematopoietic Transplantation: Preclinical Data

The hybrid resistance transplant model illustrated that NK cell alloreactions in the HvG direction mediate rejection of bone marrow grafts and play a major role in recognizing allogeneic lymphohematopoietic cells *in vivo*.[1] As the hybrid recipient mouse tolerated skin and organ allografts, NK cell alloreactivity appeared to be restricted to lymphohematopoietic targets.

The *in vivo* effects of NK cell alloreactivity also hold in the GvH direction.[2] In F1 H-2d/b $\rightarrow$ parent H-2b transplants, donor T cells are tolerant of the recipient MHC. Donor NK cells that do not express the H-2b-specific Ly49C/I inhibitory receptor (and bear H-2d-specific Ly49A/G2 receptors) are activated to kill the recipient's targets. Infusion of donor-versus-recipient alloreactive NK cells exerts several favorable effects. After host immune suppression, infused alloreactive NK cells home at all lymphohematopoietic sites of the recipient mouse and quickly ablate recipient-type lymphohematopoietic cells. Killing of recipient T lymphocytes is associated with engraftment of the MHC-mismatched bone marrow. Killing of recipient-type dendritic cells, which initiate GvHD by presenting host alloantigens to donor T cells, prevents T cell-mediated GvHD. Mice that are given alloreactive NK cells as part of the conditioning regimen are able to receive mismatched bone marrow grafts containing up to 30 times the lethal dose of allogeneic T cells without clinical or histological evidence of GvHD. Finally, alloreactive NK cells themselves do not cause GvHD. Lack of NK-mediated attack on normal tissues in the GvH direction (and in the HvG direction, as shown in the hybrid mouse transplant model; see above) indicates that healthy organ tissues, unlike lymphohematopoietic cells, do not express ligands at a level sufficient to engage activating NK cell receptors.

Donor-Versus-Recipient NK Cell Alloreactivity in Allogeneic Hematopoietic Transplantation

Donor-versus-recipient NK cell alloreactivity is mediated by a functional repertoire of donor NK cells which express inhibitory killer cell immunoglobulin-like receptor(s) (KIR) for self class I ligand(s), and sense missing expression of donor KIR ligand(s) in the recipient and mediate alloreactions.

NK cell function is regulated by a balance between activating receptors and inhibitory receptors for MHC class I molecules.[3–6] In humans, triggering of NK cell effector functions depends upon engagement of activating receptors, NKG2D and natural cytotoxicity receptors (NCRs).[7,8]

NK cell activation can also be mediated by KIR variants.[9–16] Activating KIRs have shorter cytoplasmic tails than inhibitory KIRs and a charged residue in their transmembrane domain that allows association with ITAM containing signaling polypeptides. Knowledge of the ligand specificity of activating KIRs is limited. Studies have reported only a weak interaction between KIR2DS1 and Lys80 HLA-C molecules, despite its homology to KIR2DL1, and no interaction between KIR2DS2 and Asn80 HLA-C, despite its homology to KIR2DL2 and KIR2DL3.[17,18]

In humans, the inhibitory receptors for HLA class I molecules include inhibitory KIRs and the CD94-NKG2A molecular complex. Inhibitory KIRs recognize amino acids in the COOH-terminal portion of the MHC class I α1 helix. They possess two (KIR2D) or three (KIR3D) extracellular C2-type Ig-like domains and a long cytoplasmic tail (L) containing immunoreceptor tyrosine-based inhibition motifs which recruit and activate SHP-1 and SHP-2 phosphatases for inhibitory signal transduction. KIR2DL1 recognizes HLA-C alleles characterized by a Lys80 residue (HLA-Cw4 and related, "group 2" alleles). KIR2DL2 and KIR2DL3 recognize HLA-C with an Asn80 residue (HLA-Cw3 and related, "group 1" alleles). KIR3DL1 is the receptor for HLA-B allotypes with Bw4 motifs at positions 77–83. It also recognizes HLA-Bw4 alleles except for 1301 and 1302 and some HLA-A alleles, namely 2301, 2402 and 3201. Finally, KIR3DL2 is the receptor for HLA-A3/11.

Another type of human NK cell inhibitory receptor involved in HLA recognition is CD94-NKG2A, which binds to the nonconventional class I molecule HLA-E. Several HLA class I alleles provide signal sequence peptides that bind HLA-E and allow its expression at the cell surface. Consequently, it is expressed in every individual.

HLA-class I genes educate NK cell repertoires during development. All KIR genes are randomly expressed and KIR distribution varies on NK cells. Only NK cells which express inhibitory KIRs for self HLA ligands are functionally active as they become "licensed/educated" upon interaction with self HLA molecules and thus enabled to exert alloreactivity against mismatched allogeneic targets which do not express self HLA inhibitory KIR ligands (reviewed in Refs. 6, 19–22). NK cells which express, as their only inhibitory receptor for self, a KIR whose ligand is an HLA class I group which is absent on allogeneic targets sense the missing expression of the self class I KIR ligand and mediate alloreactions (reviewed in Refs. 6, 23–26) ("missing self" recognition).[27] NK cells which do not express inhibitory receptors for self (and are thus potentially autoreactive) are tolerant to self and are retained in the NK cell repertoire in an anergic (or "hypofunctional") state.[28,29]

NK cells which express, as their only inhibitory receptor for self, a KIR for the HLA class I group which is absent on allogeneic targets sense the missing expression of the self class I KIR ligand and mediate alloreactions ("missing self" recognition) (Fig. 2).

Donor-versus-recipient NK cell alloreactions are generated between individuals who are mismatched for HLA-C allele groups and/or the HLA-Bw4 group ("KIR-ligand-mismatched").[2,23,30,31] Most donors have the potential to exert NK alloreactions as they possess a full complement of inhibitory KIR genes.[10,31,32] HLA-C group 1 receptor genes (KIR2DL2 and/or KIR2DL3) are present in 100% of individuals, and the HLA-C group 2 receptor gene (KIR2DL1) in 97%. When they were tested in large donor cohorts,[31] functional analyses detected high-frequency alloreactive NK clones against HLA-C group–mismatched allogeneic targets.

The HLA-Bw4 receptor gene (KIR3DL1) is found in ~90% of individuals. Only 2/3 of HLA-Bw4-positive individuals with the KIR3DL1

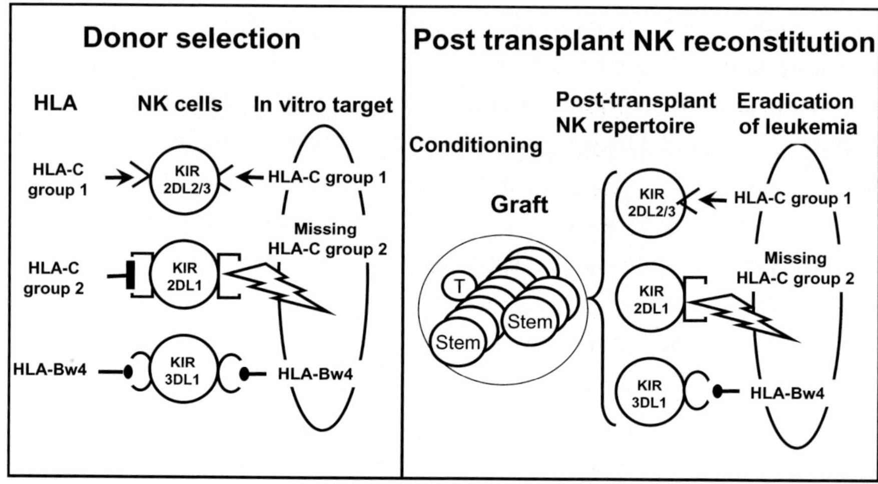

Fig. 2. Posttransplant regeneration of the donor-versus-recipient alloreactive NK cell repertoire. Left: In donors, NK cells which express inhibitory KIRs for self HLA ligands are functionally active as they become "licensed/educated" upon interaction with self HLA molecules and thus enabled to exert alloreactivity against mismatched allogeneic targets which do not express self HLA KIR ligands. Right: Engrafted stem cells give rise to the exact same donor repertoire, including alloreactive clones.

gene possess alloreactive NK clones against allogeneic HLA-Bw4-negative targets.[31] Failure to detect alloreactive NK clones may be due to their highly variable frequencies, or because certain allelic KIR3DL1 variants do not allow receptor expression at the cell membrane.[33,34]

In vitro studies on primary lymphohematopoietic lineage tumor cells showed that alloreactive NK cells kill acute and chronic myeloid leukemia, as well as T cell-acute lymphoblastic leukemia (ALL), chronic lymphocytic leukemia, non-Hodgkin's lymphoma and multiple myeloma.[26] The only nonsusceptible target was common ALL.[26,30] Alloreactive NK cells also exerted significant cytotoxicity against melanoma and renal cell carcinoma cell lines.[35]

In HLA-haplotype-mismatched ("haploidentical") hematopoietic transplantation with potential for donor-versus-recipient NK cell alloreactivity, engrafted stem cells regenerated the same repertoire as the donor's, including donor-versus-recipient alloreactive NK cells, for up to one year[30,31] (Fig. 2). In an updated analysis,[31] 112 high-risk acute myeloid leukemia (AML) patients received haploidentical transplants from NK-alloreactive ($n = 51$) or non-NK-alloreactive donors ($n = 61$). Transplantation from NK-alloreactive donors was associated with a significantly lower relapse rate in patients transplanted in complete remission (3% vs 47%) ($P < 0.003$), better event-free survival in patients transplanted not only in remission (67% vs. 18%; $P = 0.02$) but also in relapse (34% vs 6%, $P = 0.04$), and overall reduced risk of relapse or death ($P < 0.001$). The 67% probability of surviving event-free for AML patients transplanted in remission from NK-alloreactive donors is in the range of best survival rates after transplantation from unrelated donors and cord blood units. The *in vitro* resistance of common phenotype ALL to alloreactive NK killing was paralleled by lack of antileukemia effect in adult patients. However, in ALL in children, transplantation from NK-alloreactive donors was reported to decrease the risk of relapse.[36]

One recent study showed that NK cell alloreactivity provided much better protection from leukemia relapse when exerted by maternal donors (as opposed to any other donor–recipient family relationship).[36] The effect was independent of, and additional to, the beneficial effects of NK alloreactivity. The better outcome of mother-to-child transplantation may be due to maternal immune system exposure to fetal antigens during pregnancy and the ensuing memory T cell immunity against the child's paternal HLA haplotype.

Another recent study assessed NK cell alloreactivity in a large number of unrelated cord blood transplants and found that it was associated with a significantly reduced incidence of leukemia relapse ($p = 0.05$) and better leukemia-free survival (73% vs 38%; $p = 0.0016$). Benefits were significantly more marked in patients with AML.[37]

Thus, NK cell alloreactivity is effective in haploidentical and cord blood transplantation. In an attempt to explain the effectiveness in these two very different types of transplantation, one may consider that a common feature is lack of memory T cells in the graft (due to T cell depletion in haploidentical transplants and T cell naiveté in cord blood transplants).

This, apparently, permits recovery of fully functional NK cells. Evidence that T cells antagonize reconstitution of potentially alloreactive, KIR-bearing NK cells[38] derives from several other unrelated donor transplant studies, using T cell-replete grafts, including a recent one on 1489 transplants.[39–50] Most studies showed no advantage in transplantation from KIR-ligand-mismatched donors,[39–45] while a few observed an increased graft-versus-leukemia effect.[46–50] Interestingly, the study that reported the most marked survival advantage was performed in KIR-ligand-mismatched transplant recipients who received pretransplant antithymocyte globulins (ATGs) to exert *in vivo* T cell depletion.[46]

Guidelines for NK-Alloreactive Donor Selection

The search for NK-alloreactive donors, which may require extension beyond the immediate family, increases the chance of finding a "perfect mismatch" from the random 30% to >60%. First, the transplantation candidate is HLA-typed. Those who express class I alleles belonging to the three class I groups recognized by KIRs (HLA-C group 1, HLA-C group 2, and HLA-Bw4 alleles) will block all NK cells from every donor and belong to the one-third of the population that is resistant to alloreactive NK killing. Patients who express only one or two of these allele groups may find NK-alloreactive donors.

Donor HLA typing will identify the family member who does not express the class I group(s) expressed by the patient and has, therefore, the potential for NK alloreactivity. Not all inhibitory KIRs are present in 100% of the population. Although KIR2DL2/3, the receptors for HLA-C group 1, are present in all, KIR2DL1, the receptor for HLA-C group 2, is found in 97% of individuals and KIR3DL1, the receptor for HLA-Bw4 alleles, is found in ~90%. Donor KIR genotyping ensures the donor possesses the relevant NK cells.

In HLA-Bw4 mismatches, even when the KIR3DL1 gene is present, NK repertoire studies showed alloreactive NK cells in ~2/3 of individuals. This may be because they occur at highly variable frequencies, or because allelic KIR3DL1 variants may not allow receptor expression at the cell membrane. Thus, for HLA-Bw4 mismatches, direct assessment of the donor NK repertoire is necessary.

References

1. Cudkowicz G, Bennett M. (1972) Peculiar immunobiology of bone-marrow allografts. II. Rejection of parental grafts by resistant F1 hybrid mice. *J Exp Med* **135**: 1028–1036.
2. Ruggeri L, Capanni M, Urbani E *et al.* (2002) Effectiveness of donor natural killer cell alloreactivity in mismatched hematopoietic transplants. *Science* **295**: 2097–2100.
3. Rosen DB, Cao W, Avery DT *et al.* (2008) Up on the tightrope: Natural killer cell activation and inhibition. *Nat Immunol* **9**: 495–502.
4. Gasser S, Raulet DH. (2006) Activation and self-tolerance of natural killer cells. *Immunol Rev* **214**: 130–142.
5. Yokoyama WM, Kim S. (2006) Licensing of natural killer cells by self-major histocompatibility complex class I. *Immunol Rev* **214**: 143–154.
6. Parham P. (2006) Taking license with natural killer cell maturation and repertoire development. *Immunol Rev* **214**: 155–160.
7. Moretta L, Bottino C, Pende D *et al.* (2004) Different checkpoints in human NK cell activation. *Trends Immunol* **25**: 670–676.
8. Lanier LL. (2005) NK cell recognition. *Annu Rev Immunol* **23**: 225–274.
9. Colonna M, Samaridis J. (1995) Cloning of immunoglobulin-superfamily members associated with HLA-C and HLA-B recognition by human natural killer cells. *Science* **268**: 405–408.
10. Uhrberg M, Valiante NM, Shum BP *et al.* (1997) Human diversity in killer-cell inhibitory receptor genes. *Immunity* **7**: 753–763.
11. Vilches C, Parham P. (2002) KIR: Diverse, rapidly evolving receptors of innate and adaptive immunity. *Ann Rev Immunol* **20**: 217–251.
12. Moretta A, Sivori S, Vitale M *et al.* (1995) Existence of both inhibitory (p58) and activatory (p50) receptors for HLA-C molecules in human natural killer cells. *J Exp Med* **182**: 875–884.

13. Biassoni R, Pessino A, Malaspina A *et al.* (1997) Role of amino acid position 70 in the binding affinity of p50.1 and p58.1 receptors for HLA-Cw4 molecules. *Eur J Immunol* **27**: 3095–3099.

14. Vales-Gomez M, Reyburn HT, Erskine RA, Strominger JL. (1998) Differential binding to HLA-C of p50-activating and p58-inhibitory natural killer cell receptors. *Proc Natl Acad Sci USA* **95**: 14326–14331.

15. Winter CC, Gumperz JE, Parham P *et al.* (1998) Direct binding and functional transfer of NK cell inhibitory receptors reveal novel patterns of HLA-C allotype recognition. *J Immunol* **161**: 571–577.

16. Parham P. (2005) MHC class I molecules and KIRs in human history, health and survival. *Nat Rev Immunol* **5**: 201–214.

17. Saulquin X, Gastinel LN, Vivier E. (2004) Crystal structure of the human natural killer cell activating receptor KIR2DS2 (CD158j). *J Exp Med* **197**: 933–938.

18. Stewart CA, Laugier-Anfossi F, Vély F *et al.* (2005) Recognition of peptide–MHC class I complexes by activating killer immunoglobulin-like receptors. *Proc Natl Acad Sci USA* **102**: 13224–13229.

19. Joncker NT, Raulet DH. (2008) Regulation of NK cell responsiveness to achieve self-tolerance and maximal responses to diseased target cells. *Immunol Rev* **224**: 85–97 .

20. Yawata M, Yawata N, Draghi M *et al.* (2008) MHC class I–specific inhibitory receptors and their ligands structure diverse human NK-cell repertoires toward a balance of missing self-response. *Blood* **112**: 2369–2380.

21. Jonsson AH, Yokoyama WM. (2009) Natural killer cell tolerance licensing and other mechanisms. *Adv Immunol* **101**: 27–79.

22. Brodin P, Kärre K, Höglund P. (2009) NK cell education: Not an on–off switch but a tunable rheostat. *Trends Immunol* **30**: 143–149.

23. Kärre K. (2002) A perfect mismatch. *Science* **295**: 2029–2031.

24. Farag SS, Fehniger TA, Ruggeri L *et al.* (2002) Natural killer cell receptors: New biology and insights into the graft versus leukemia effect. *Blood* **100**: 1935–1947.

25. Velardi A, Ruggeri L, Moretta A, Moretta L. (2002) NK cells: A lesson from mismatched haematopoietic transplantation. *Trends Immunol* **23**: 438–444.

26. Ruggeri L, Aversa F, Martelli MF, Velardi A. (2006) Allogeneic hematopoietic transplantation and natural killer cell recognition of missing self. *Immunol Rev* **214**: 202–218.

27. Kärre K. (1995) Express yourself or die: Peptides, MHC molecules, and NK cells. *Science* **267**: 978–979.

28. Fernandez NC, Treiner E, Vance RE *et al.* (2005) A subset of natural killer cells achieves self-tolerance without expressing inhibitory receptors specific for self-MHC molecules. *Blood* **105**: 4416–4423.

29. Anfossi N, André P, Guia S *et al.* (2006) Human NK cell education by inhibitory receptors for MHC class I. *Immunity* **25**: 331–342.

30. Ruggeri L, Capanni M, Casucci M *et al.* (1999) Role of natural killer cell alloreactivity in HLA-mismatched hematopoietic stem cell transplantation. *Blood* **94**: 333–339.

31. Ruggeri L, Mancusi A, Capanni M *et al.* (2007) Donor natural killer cell allorecognition of missing self in haploidentical hematopoietic transplantation for acute myeloid leukemia: Challenging its predictive value. *Blood* **110**: 433–440.

32. Hsu KC, Chida S, Geraghty DE, Dupont B. (2002) The killer cell immunoglobulin-like receptor (KIR) genomic region: Gene-order, haplotypes and allelic polymorphism. *Immunol Rev* **190**: 40–52.

33. Pando MJ, Gardiner CM, Gleimer M *et al.* (2003) The protein made from a common allele of KIR3DL1 (3DL*004) is poorly expressed at cell surfaces due to substitution at position 86 in Ig domain 0 and 182 in Ig domain 1. *J Immunol* **171**: 6640–6647.

34. Thomas R, Yamada E, Alter G *et al.* (2008) Novel KIR3DL1 alleles and their expression levels on NK cells: Convergent evolution of KIR3DL1 phenotype variation? *J Immunol* **180**: 6743–6750.

35. Igarashi T, Wynberg J, Srinivasan R *et al.* (2004) Enhanced cytotoxicity of allogeneic NK cells with killer immunoglobulin-like receptor ligand incompatibility against melanoma and renal cell carcinoma cells. *Blood* **104**: 170–177.

36. Stern M, Ruggeri L, Mancusi A *et al.* (2008) Survival after T cell-depleted haploidentical stem cell transplantation is improved with mothers as donors. *Blood* **112**: 2990–2995.

37. Willemze R, Rodrigues CA, Labopin M *et al.* (2009) KIR-ligand incompatibility in the graft-versus-host direction improves outcomes after umbilical cord blood transplantation for acute leukemia. *Leukemia* **23**: 492–500.

38. Cooley S, McCullar V, Wangen R *et al.* (2005) KIR reconstitution is altered by T cells in the graft and correlates with clinical outcomes after unrelated donor transplantation. *Blood* **106**: 4370–4376.

39. Davies SM, Ruggeri L, DeFor T *et al.* (2002) Evaluation of KIR ligand incompatibility in mismatched unrelated donor hematopoietic transplants. *Blood* **100**: 3825–3827.

40. Lowe EJ, Turner V, Handgretinger R *et al.* (2003) T cell alloreactivity dominates natural killer cell alloreactivity in minimally T cell-depleted HLA-non-identical paediatric bone marrow transplantation. *Br J Haematol* **123**: 323–326.

41. Bornhauser M, Schwerdtfeger R, Martin H *et al.* (2004) Role of KIR ligand incompatibility in hematopoietic stem cell transplantation using unrelated donors. *Blood* **103**: 2860–2861.

42. Farag SS, Bacigalupo A, Eapen M *et al.* (2006) The effect of KIR ligand incompatibility on the outcome of unrelated donor transplantation: A report from the Center for International Blood and Marrow Transplant Research, the European Blood and Marrow Transplant Registry, and the Dutch Registry. *Biol Blood Marrow Transplant* **12**: 876–884.

43. Hsu KC, Gooley T, Malkki M *et al.* (2006) KIR ligands and prediction of relapse after unrelated donor hematopoietic cell transplantation for hematologic malignancy. *Biol Blood Marrow Transplant* **12**: 828–836.

44. Kröger N, Binder T, Zabelina T *et al.* (2006) Low number of donor activating killer immunoglobulin-like receptors (KIR) genes but not KIR-ligand mismatch prevents relapse and improves disease-free survival in leukemia patients after *in vivo* T-cell depleted unrelated stem cell transplantation. *Transplantation* **82**: 1024–1030.

45. Yabe T, Matsuo K, Hirayasu K *et al.* (2008) Japan Marrow Donor Program. Donor killer immunoglobulin-like receptor (KIR) genotype-patient cognate KIR ligand combination and antithymocyte globulin preadministration are critical factors in outcome of HLA-C-KIR ligand-mismatched T cell-replete unrelated bone marrow transplantation. *Biol Blood Marrow Transplant* **14**: 75–87.
46. Giebel S, Locatelli F, Lamparelli T *et al.* (2003) Survival advantage with KIR ligand incompatibility in hematopoietic stem cell transplantation from unrelated donors. *Blood* **102**: 814–819.
47. Beelen DW, Ottinger HD, Ferencik S *et al.* (2005) Genotypic inhibitory killer immunoglobulin-like receptor ligand incompatibility enhances the long-term antileukemic effect of unmodified allogeneic hematopoietic stem cell transplantation in patients with myeloid leukemias. *Blood* **105**: 2594–2600.
48. Elmaagacli AH, Ottinger H, Koldehoff M *et al.* (2005) Reduced risk for molecular disease in patients with chronic myeloid leukemia after transplantation from a KIR-mismatched donor. *Transplantation* **79**: 1741–1747.
49. Kröger N, Shaw B, Iacobelli S *et al.* (2005) Comparison between antithymocyte globulin and alemtuzumab and the possible impact of KIR-ligand mismatch after dose-reduced conditioning and unrelated stem cell transplantation in patients with multiple myeloma. *Br J Haematol* **129**: 631–643.
50. Dawson MA, Spencer A. (2005) Successful use of haploidentical stem-cell transplantation with KIR mismatch as initial therapy for poor-risk myelodysplastic syndrome. *J Clin Oncol* **23**: 4473–4474.

Chapter 8

Adoptive Immunotherapy for Prophylaxis and Therapy of Infectious Complications After Allogeneic Hematopoietic Stem Cell Transplantation

Markus Kapp, Hermann Einsele* and Götz Ulrich Grigoleit*,†*

Introduction

Allogeneic hematopoietic stem cell transplantation (HSCT) is associated with high rates of viral or fungal infections, and these problems often increase after T cell depletion. These complications are associated with severe T cell lymphopenia and lack of restoration of pathogen-specific immunity. Therefore, a need for adoptive T cell therapies after HSCT became evident.

Infections After Allogeneic-HSCT

Cytomegalovirus

Cytomegalovirus (CMV) usually causes an asymptomatic infection in immunocompetent individuals. It is latent in approximately 70% of

*Medizinische Klinik und Poliklinik II, Julius Maximilians University of Würzburg, Germany.
†Medizinische Klinik und Poliklinik II, Building C11, Josef-Schneider-Strasse 2, 97080 Würzburg, Germany, e-mail: grigoleit_g@klinik.uni-wuerzburg.de.

healthy adults and replicates in epithelial cells, fibroblasts and monocytes. Immunocompromised patients, especially those undergoing allogeneic HSCT, carry a high risk of CMV disease.

Reactivation in the stem cell recipient can result in clinical manifestations such as interstitial pneumonitis, gastroenteritis, fever, hepatitis, encephalitis and retinitis.[1] CMV-specific T cells in the graft are a major requirement for subsequent recovery of a protective T cell response and play an important role in immune protection after both primary infection and reactivation of latent disease.

Prophylactic administration of antiviral agents such as ganciclovir or foscavir have proven to reduce the rate of CMV infection and disease markedly, but at the cost of a higher incidence of secondary bacterial and mainly fungal infections due to secondary neutropenia and possible ganciclovir-associated immunosuppression or renal failure. Hence, there is no added survival benefit.[2]

Epstein–Barr Virus

Epstein–Barr virus (EBV) infects more than 95% of the world's population. Primary infection usually produces a mild self-limiting disease, which is followed by latent infection in B cells and productive replication in B cells and mucosal epithelium.

In immunocompromised hosts, the outgrowth of B cells, which are highly susceptible to virus-specific T cells, may lead to the development of posttransplant lymphoproliferative disease (PTLD).

PTLD after HSCT is a rare disease (less than 1%) but the incidence is increased in immunocompromised patients, especially recipients of stem cells from unrelated or human leukocyte antigen (HLA)–mismatched donors receiving T cell-depleted grafts to prevent graft-vs-host disease (GvHD).[3–5]

A promising option for prophylaxis and treatment of PTLD after HSCT is rituximab, a monoclonal antibody against CD20, the B cell phenotypic antigen. Response rates to rituximab between 55% and 100% have been demonstrated.[5–7] However, rituximab produces a depletion of normal B cells for more than six months, which might enhance and prolong susceptibility to infections posttransplant.

Adenovirus

Adenovirus (ADV) is a DNA virus and generally infects mucosal epithelium. Acute infection is rarely fatal in healthy adults, but it can cause significant morbidity and mortality in immunocompromised individuals with a wide range of clinical symptoms (pneumonia, hemorrhagic cystitis, nephritis, colitis, hepatitis, encephalitis). Especially after pediatric HSCT, adenovirus shows quite a high incidence.[8]

Clearance of adenovirus infection has been associated with the detection of adenovirus-specific T cells[9,10] and the recovery is significantly delayed in recipients of matched, unrelated donor and haploidentical transplant with intensive immunosuppression (e.g. Campath).[10]

Fungal Infections

Among fungal infections in the immunocompromised host, *Aspergillus spp.* represent one of the most common causes of infection-related mortality. In addition, therapy with antifungal drugs does not always lead to satisfactory effects. Late infections are observed even after neutrophil recovery and their incidence is increased by GvHD and its immune-suppressive treatment.[11,12] Furthermore, patients with *Aspergillus* infection posttransplant, showing an antigen-specific T cell proliferation posttransplant with a predominantly *Aspergillus*-specific T_{H1} response, have an improved outcome.[13]

Adoptive T Cell Therapy

Donor Lymphocyte Infusions

Unmanipulated T cells contained in donor lymphocyte infusions (DLIs) have been shown to induce remissions of relapsed leukemia after stem cell transplantation and to enhance viral-specific immunity. But, in addition, the T cells may induce potentially life-threatening GVHD.[14] This is unacceptable for patients who are simply at risk for relapse or for those with viral infections.

Depletion of Alloreactive T Cells

To eliminate GvHD while preserving the T cells requires ensuring that adequate immune reconstitution may be achieved by the selective depletion of alloreactive T cells from HSCT grafts.

T cell activation markers, such as CD25, CD69, CD137 and CD8,[15–18] may serve as target molecules for selective allodepletion: donor cells (e.g. bone marrow or leukapheresis products) may be exposed to recipients' cells. Thereby, alloreactive T cells in the graft are activated and can be targeted by antibodies directed at activation-associated markers.

Some studies have used immunotoxins or magnetic depletion of cells which express CD25.[18,19]

Initial laboratory studies showed the abrogation of recognition of recipient cells after $CD25^+$ allodepletion, whereas reactivity with viral antigens (e.g. derived from CMV and EBV) or tumor-associated antigens [e.g. proteinase-1 and histocompatibility antigen (HA)-1][20] was conserved. In clinical trials, it could be shown that using this approach immune reconstitution, even after haploidentical HSCT, can be improved without induction of significant GvHD.[18] A potential disadvantage of CD25-based allodepletion could be an anticipated increased risk for the emergence of autoimmune disorders or GvHD due to depletion of T_{regs} mediating suppression of alloreactivity *in vivo.*

Another activation marker which is applied for selective allodepletion is CD69. This is an inducible cell surface glycoprotein representing a very early marker during activation of lymphocytes. As with CD25 allodepletion, maintenance of CMV-specific and EBV-specific cytotoxic T lymphocytes has been shown after $CD69^+$ deletion.[15] It is important to note that T_{regs} are not touched by this approach since they retain CD69 negativity after allogeneic stimulation.

Some other groups also tried to separate useful immune reactions posttransplant from alloreactions by depletion of all CD8[+] T cells,[21–23] driven by the idea that the remaining CD4[+] subsets may be sufficient to allow immune reconstitution.

Some studies initially suggested a separation of GvHD from GvL[16,21] but overall partial CD8[+] depletion was insufficient to prevent GvHD. Therefore, CD8[+] depletion is probably less suitable for engineering the graft for a safe and efficient immune recovery.

Another strategy for selective depletion of alloreactive T cells while retaining disease-related immune responses is photodepletion targeting the impaired ability of activated T cells to efflux a phototoxic rhodamide-like dye (TH9402) due to changes in their multidrug resistance pump p-glycoprotein (MDR1). Mielke *et al.*[24] improved the efficiency and reliability of selective allodepletion using a TH9402-based photodepletion method as an alternative strategy to surface marker targeting.

The use of expanded lymphocytes as antigen-presenting cells (APCs) allowed the generation of large numbers of allodepleted T cells in clinical scale cell volumes under good manufacturing practice (GMP) conditions. The established process was capable of highly efficient removal of alloreactive lymphocytes from mismatched and matched cocultures, and maintained desirable third party responses, including antiviral and antibacterial responses, and therefore represents a promising alternative to the methods described above.

Enrichment of Antigen-specific T Cells

Viral infections that are caused by delayed immune reconstitution can be prevented by application of antigen-specific CTLs following HSCT.

To date, various strategies for generating virus-specific T lymphocytes have been characterized. Some of these protocols rely on the use of CMV-infected fibroblasts or EBV-infected B cell lines to induce specific T cells *ex vivo.*[25–28] These procedures are effective but the application of replicative virus during the stimulation does not meet the criteria of T cell stimulation under current GMP standards because of the potential biological risk resulting from the use of live virus particles.

Other approaches use CMV peptide-pulsed dendritic cells (DCs),[29,30] CMV antigen-pulsed DCs[26,31] or genetically modified antigen-presenting cells (APCs)[27,28] to generate CMV-specific T cells. Even though these methods are very effective, they are expensive and time-consuming. Hence, alternative strategies to generate CMV-specific T cell responses for adoptive transfer are highly warranted.

The use of peptide-HLA multimers facilitates the visualization and isolation of antigen-specific CTLs.[32] CD8[+] T cells that bind multimeric HLA complexes can be isolated to high purity using magnetic beads or FACS sorting.[33–35] A new kind of multimeric HLA complex, binding reversible to the T cell receptor, offers the opportunity to select nearly untouched antigen-specific CTLs.[36] Thus, phenotypical analysis with MHC-peptide multimers, functional assays as well as multimer-based enrichment protocols can now be used in the setting of adoptive T cell therapy. The transfer of CMV-specific CTLs freshly isolated from peripheral blood might be superior to the *in vitro* expansion and manipulation of T cells. The *in vitro* expansion may increase the expression of the proapoptotic FAS molecule (CD95) and reduce the telomere length of specific T cells, leading to shorter survival of the adoptive transferred T cells.[37] Furthermore, there is both a remarkable increase to contaminate the CTL preparation during *in vitro* expansion procedures and an increase in the costs of adoptive immunotherapy.

A variation of the selection based upon the expression of surface markers as discussed for the allodepletion (see above) is the capture of cells that respond with production of effector cytokines such as interferon-γ to stimulations with a respective infectious agent. Our group conducted a study to evade the restrictions in the generation of virus-specific T cell lines for adoptive transfer into allogeneic SCT recipients without affecting the function of the generated T cell lines.[38]

Adenovirus-specific CTLs and *Aspergillus*-specific T_H cells can also be obtained in this way after *in vitro* stimulation with a respective antigen.

These cells showed both markedly reduced alloreactivity and antigen-specific effector functions *in vitro*.[39–42]

Clinical Trials

Cytomegalovirus

Riddell *et al.*[25] conducted the first trial that demonstrated a successful transfer of CMV-specific CTLs isolated from bone marrow donors, propagated *in vitro*, and adoptively transferred to immunodeficient bone marrow transplant recipients. The approach was very safe, with evidence of a persistent reconstitution of CMV-specific CTLs.

In another study, the Seattle group treated 14 patients after allogeneic SCT with intravenous infusions of CMV-specific T cell clones from their donors, beginning 30–40 days after marrow transplantation.[43] In total, 56 infusions (4/patient) of CMV-specific cytotoxic T lymphocyte clones were performed without any major toxic effects, and CMV viremia and CMV disease were absent in all 14 patients receiving adoptive immunotherapy.

Our group demonstrated a few years later that CMV load drops significantly after infusion of donor-derived CMV-specific $CD4^+$ polyclonal T cell lines.[44] Anti-CMV cellular therapy was successful in 5 of 7 patients, whereas in 2 of 7 patients, who received an intensified immune suppression at the time of or after T cell therapy, only transient reductions in virus load were obtained.

A similar strategy was chosen by Peggs *et al.*,[45] who treated 16 patients. A massive *in vivo* expansion of CMV-specific CTLs was observed, leading to a recovery of viral immunity. 50% of the treated patients (8/16) did not require further treatment with antiviral drugs.

Cobbold *et al.*[34] showed reduction of CMV viremia in all patients treated with CMV-specific CTLs isolated directly by using HLA-peptide multimeric complexes. A complete clearance of CMV infection in 8 patients, including 1 who had a prolonged history of CMV infection that was refractory to antiviral therapy, was documented.

Epstein–Barr Virus

Heslop *et al.* have shown that EBV-specific CTLs can survive for up to 8 years after infusion. These cells could even expand up to 2–4 logs after infusion and high virus load was reduced in about 20% of patients.[46,47] In a clinical trial with high-risk patients receiving T-cell-depleted marrow, none of the 58 patients who received EBV-specific CTLs as prophylaxis developed PTLD.[48]

Of the 6 patients with active PTLD at the time of infusion, donor-derived EBV-specific CTL lines induced remission in 5.[49] Other studies have also confirmed the activity of EBV-specific CTLs posttransplant even in the haploidentical setting.[7,50]

Adenovirus

Feuchtinger *et al.*[40] undertook a study in which they infused $1.2–50 \cdot 10^3$/kg ADV-specific CTLs selected by interferon-γ secretion assay and after short *in vitro* stimulation into 9 pediatric patients with systemic ADV infection following allogeneic HSCT. Infusions were tolerated by all patients, and *in vivo* expansion of ADV-specific CTLs was associated with a decrease in viral load in 5 out of 6 evaluable patients. Nevertheless, therapeutic efficacy was not dependent on T cell number, suggesting an *in vivo* expansion of the transferred cells.

Fungus-specific T Lymphocytes

Neutropenia post-HSCT is still an important risk factor for opportunistic invasive fungal infections. However, most cases develop after taking neutrophils during potent immunosuppressive therapy for GvHD prevention or treatment, implicating a contribution of deficient T cells.

Aspergillus spp. causes the most devastating of fungal disorders. The *Aspergillus* antigen Asp f16 was loaded on dendritic cells as antigen-presenting cells and thereby specific T cells could be generated in healthy donors.[51,52] Another approach was the selection of *Aspergillus*-specific

T_{H1} cells by using the interferon-γ secretion assay after stimulation with *Aspergillus* antigen.[42] In addition, Perruccio *et al.*[53] transferred these T cells in patients post-HSCT: 10 patients with *Aspergillus* pneumonia and positive galactomannan antigenemia were treated with *Aspergillus*-derived T cell clones. In all patients galactomannan antigenemia fell to normal within 6 weeks, with 9 patients clearing their *Aspergillus* infection.

Conclusions

Antigen-specific T cells are essential for controlling reactivation or primary infection with viral or fungal infections, as outlined above. Adoptive immunotherapy offers an elegant possibility of improving immune reconstitution in such patients, leading to control of pathogen replication without apparent side effects. This may represent an essential benefit for the patients, since the use of potentially toxic antiviral and/or antifungal drugs (e.g. myelo- or nephrotoxicity) may be reduced and the already-reported problems of drug resistance may be circumvented.

Stimulation and expansion conditions have to be improved to generate T cell lines containing not only terminally differentiated effector cells but also central-memory T cells, which are essential for building up a memory T cell response in the recipient.[54] Further controlled trials with adoptive transfer of pathogen-specific T cells versus drug administration are needed to clarify the role of cellular immunotherapy in routine treatment algorithms of infections in the immunocompromised host.

References

1. Boeckh M, Nichols WG, Papanicolaou G *et al.* (2003) Cytomegalovirus in hematopoietic stem cell transplant recipients: Current status, known challenges, and future strategies. *Biol Blood Marrow Transplant* **9**: 543–558.
2. Einsele H, Bertz H, Beyer J *et al.* Infectious Diseases Working Party (AGIHO) of the German Society of Hematology and Oncology

(DGHO). (2003) Infectious complications after allogeneic stem cell transplantation: Epidemiology and interventional therapy strategies — guidelines of the Infectious Diseases Working Party (AGIHO) of the German Society of Hematology and Oncology (DGHO). *Ann Hematol* **82**: 175–185.

3. Curtis RE, Travis LB, Rowlings PA *et al.* (1999) Risk of lymphoproliferative disorders after bone marrow transplantation: A multi-institutional study. *Blood* **94**: 2208–2216.

4. Cohen JM, Cooper N, Chakrabarti S *et al.* (2007) EBV-related disease following haematopoietic stem cell transplantation with reduced intensity conditioning. *Leuk Lymphoma* **48**: 256–269.

5. Brunstein CG, Weisdorf DJ, DeFor T *et al.* (2006) Marked increased risk of Epstein–Barr virus-related complications with the addition of antithymocyte globulin to a nonmyeloablative conditioning prior to unrelated umbilical cord blood transplantation. *Blood* **108**: 2874–2880.

6. Kuehnle I, Huls MH, Liu Z *et al.* (2000) CD20 monoclonal antibody (rituximab) for therapy of Epstein–Barr virus lymphoma after hemotopoietic stem-cell transplantation. *Blood* **95**: 1502–1505.

7. Comoli P, Basso S, Zecca M *et al.* (2007) Preemptive therapy of EBV-related lymphoproliferative disease after pediatric haploidentical stem cell transplantation. *Am J Transplant* **7**: 1648–1655.

8. Myers GD, Krance RA, Weiss H *et al.* (2005) Adenovirus infection rates in pediatric recipients of alternate donor allogeneic bone marrow transplants receiving either antithymocyte globulin (ATG) or alemtuzumab (Campath). *Bone Marrow Transplant* **36**: 1001–1008.

9. Feuchtinger T, Lucke J, Hamprecht K *et al.* (2005) Detection of adenovirus-specific T cells in children with adenovirus infection after allogeneic stem cell transplantation. *Br J Haematol* **128**: 503–509.

10. Myers GD, Bollard CM, Wu MF *et al.* (2007) Reconstitution of adenovirus-specific cell-mediated immunity in pediatric patients after hematopoietic stem cell transplantation. *Bone Marrow Transplant* **39**: 677–686.

11. Wingard JR. (1999) Fungal infections after bone marrow transplant. *Biol Blood Marrow Transplant* **5**: 55–68.

12. Sable CA, Donovan GR. (1994) Infections in bone marrow transplant recipients. *Clin Infect Dis* **18**: 273–284.

13. Hebart H, Bollinger C, Fisch P *et al.* (2002) Analysis of T-cell responses to *Aspergillus fumigatus* antigens in healthy individuals and patients with hematologic malignancies. *Blood* **100**: 4521–4528.

14. Mackinnon S, Papadopoulos EB, Carabasi MH *et al.* (1995) Adoptive immunotherapy using donor leukocytes following bone marrow transplantation for chronic myeloid leukemia: Is T cell dose important in determining biological response? *Bone Marrow Transplant* **15**: 591–594.

15. Hartwig UF, Nonn M, Khan S *et al.* (2006) Depletion of alloreactive T cells via CD69: Implications on antiviral, antileukemic and immunoregulatory T lymphocytes. *Bone Marrow Transplant* **37**: 297–305 [Context Link].

16. Alyea EP, Canning C, Neuberg D *et al.* (2004) CD8$^+$ cell depletion of donor lymphocyte infusions using CD8 monoclonal antibody-coated high-density microparticles (CD8-HDM) after allogeneic hematopoietic stem cell transplantation: A pilot study. *Bone Marrow Transplant* **34**: 123–128.

17. Wehler TC, Nonn M, Brandt B *et al.* (2007) Targeting the activation-induced antigen CD137 can selectively deplete alloreactive T cells from antileukemic and antitumor donor T-cell lines. *Blood* **109**: 365–373.

18. Amrolia PJ, Mucioli-Casadei G, Huls H *et al.* (2005) Add-back of allodepleted donor T cells to improve immune reconstitution after haplo-identical stem cell transplantation. *Cytotherapy* **7**: 116–125.

19. Solomon SR, Mielke S, Savani BN *et al.* (2005) Selective depletion of alloreactive donor lymphocytes: A novel method to reduce the severity of graft-versus-host disease in older patients undergoing matched sibling donor stem cell transplantation. *Blood* **106**: 1123–1129.

20. Amrolia PJ, Muccioli-Casadei G, Huls H *et al.* (2006) Adoptive immunotherapy with allodepleted donor T-cells improves immune reconstitution after haploidentical stem cell transplantation. *Blood* **108**: 1797–1808.

21. Ho VT, Kim HT, Li S *et al.* (2004) Partial CD8[+] T-cell depletion of allogeneic peripheral blood stem cell transplantation is insufficient to prevent graft-versus-host disease. *Bone Marrow Transplant* **34**: 987–994.

22. Mohty M, Bagattini S, Chabannon C *et al.* (2004) CD8[+] T cell dose affects development of acute graft-vs.-host disease following reduced-intensity conditioning allogeneic peripheral blood stem cell transplantation. *Exp Hematol* **32**: 1097–1102.

23. Kalaycio M, Rybicki L, Pohlman B *et al.* (2005) CD8[+] T-cell-depleted, matched unrelated donor, allogeneic bone marrow transplantation for advanced AML using busulfan-based preparative regimens. *Bone Marrow Transplant* **35**: 247–252.

24. Mielke S, Nunes R, Rezvani K *et al.* (2008) A clinical-scale selective allodepletion approach for the treatment of HLA-mismatched and matched donor–recipient pairs using expanded T lymphocytes as antigen-presenting cells and a TH9402-based photodepletion technique. *Blood* **111**: 4392–4402.

25. Riddell SR, Watanabe KS, Goodrich JM *et al.* (1992) Restoration of viral immunity in immunodeficient humans by the adoptive transfer of T-cell clones. *Science* **257**: 238–241.

26. Szmania S, Galloway A, Bruorton M *et al.* (2001) Isolation and expansion of cytomegalovirus-specific cytotoxic T lymphocytes to clinical scale from a single blood draw using dendritic cells and HLA-tetramers. *Blood* **98**: 505–512.

27. Koehne G, Gallardo HF, Sadelain M *et al.* (2000) Rapid selection of antigen-specific T lymphocytes by retroviral transduction. *Blood* **96**: 109–117.

28. Kondo E, Topp MS, Kiem HP *et al.* (2002) Efficient generation of antigen-specific cytotoxic T cells using retrovirally transduced CD40-activated B cells. *J Immunol* **169**: 2164–2171.

29. Kleihauer A, Grigoleit U, Hebart H *et al.* (2001) *Ex vivo* generation of human cytomegalovirus-specific cytotoxic T-cells by peptide-pulsed dendritic cells. *Brit J Haematol* **113**: 231–239.

30. Vannucchi AM, Glinz S, Bosi A *et al.* (2001) Selective *ex vivo* expansion of cytomegalovirus-specific CD4$^+$ and CD8$^+$ T lymphocytes using dendritic cells pulsed with a human leucocyte antigen A*0201-restricted peptide. *B J Haematol* **113**: 479–482.

31. Peggs KS, Preiser W, Kottaridis PD *et al.* (2001) Induction of cytomegalovirus (CMV)-specific T-cell responses using dendritic cells pulsed with CMV antigen: A novel culture system free of live CMV virions. *Blood* **97**: 994–1000.

32. Altman JD, Moss PA, Goulder PJ *et al.* (1996) Phenotypic analysis of antigen-specific T lymphocytes. *Science* **274**: 94–96.

33. Keenan RD, Ainsworth J, Khan N *et al.* (2001) Purification of cytomegalovirus-specific CD8 T cells from peripheral blood using HLA–peptide tetramers. *Br J Haematol* **115**: 428–434.

34. Cobbold M, Khan N, Pourgheysari B *et al.* (2005) Adoptive transfer of cytomegalovirus-specific CTL to stem cell transplant patients after selection by HLA-peptide tetramers. *J Exp Med* **202**: 379–386.

35. Bunde T, Kirchner A, Hoffmeister B *et al.* (2005) Protection from cytomegalovirus after transplantation is correlated with immediate early 1-specific CD8 T cells. *J Exp Med* **201**: 1031–1036.

36. Knabel M, Franz TJ, Schiemann M *et al.* (2002) Reversible MHC multimer staining for functional isolation of T-cell populations and effective adoptive transfer. *Nat Med* **8**: 631–637.

37. Tan R, Xu X, Ogg GS *et al.* (1999) Rapid death of adoptively transferred T cells in acquired immunodeficiency syndrome. *Blood* **93**: 1506–1510.

38. Rauser G, Einsele H, Sinzger C *et al.* (2004) Rapid generation of combined CMV-specific CD4$^+$ and CD8$^+$ T-cell lines for adoptive transfer into recipients of allogeneic stem cell transplants. *Blood* **103**: 3565–3572.

39. Feuchtinger T, Lang P, Hamprecht K *et al.* (2004) Isolation and expansion of human adenovirus-specific CD4$^+$ and CD8$^+$ T cells

according to IFN-gamma secretion for adjuvant immunotherapy. *Exp Hematol* **32**: 282–289.

40. Feuchtinger T, Matthes-Martin S, Richard C *et al.* (2006) Safe adoptive transfer of virus-specific T-cell immunity for the treatment of systemic adenovirus infection after allogeneic stem cell transplantation. *Br J Haematol* **134**: 64–76.

41. Chatziandreou I, Gilmour KC, McNicol AM *et al.* (2007) Capture and generation of adenovirus specific T cells for adoptive immunotherapy. *Br J Haematol* **136**: 117–126.

42. Beck O, Topp MS, Koehl U *et al.* (2006) Generation of highly purified and functionally active human TH1 cells against *Aspergillus fumigatus*. *Blood* **107**(6): 2562–2569.

43. Walter EA, Greenberg PD, Gilbert MJ *et al.* (1995) Reconstitution of cellular immunity against cytomegalovirus in recipients of allogeneic bone marrow by transfer of T-cell clones from the donor. *N Engl J Med* **333**: 1038–1044.

44. Einsele H, Roosnek E, Rufer N *et al.* (2002) Infusion of cytomegalovirus (CMV)-specific T-cells for the treatment of CMV infection not responding to antiviral chemotherapy. *Blood* **99**: 3916–3922.

45. Peggs KS, Verfuerth S, Pizzey A *et al.* (2003) Adoptive cellular therapy for early cytomegalovirus infection after allogeneic stem-cell transplantation with virus-specific T-cell lines. *Lancet* **362**: 1375–1377.

46. Rooney CM, Smith CA, Ng C *et al.* (1995) Use of gene-modified virus-specific T-lymphocytes to control Epstein–Barr virus-related lymphoproliferation. *Lancet* **345**: 9–13.

47. Heslop HE, Ng CYC, Li C *et al.* (1996) Long-term restoration of immunity against Epstein–Barr virus infection by adoptive transfer of gene-modified virus-specific T lymphocytes. *Nat Med* **2**: 551–555.

48. Gottschalk S, Rooney CM, Heslop HE. (2005) Post-transplant lymphoproliferative disorders. *Annu Rev Med* **56**: 29–44.

49. Gottschalk S, Ng CYC, Smith CA *et al.* (2001) An Epstein–Barr virus deletion mutant that causes fatal lymphoproliferative disease unresponsive to virus-specific T cell therapy. *Blood* **97**: 835–843.

50. Gustafsson A, Levitsky V, Zou JZ *et al.* (2000) Epstein–Barr virus (EBV) load in bone marrow transplant recipients at risk to develop posttransplant lymphoproliferative disease: prophylactic infusion of EBV-specific cytotoxic T cells. *Blood* **95**: 807–814.

51. Ramadan G. (2004) Generation of *Aspergillus*-specific T lymphocytes with cytotoxic activity. *Egypt J Immunol* **11**: 59–70.

52. Ramadan G, Konings S, Kurup VP, Keever-Taylor CA. (2004) Generation of *Aspergillus*- and CMV-specific T-cell responses using autologous fast DC. *Cytotherapy* **6**: 223–234.

53. Perruccio K, Tosti A, Burchielli E *et al.* (2005) Transferring functional immune responses to pathogens after haploidentical hematopoietic transplantation. *Blood* **106**: 4397–4406.

54. Berger C, Jensen MC, Lansdorp PM *et al.* (2008) Adoptive transfer of effector CD8 T cells derived from central memory cells establishes persistent T cell memory in primates. *J Clin Invest* **118**: 294–305.

Chapter 9

The Challenge in Hematopoietic Stem Cell Transplantation: Shortening the Immunodeficiency Period

*Liliane Dal Cortivo[†], Salima Hacein-Bey-Abina[†],
Yamina Hamel[‡], Alain Fischer[‡,§], Isabelle André-Schmutz[‡]
and Marina Cavazzana-Calvo*[,†]*

Introduction

Since the discovery of T lymphocytes as the cells responsible for the occurrence of acute graft-versus-host disease (GvHD), T cell depletion of the graft has enabled the performance of allogeneic hematopoietic stem cell transplantation (HSCT) even when an HLA-genoidentical or phenoidentical healthy donor is not available. Unfortunately, this procedure has not significantly extended the use of partially HLA-compatible HSCT, with the exception of the treatment of severe combined immunodeficiencies (SCIDs), because even though these donor T cells cause GvHD, they also promote hematopoietic engraftment, reconstitution of T cell immunity (particularly in adults with reduced thymic function), and mediate a potent beneficial antitumor phenomenon known as the

---

*Corresponding author.

[†]Department of Biotherapy, Hopital Necker Enfants-Malades, AP-HP, Université Paris Descartes, Paris, France.

[‡]Unité U768, Institut National Scientifique d'Etude et de Recherche Médicale (INSERM), Hopital Necker Enfants-Malades, Paris, France.

[§]Pediatric Immunology and Hematology Unit, Hopital Necker Enfants-Malades, AP-HP, Université Paris Descartes, Paris, France. E-mail: m.cavazzana@nck.aphp-fr.

graft-versus-leukemia (GvL) effect. Thus, optimal GvHD prevention is counterbalanced by serious complications that hamper the achievement of a successful outcome of haploidentical HSCT. Establishing a method for accelerating the immune reconstitution of these patients means removing this major obstacle to the extended use of partially HLA-compatible HSCT.

In this chapter, we summarize our research work on improving the outcome of this particularly difficult setting of HSCT. Three main procedures are under investigation by our group and one cannot rule out the possibility that a combination of these different methods may be required, depending on the patient's age and the underlying disease. A form of "*à la carte*" transplantation is highly warranted in order to solve today's two main problems in HSC transplantation: immune reconstitution and thymic involution.

Depletion of Alloreactive T Cells

In the 1980s, discovery of the sequential appearance of specific activation markers on the T cell surface led to the development of a strategy based on the *ex vivo* depletion of specifically antihost-activated T cells. The first reports used monoclonal antibodies directed against the high-affinity IL-2 receptor (CD25) or CD69 and coupled to either a toxin or magnetic beads. Successful antihost T cell depletion was confirmed by nonreactivity in a mixed lymphocyte reaction (MLR) assay between fully HLA haploincompatible or phenoidentical donor/recipient pairs[1–6] or in HLA genoidentical siblings, where minor HLA Ag disparities occur.[7] In the HLA-mismatched setting, the addition of anti-CD25 ricin immunotoxin in a two-day MLR led to a reduction of over 98% in the residual proliferation for recipient cells.[1,4] Differences in the techniques used (such as the use of an immunotoxin or magnetic beads for depletion) and the type of stimulator cells account for the variability in residual proliferation, which has been reported as ranging from 8% to 26%.[2,3,5,6,8] *In vivo* studies in a murine model showed that T cell depletion was at least partially effective in preventing both graft rejection and GvHD in a one-haplotype-mismatched combination.[10] In a phase I/II study, $1–8 \times 10^5$ allodepleted T cells/kg were infused (at between 15 and 47 days post-HSCT) into 15 pediatric patients with acquired or congenital hematopoietic disorders.[11] No cases of severe (> grade II) GvHD occurred. Grade I or II GvHD (which developed in four patients) was cured by treatment with steroids in three cases and with Leucotac® (Biotest, Buc, France) treatment in the fourth. It is noteworthy that in all four cases, antihost residual proliferation was greater than 1%. Evidence for early T cell expansion was shown in three patients with ongoing viral infections. Specific antiviral responses occurred at a time when such responses are not normally detected following T cell-depleted HSCT. These results demonstrate that *ex vivo* selective depletion of GvHD-causing T cells is feasible and efficient, even in a haploidentical setting. Infusion of HSCT patients with T cells allodepleted by an anti-CD25 ricin α chain immunotoxin has been tested by two other groups, with similar results.[12,13]

Magnetic cell sorting presents several advantages over the use of immunotoxins, such as higher recovery rates and greater potential for clinical use. The technique is based on existing clinical grade devices and the ability to use the cells immediately after the procedure.[3,8] In terms of the immune competence of allodepleted T cells, it has been shown that the numbers of cytotoxic precursor cells (as evaluated by a limiting dilution assay specific for cytomegalovirus-infected fibroblasts and Epstein–Barr virus–transformed cell lines) are not affected by depletion treatment with anti-CD25 immunotoxins.[4]

In an attempt to improve the allodepletion procedure and infuse higher numbers of cells, we have turned to magnetic beads for allodepleting CD25-expressing T cells. Results in terms of efficiency and specificity have been similar to those obtained with the anti-CD25 ricin α chain immunotoxin (our unpublished observations). Allodepleted T cells can be prepared and then frozen until safety screening tests have been completed, without any significant changes in their anti-infectious activity measured *in vitro*. This procedure is currently being tested in a phase I/II clinical trial in which a total of 25 pediatric patients with inherited immune system disorders are due to be enrolled. However, half of the 18 procedures already performed did not fulfill the validation criteria for injection into the patients. The main reason was insufficient activation (as evidenced by

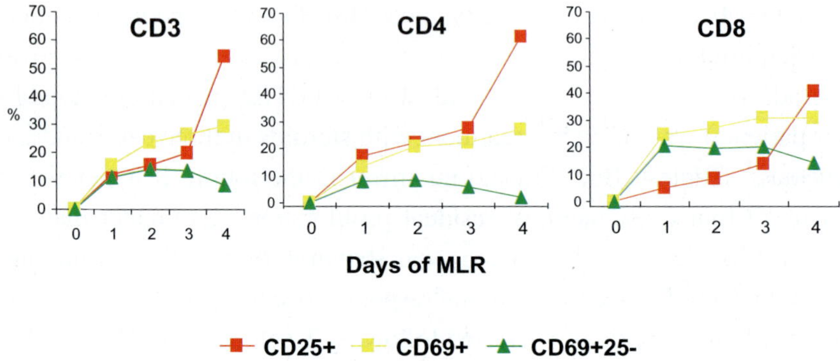

Figure 1. The kinetics of CD25 and CD69 expression on T lymphocytes was measured throughout a 2–4-day MLR by immunofluorescence analysis.

CD25 expression), thereafter preventing optimal magnetic elimination. The following factors may influence activation:

(1) The MLR duration: CD25 is better expressed after four days of coculture (Fig. 1) than after three days as initially scheduled.

(2) The MLR container: the CD3/CD25 expression level was raised in culture conditions promoting cell–cell contact; in fact, MLR-induced T cell activation performed in different containers (i.e. microwell plates, flasks or vertical bags) (Fig. 2) was better in vertical bags but did not seem to be influenced by the effector:stimulator ratio (Fig. 3).

Three patients received 0.5 to 3×10^5 immunomagnetically depleted lymphocytes per kg. One of them cleared a CMV infection two weeks after cell infusion, as evidenced (Fig. 4) by the decrease in the CMV viral load (measured by PCR) concomitantly with an increased blood count of interferon-gamma (IFN-γ)–secreting T lymphocytes. However, this effect could not be seen in the other patients and grade II GvH was observed in both cases — showing the lack of reproducibility and the need to better assess the extent of alloreactivity depletion.

Taken as a whole, these results show the need to improve this allodepletion technology. To this end, other protocols for *ex vivo* elimination

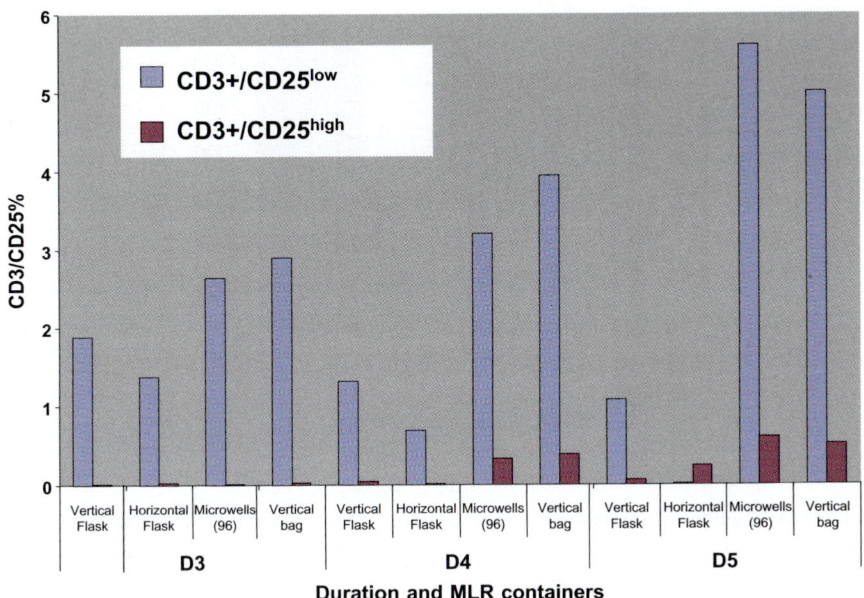

Figure 2. The kinetics of CD25 expression on T lymphocytes was measured by immuno-fluorescence analysis throughout a 2–5-day MLR performed in 96-microwell plates/flasks/bags (horizontal and vertical).

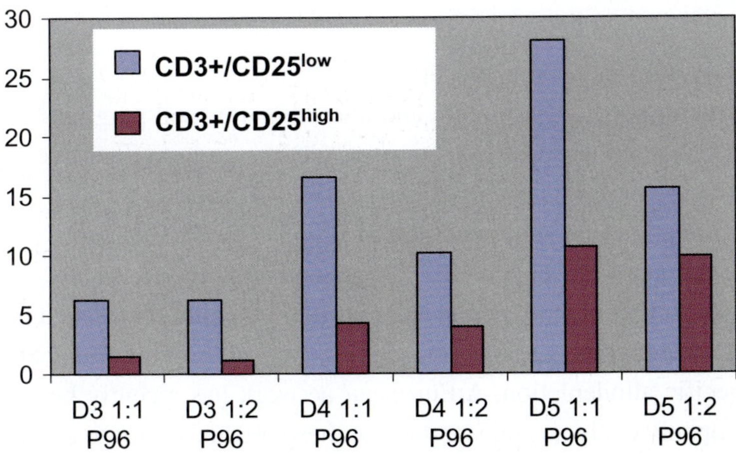

Figure 3. CD3+25+cell % expression during MLR in microwells as a function of the effector:stimulator ratio (1:1 and 1:2).

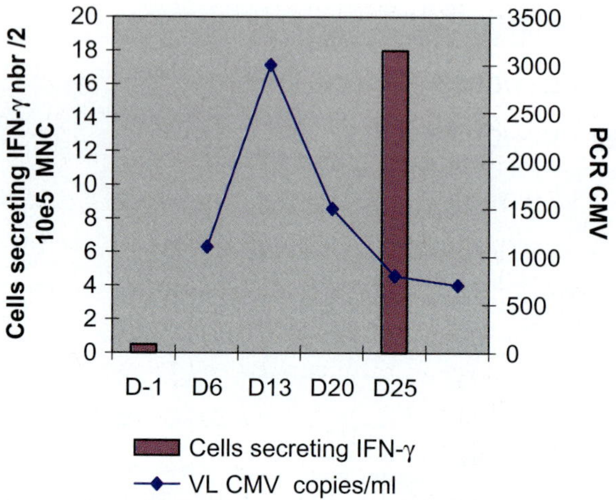

Figure 4. Number of the patient's cells secreting IFN-γ, and CMV PCR viral load (VL) before and 30 days after lymphocyte infusion. The histogram indicates the number of peripheral blood cells secreting IFN-γ before and 30 days after lymphocyte infusion assessed by Elispot. The blue curve indicates the decrease overtime of the CMV VL measured by PCR.

of activated antihost alloreactive T cells have been developed in the recent past, based on:

- Activation-induced cell death;[14]
- Targeting of P glycoprotein and photodynamic cell purging;[15,16]
- FACS-based positive selection of CD25[+] carboxyfluorescein diacetate succinimidyl ester (CFSE)–positive T cells;[17]
- Elimination of a subpopulation of CD38[+] CD[high] T cells;[18]
- Selection of memory cells:[19–21] recently published results seem to indicate that photodynamic cell purging[19,20] could represent a promising technology capable of significantly improving the extent of specific allodepletion. A European network has recently been set up to openly evaluate and standardize these methods prior to any clinical application.

Antivirus-Specific Immunotherapy

Adoptive immunotherapy — consisting of infusion of antivirus-specific cytotoxic T cells (CTLs) generated *ex vivo* from the seropositive donor — has formally demonstrated its efficacy in the treatment of life-threatening viral infections in the immunocompromised host. Nevertheless, its large-scale clinical application was rapidly compromised by several limitations that rapidly arose, such as (i) the absence of sustained response if only $CD8^+$ T cells are infused, (ii) the need to generate specific CTLs using independent antigen-presenting cells (APCs) for each virus and (iii) the overall duration of the procedure prior to infusion into patients. Moreover, *in vitro* clonal expansion can be associated with expression of the proapoptotic molecule CD95 by cultured cells, thus limiting their *in vivo* survival.[22] The use of a single APC presenting more than one set of viral antigens to generate polyspecific CTLs can partially circumvent at least one of these obstacles. The feasibility and specificity of this strategy have been shown. Indeed, by using a single APC transduced with a replication-defective adenovirus vector (rAd) encoding the immunodominant antigen for the CMV and EBV viruses (i.e. CMVpp65 and EBV EBNA-3C), combined CMV and adenovirus-specific or EBV- and adenovirus-specific T cytotoxic cells can be generated efficiently.[23] Nevertheless, the need to generate donor APCs and combine gene and cell therapies (together with the culture time needed to generate them) makes this strategy extremely burdensome. Overall, these aspects have prompted us to prefer the adoptive transfer of directly isolated peripheral blood antigen-specific CTLs to the infusion of CTLs that have undergone prolonged *in vitro* culture. We have focused our attention on two methods, i.e. cytokine secretion capture columns and peptide-HLA tetramers.

The capture of T cells that secrete IFN-γ in response to stimulation by viral antigens enables rapid T cell selection under GMP conditions, as demonstrated for adenovirus-specific T cells.[24] The advantage of this strategy is that previous knowledge of viral epitopes is not required and there is no HLA restriction; the down side is that it produces small numbers of selected cells. Despite the possibility of amplifying the cells *in vitro* before injection, a certain degree of contamination by remaining alloreactive T cells could hamper the wide use of this technique in partially HLA-compatible settings. Precisely quantifying this contamination is a key challenge for the extended use of this technique.

In addition to specificity, the main challenge for specific T cell immunotherapy is the reduction of alloreactivity and, consequently, the risk of GvHD induction. With this technology, alloreactive T cells (even though fewer in number) are still detectable when isolated human adenovirus (HadV)-specific T cells are cultured with HLA-mismatched cells in a mixed lymphocyte culture, whereas a huge reduction in alloreactive T cells is detectable when an HLA-matched mixed lymphocyte culture is performed. One way of circumventing this obstacle (or at least of reducing the GvHD risk) is to inject low doses of these specific T cells since, on the basis of previously published experiments, the latter are able to greatly expand *in vivo* in the presence of viremia. In addition, the study reported by Feuchtinger *et al.*[24] suggests that the efficacy of the adoptive transfer of T cell immunity is independent of the infused cell dose but probably dependent on the viral load. Starting from these encouraging results, we are setting up a similar protocol for CMV and/or AdV donor adoptive immunotherapy in infected HSCT recipients. Preliminary results in our laboratory show that the obtained CTLs are virus-specific: in an IFN-γ Elispot assay, the number of secreting cells was 16-fold higher after selection. In a ^{51}Cr release cytotoxicity assay, 40% lysis of pulsed phytohemagglutinin (PHA) blasts was observed at a ratio of 20:1 (Fig. 5). Residual proliferation — evaluated by ^{3}H thymidine uptake before and after a three-day MLR performed with autologous peripheral blood mononuclear cells (PBMCs) and allogenic PBMCs — revealed a decrease in alloreactivity of up to 80% among the isolated cells (Fig. 6).

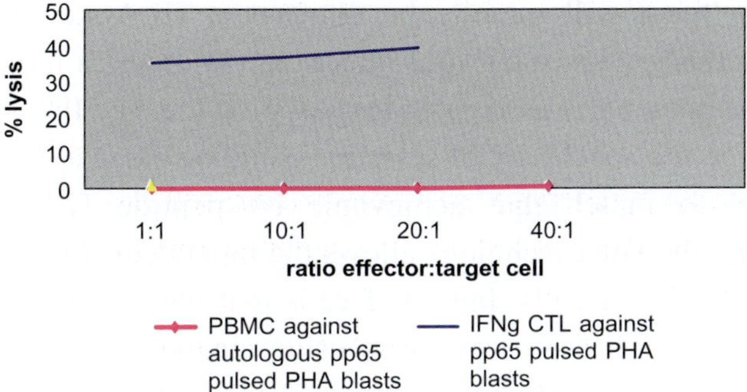

Figure 5. HLA-restricted cytotoxicity of PBMCs before and after selection was tested against autologous PHA blasts, pulsed with pp65 peptide in a 4 h standard chromium release assay.

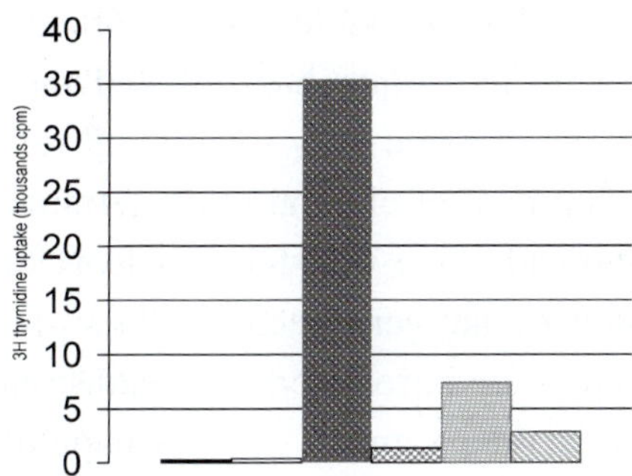

Figure 6. Alloreactivity of autologous PBMCs before and after IFN-γ selection (Miltenyi Biotec) was tested (^{3}H thymidine uptake) against autologous PBMC and third party PBMC (C) after 3 day MLC.

^{3}H thymidine uptake was measured after a three day culture of:

- Autologous PBMC alone before selection (■)
- Third party PBMC alone (□)
- Autologous PBMC before selection against irradiated third party (▨)
- Autologous PBMC before selection against autologous PBMC before selection (▨)
- Autologous PBMC after selection against irradiated third party (▨)
- Autologous PBMC after selection against irradiated autologous PBMC before selection (▨).

This protocol will initially be targeted at HLA-matched patients with chemotherapy-resistant viral infections, in order to more carefully evaluate the potentially associated toxicity risk (i.e. GvHD occurrence).

However, the specificity of selection using cytokine secretion assays is unlikely to match that achievable by peptide HLA tetramers. Furthermore, the latter technique allows the rapid detection and isolation of antigen-specific T cells. Indeed, T cells that bind the tetramer can be isolated with a high degree of purity using magnetic beads coated with antibody specific for the phycoerythrin fluorochrome (which is used to label the tetramer).[25] Starting with a 250 ml blood sample or leuka-pheresis specimen from the donor, Moss and collaborators[26] have shown that it is possible to select CMV-specific CTLs with a purity of over 95%. Moreover, these cells are viable, can proliferate *in vitro* and show functional activity. This technique has enabled the treatment of nine patients and has generated some very interesting results.[26] We are now working on the development of clinical grade tetramers.

The advantages of adoptive transfer protocols that allow the rapid selection and infusion of antigen-specific CTLs are clear. If adoptive transfer procedures are to be introduced into mainstream clinical practice and significantly change the prognosis of HLA-haploidentical transplants, they must offer speed, flexibility and relative ease of delivery.

Ex Vivo Expansion of a Human Progenitor Committed to the T Cell Lineage and Able to Seed the Thymus

Despite all the above-mentioned technical improvements, T-cell-based therapies are still associated with several problems, including the limited availability of suitable cells, the occurrence of GvHD when allogeneic T cells are used and a requirement for *in vitro* and *in vivo* cytokines to guarantee the survival and/or expansion of the cell product. An alternative strategy for shortening the length of the immunodeficient period follow-ing HSCT consists in speeding up thymopoiesis and thus the production of mature T cells. Several groups (including ours) have attempted to optimize thymopoiesis by treating HSCT recipients (only in preclinical murine models, up to now) with cytokines such as IL-7, IL-15 and KGF.[27–30] The experiments generated contradictory results and these treatments will require further study before clinical applications can be envisaged. Alternatively, speeding up thymopoiesis by injecting *ex-vivo*-generated T cell precursors has been made possible thanks to two recent major advances: the establishment of a Notch-signaling-based culture system capable of inducing and maintaining T cell differentiation, and the characterization of early steps of lymphopoiesis in humans (including the identification of a postnatal thymus seeding candidate). The first improvement showed that when OP9 cell lines (derived from murine bone marrow) were transduced with the Notch ligand Delta-like-1 (one of three mammalian delta-like Notch ligands), the resulting OP9-DL1 cells promoted T lymphopoiesis by both murine and human cord blood (CB) and bone marrow hematopoietic stem cells (for a review, see Ref. 31). Nevertheless, until recently, the OP9-DL1 coculture system was not efficient enough to allow quantification of human T cell potential and thus the comparison of various progenitor compartments — a prerequisite for identification of the genuine T cell precursor population. By optimizing this technique, we performed an efficient quantitative and qualitative analysis of the T cell potential of human progenitors (manuscript in preparation) and then identified a thymus-seeding progenitor during the postnatal period in humans.[32]

In particular, we have recently described a CD34$^+$ CD10$^+$ lin$^-$ human lymphoid progenitor which is present not only in the CB and bone marrow but also in the blood and the thymus at all ages. This lymphoid progenitor can be divided into two subsets: a CD24-expressing, B cell committed population and a CD24$^-$ population which is able to differentiate into all the various lymphoid subpopulations, as well as into dendritic cells. Moreover, this CD10$^+$ CD24$^-$ cell fraction expresses the IL-7Rα and γc subunit receptors, as described for the murine common lymphoid progenitor (for a review, see Ref. 33). *In vitro*, this cell population displays a high T cell differentiation potential once cultured on OP9-Delta-1 stroma cell lines.[32] At present, we are concentrating our efforts on identifying the mechanism involved in thymus homing in this population.

This work forms the basis for identifying a clinically suitable technology capable of irreversibly expanding *in vitro* human hemotopoietic stem cells (HSCs) toward the T cell compartment. This expanded T cell population could be injected (together with the nonmanipulated, immunoselected CD34$^+$ graft) and would significantly shorten the immunodeficient period that characterizes the first six months following partially HLA-incompatible bone marrow transplantation.

Three reports have provided evidence to suggest that brief exposure to Notch ligands is enough to induce T cell differentiation and increase the T cell potential of murine and human HSCs.[34–36] Zakrzewski *et al.* cocultured T cell-depleted murine HSCs with OP9-DL1 cells, in order to amplify allogeneic lymphoid precursors.[34] Following injection into lethally irradiated mice, the cocultured cells (i) increased host thymic cellularity and donor T cell chimerism, (ii) gave rise to host-tolerant CD4$^+$ and CD8$^+$ populations with normal T cell properties, and (iii) improved resistance to *Listeria* infection. Moreover, the cells significantly mediated GvL activity. No GvHD was observed. More recently, the same group showed that murine allogenic T cell precursors can be applied irrespective of major histocompatibility complex (MHC) disparities and even in the absence of stem cell rescue.[35] The *ex-vivo*-generated progenitor cells gave rise to host-MHC-restricted and host-tolerant, functional allogeneic T cells. The procedure improved survival and antitumor responses in the absence of GvHD in the recipients. To further enhance antitumor activity, T cell precursors were transduced to express a chimeric receptor that targets the human CD19 expressed by A20-TGL lymphoma cells. When challenged with A20-TGL lymphoma cells, recipients showed a significant additional antitumor activity and no increase in GvHD incidence. This study provided the first evidence that genetic manipulation of *ex-vivo*-enhanced T cell precursors can be used to generate antigen-specific T cells that can be applied to any recipient, irrespective of MHC disparities and independently of HSCT.

Lefort and colleagues provided the first evidence that this strategy may be applicable to human progenitors by showing that brief *in vitro* stimulation of CD34$^+$ CB cells with the Notch ligand Delta-4 (DL4) was sufficient to promote T cell differentiation *in vitro*.[36] In this study, DL4 triggered immunophenotypic changes (CD7$^+$cytCD3$^+$ cells) and molecular changes (*de novo* expression of several T cell-related transcription factors and TCR-gamma rearrangement) consistent with early T cell lineage differentiation. Conversely, B cell transcripts were simultaneously silenced. These early changes were shown to mediate long-term effects on the further differentiation potential of these T cells. Priming with DL4 led to an acceleration of T cell development *in vitro* (including completion of the TCR rearrangement in culture systems suitable for T cell development), whereas B cell development was inhibited.

Some basic questions remain to be formally resolved prior to any clinical application. These questions notably relate to:

- Optimization of the culture conditions during exposure to DL4;
- Optimization of the length of the culture period, in order to avoid the appearance of complete TCR rearrangements in the absence of proper thymic stroma, which would potentially cause autoimmune disease or prevent functional responses to infectious agents *in vivo*;
- Proof that the expanded progenitors are still able to efficiently seed the thymus (by transferring them to NOD/SCID/γc recipients);
- Characterization of the functionality of the T cells produced in NOD/SCID/γc recipients by monitoring the immune response to various infectious agents.

These experiments are now in progress in our laboratory and will hopefully provide further information on whether an adoptive transfer of T precursor cells can enhance T cell reconstitution after HSCT, which represents an important condition for the further development of this new immunotherapy. If these objectives are met, a clinical trial with *in-vitro-*generated T cell precursors could be designed, in order to establish whether the above-mentioned technique can improve the long-term survival curve in these very problematic HSC transplants.

References

1. Cavazzana-Calvo M, Fromont C, Le Deist F *et al.* (1990) Specific elimination of alloreactive T cells by an anti-interleukin-2 receptor B chain-specific immunotoxin. *Transplantation* **50**(1): 1–7.

2. Mavroudis DA, Jiang YZ, Hensel N *et al.* (1996) Specific depletion of alloreactivity against haplotype mismatched related individuals by a recombinant immunotoxin: A new approach to graft-versus-host disease prophylaxis in haploidentical bone marrow transplantation. *Bone Marrow Transplant* **17**(5): 793–799.

3. Garderet L, Snell V, Przepiorka D *et al.* (1999) Effective depletion of alloreactive lymphocytes from peripheral blood mononuclear cell preparations. *Transplantation* **67**(1): 124–130.

4. Montagna D, Yvon E, Calcaterra V *et al.* (1999) Depletion of alloreactive T cells by a specific anti-interleukin-2 receptor p55 chain immunotoxin does not impair *in vitro* antileukemia and antiviral activity. *Blood* **93**(10): 3550–3557.

5. Fehse B, Frerk O, Goldmann M *et al.* (2000) Efficient depletion of alloreactive donor T lymphocytes based on expression of two activation-induced antigens (CD25 and CD69). *Br J Haematol* **109**(3): 644–651.

6. Datta AR, Barrett AJ, Jiang YZ *et al.* (1994) Distinct T cell populations distinguish chronic myeloid leukaemia cells from lymphocytes in the same individual: A model for separating GVHD from GVL reactions. *Bone Marrow Transplant* **14**(4): 517–524.

7. Mavroudis DA, Dermime S, Molldrem J *et al.* (1998) Specific depletion of alloreactive T cells in HLA-identical siblings: A method for separating graft-versus-host and graft-versus-leukaemia reactions. *Br J Haematol* **101**(3): 565–570.

8. Koh MB, Prentice HG, Lowdell MW. (1999) Selective removal of alloreactive cells from haematopoietic stem cell grafts: Graft

engineering for GVHD prophylaxis. *Bone Marrow Transplant* **23**(10): 1071–1079.

9. Engert A, Martin G, Amlot P *et al.* (1991) Immunotoxins constructed with anti-CD25 monoclonal antibodies and deglycosylated ricin A-chain have potent anti-tumour effects against human Hodgkin cells *in vitro* and solid Hodgkin tumours in mice. *Int J Cancer* **49**(3): 450–456.

10. Cavazzana-Calvo M, Stephan JL, Sarnacki S *et al.* (1994) Attenuation of graft-versus-host disease and graft rejection by *ex vivo* immuno-toxin elimination of alloreactive T cells in an H-2 haplotype disparate mouse combination. *Blood* **83**(1): 288–298.

11. André-Schmutz I, Le Deist F, Hacein-Bey H *et al.* (2002) Preventing GVHD while improving immune reconstitution in allogeneic stem cell transplantation by infusion of donor T lymphocytes after *ex vivo* depletion of CD25$^+$ alloreactive cells with an immunotoxin. *Lancet* **360**: 130–137.

12. Mielke S, Solomon SR, Barrett AJ. (2005) Selective depletion strategies in allogeneic stem cell transplantation. *Cytotherapy* **7**(2): 109–115.

13. Amrolia PJ, Mucioli-Casadei G, Huls H *et al.* (2005) Add-back of allodepleted donor T cells to improve immune reconstitution after haplo-identical stem cell transplantation. *Cytotherapy* **7**(2): 116–125.

14. Hartwig UF, Robbers M, Wickenhauser C, Huber C. (2002) Murine acute graft-versus-host disease can be prevented by depletion of alloreactive T lymphocytes using activation-induced cell death. *Blood* **99**(8): 3041–3049.

15. Guimond M, Balassy A, Barrette M *et al.* (2002) P-glycoprotein targeting: A unique strategy to selectively eliminate immunoreactive T cells. *Blood* **100**(2): 375–382.

16. Chen BJ, Cui X, Liu C, Chao NJ. (2002) Prevention of graft-versus-host disease while preserving graft-versus-leukemia effect after selective depletion of host-reactive T cells by photodynamic cell purging process. *Blood* **99**(9): 3083–3088.

17. Godfrey WR, Krampf MR, Taylor PA, Blazar BR. (2004) *Ex vivo* depletion of alloreactive cells based on CFSE dye dilution, activation antigen selection, and dendritic cell stimulation. *Blood* **103**(3): 1158–1565.

18. Martins SL, St John LS, Champlin RE *et al.* (2004) Functional assessment and specific depletion of alloreactive human T cells using flow cytometry. *Blood* **104**(12): 3429–3436.

19. Boumedine RS, Roy DC. (2005) Elimination of alloreactive T cells using photodynamic therapy. *Cytotherapy* **7**(2): 134–143.

20. Le NT, Chen BJ, Chao NJ. (2005) Selective elimination of alloreactivity from immunotherapeutic T cells by photodynamic cell purging and memory T-cell sorting. *Cytotherapy* **7**(2): 126–133.

21. Anderson BE, McNiff J, Yan J *et al.* (2003) Memory CD4[+] T cells do not induce graft-versus-host disease. *J Clin Invest* **112**(1): 101–108.

22. Tan R, Xu X, Ogg GS *et al.* (1999) Rapid death of adoptively transferred T cells in acquired immunodeficiency syndrome. *Blood* **93**(5): 1506–1510.

23. Hamel Y, Blake N, Gabrielsson S *et al.* (2002) Adenovirally transduced dendritic cells induce bispecific cytotoxic T lymphocyte responses against adenovirus and cytomegalovirus pp65 or against adenovirus and Epstein–Barr virus EBNA3C protein: A novel approach for immunotherapy. *Hum Gene Ther* **13**(7): 855–866.

24. Feuchtinger T, Matthes-Martin S, Richard C *et al.* (2006) Safe adoptive transfer of virus-specific T-cell immunity for the treatment of systemic adenovirus infection after allogeneic stem cell transplantation. *Br J Haematol* **134**(1): 64–76.

25. Keenan RD, Ainsworth J, Khan N *et al.* (2001) Purification of cytomegalovirus-specific CD8 T cells from peripheral blood using HLA-peptide tetramers. *Br J Haematol* **115**(2): 428–434.

26. Cobbold M, Khan N, Pourgheysari B *et al.* (2005) Adoptive transfer of cytomegalovirus-specific CTL to stem cell transplant patients after selection by HLA-peptide tetramers. *J Exp Med* **202**(3): 379–386.

27. André-Schmutz I, Bonhomme D, Yates F *et al.* (2004) IL-7 effect on immunological reconstitution after HSCT depends on MHC incompatibility. *Br J Haematol* **126**(6): 844–851.

28. Alpdogan O, Eng JM, Muriglan SJ *et al.* (2005) Interleukin-15 enhances immune reconstitution after allogeneic bone marrow transplantation. *Blood* **105**(2): 865–873.

29. Alpdogan O, Muriglan SJ, Eng JM *et al.* (2003) IL-7 enhances peripheral T cell reconstitution after allogeneic hematopoietic stem cell transplantation. *J Clin Invest* **112**(7): 1095–1107.

30. Rossi S, Blazar BR, Farrell CL *et al.* (2002) Keratinocyte growth factor preserves normal thymopoiesis and thymic microenvironment during experimental graft-versus-host disease. *Blood* **100**(2): 682–691.

31. de Pooter R, Zúñiga-Pflücker JC. (2007) T-cell potential and development *in vitro*: The OP9-DL1 approach. *Curr Opin Immunol* **19**(2): 163–168.

32. Six EM, Bonhomme D, Monteiro M *et al.* (2007) A human postnatal lymphoid progenitor capable of circulating and seeding the thymus. *J Exp Med* **204**(13): 3085–3093.

33. Bhandoola A, von Boehmer H, Petrie HT, Zúñiga-Pflücker JC. (2007) Commitment and developmental potential of extrathymic and intrathymic T cell precursors: Plenty to choose from. *Immunity* **26**(6): 678–689.

34. Zakrzewski JL, Kochman AA, Lu SX *et al.* (2006) Adoptive transfer of T-cell precursors enhances T-cell reconstitution after allogeneic hematopoietic stem cell transplantation. *Nat Med* **12**(9): 1039–1047.

35. Zakrzewski JL, Suh D, Markley JC *et al.* (2008) Tumor immunotherapy across MHC barriers using allogeneic T-cell precursors. *Nat Biotechnol* **26**(4): 453–461.

36. Lefort N, Benne C, Lelievre JD *et al.* (2006) Short exposure to Notch ligand Delta-4 is sufficient to induce T-cell differentiation program and to increase the T cell potential of primary human CD34$^+$ cells. *Exp Hematol* **34**(12): 1720–1729.

Chapter 10

Treatment of Adenovirus Infection After Haploidentical Stem Cell Transplantation in Children

*Tobias Feuchtinger, Rupert Handgretinger and Peter Lang**

Introduction

Mismatched related (haploidentical) hematopoietic stem cell transplantation (HSCT) has emerged as a standard procedure in the management of malignant and nonmalignant diseases. However, viral infections remain one of the major causes of morbidity and mortality in patients who receive T cell-depleted grafts from mismatched donors.[1–3] In most cases, viral infections result from reactivation of latent viruses such as cytomegalovirus (CMV), human adenovirus (ADV) and Epstein–Barr virus (EBV). In children adenovirus has become a major viral pathogen, responsible for significant posttransplantation morbidity and mortality.[4–6] Increased frequencies of severe ADV infections have also been detected in solid organ transplant recipients and human immune deficiency virus (HIV)–positive patients. Importantly, an increased risk of adenovirus infection can be correlated with the lack of endogenous T cell immunity, capable of controlling such infectious agents.[7–9] Here, we focus on current treatment options for adenovirus infections after transplantation from mismatched related (haploidentical) donors.

*Corresponding author. Peter Lang, Children's University Hospital, University of Tuebingen, Hoppe-Seyler-Str. 1, D-72072 Tuebingen, Germany. E-mail: peter.lang@ med.uni-tuebingen.de

Table 1. Adenovirus Classification

Species	Serotypes	Clinical Features
A	12, 18, 31	Pneumonia, enteritis
B	3, 7, 11, 14, 16, 21, 34, 35, 50	Hemorrhagic cystitis
C	1, 2, 5, 6	Hepatitis, pneumonia, dissemination; high frequency post-HSCT
D	8–10, 13, 15, 17, 19, 20, 22–30, 32, 33, 36–39, 42–49, 51	Eye, gastrointestinal tract
E	4	Respiratory tract
F	40, 41	Gastrointestinal tract

Structure of Adenovirus

Human adenoviruses (ADV) are nonenveloped, ubiquitous, lytic double-stranded DNA viruses. Taxonomy distinguishes 51 different human serotypes, divided into 6 species, A–F (Table 1). Serotypes from all species can cause disease in both immunocompetent and immunocompromised subjects, although only approximately half of these strains have been associated with human disease with a variant symptom spectrum in different strains (Table 1).[10] Adenoviruses have a characteristic morphology, with an icosahedral capsid consisting of three major proteins — hexon, penton base, and a knobbed fiber — along with a number of minor proteins.[11] ADV has a wide tropism and can infect most human body cells. Primary binding of the virus capsid to the target cell occurs by binding between the fiber protein on the virus capsid and the Coxsackie–adenovirus receptor (CAR)[12] with the exception of species B viruses, which interact with target cells through CD46,[13] and species D viruses (serotypes 8, 19a, and 37) which bind to sialic acid residues rather than to CAR on target cells.[14] After internalization the virus travels to endosomes and the cytosol and translocates the viral genomes to the nucleus for expression of viral genes. During this process proteins of the virion gain access to major histocompatibility complex (MHC) class I and II processing pathways, so that infected cells can be recognized by the adenovirus-specific T cell receptor even in the absence of subsequent virus gene expression. The viral gene expression of nonstructural proteins can be divided into early and late gene products. Early viral gene products mediate viral gene expression and DNA replication, induce cell cycle progression, block apoptosis, and antagonize various host antiviral measures, whereas late gene products promote virus assembly and escape.

Transmission of ADV is by either the respiratory droplet or the oral–fecal route. Primary infection is usually early in life during infancy and childhood,[15] with either asymptomatic or trivial respiratory or gastrointestinal symptoms. After primary infection, ADV establishes latency in lymphoid tissue[16] with persistent infection. Although primary infections are self-limited, species C viruses display prolonged fecal excretion months, and even years, although the virus is no longer detected in nasopharyngeal washings.[17] Restriction analysis of viruses isolated up to four years after initial infection suggested chronic persistent infection rather than reinfection with the same serotype. Viral DNA could have been detected in mucosa/adenoidal T lymphocytes as the source of persistence, decreasing with age.[18]

The Role of T Cells in Adenovirus-Specific Immunity

The kinetics and specificity of ADV-directed immune responses have been sparsely investigated until recent years, whereas for adenoviral vectors complex mechanisms of immune responses and mechanisms of immune evasion for both the innate and adaptive immune systems have been described. The gene products of the E1A, E1B, and E3 region are involved in processes that prevent recognition and lysis of infected cells by cytotoxic T lymphocytes. Both innate and adaptive immune mechanisms respond to ADV infection. The innate immune response represents the first line of defense against the invading pathogens. Neutrophils and antigen-presenting cells internalize the virus and act as a part of the innate and adaptive immune response. NK cells mount an acute response to adenoviral vector transduction and play a role in the antiviral response during the early phase after T cell-depleted stem cell transplantation.[1,19]

Antigen-specific T cells are known to be an essential part of the immune responses required to control viral infection. The frequencies of these T cells may extensively increase in response to an acute infection and normally decline after successful control of the virus. Although the immune response to adenoviral vectors has been studied extensively,[20] little is known about the cellular immune response in the control of human "wild-type" adenoviruses *in vivo*. Proliferative responses of CD4[+] T cells in healthy donors suggested cross-reactive livelong persistence ADV-specific T cell immunity, but follow an age-dependent decrease over decades, as documented in blood samples of solid organ transplant recipients and healthy individuals.[16] T cells generated by using ADV antigen pulsed dendritic cells were found to contain a mixture of effector cells that recognize virus antigens in the context of both class I and class II antigens.[21] Additionally, T cells prepared *in vitro* against one ADV subtype showed extensive crossreactivity to other subtypes.[22,23] Recently, we have shown that the presence of ADV-specific T cells in peripheral blood post-HSCT is associated with a favorable prognosis, whereas ADV-viremia in the absence of specific T cells leads to ADV-associated mortality in both matched and mismatched donor transplantations.[8] The specificity of the T cell response is mainly directed against capsid proteins[20] with the adenoviral hexon protein as an immunodominant region.[24] The amino acid sequence of the hexon protein can be subdivided into hypervariable and conserved regions among adenovirus species and subtypes.[25] MHC-II-restricted peptide epitopes within the hexon protein have been described,[26,27] as well as MHC-I-restricted peptides for HLA-A1, -A2, -B7, and HLA-A24,[28,29] and some of the epitopes induce T cells that are cross-reactive among subgroups. Reactivity to other epitopes is specific to one or two subgroups, demonstrating that ADV-specific T cells can be either broadly cross-reactive or reactive to a restricted spectrum of viral strains.[28]

Incidence and Risk Factors of Adenovirus Infection Post-HSCT

Following initial reports on the relevance of ADV infections after stem cell transplantation,[6,10] an increasing incidence of ADV infections has been described over the last decades, which has been attributed to the increased use of T cell-depleted HSCT. However, the tremendous improvement of diagnostic methods and surveillance strategies limits the comparison with historical control groups. The cumulative risk of infection ranged between 8.5% and 29%.[6,30–34] Recipients of allogeneic stem cells, as opposed to autologous stem cell recipients, are more likely to have ADV infection and disease.[30,31,34] The incidence is higher in unrelated donor versus matched sibling donor transplants (26% versus 9%).[32] Pediatric patients were also more likely than adults to have an infection.[31,32,35] The highest incidence (84%) was found in young children up to five years of age, transplanted with T cell-depleted grafts other than an HLA-genotypically-identical related donor.[33] Isolation from two or more sites is correlated with a poor outcome.[31,32] Significant risk factors associated with ADV infections among allogeneic recipients included younger age, grade II–IV graft-vs-host disease, alemtuzumab treatment, and a second allogeneic HSCT.[6,36] In our own experience with haploidentical transplantations in children, viral infections remained a significant cause of mortality. The cumulative incidence of lethal viral infections of a cohort of 63 patients transplanted between 1995 and 2004 with CD34-positive selected haploidentical stem cells was 16% for all infections (caused by ADV, CMV or HSV) and 8.5% for the subgroup of infections caused by ADV. HADV and CMV were identified by PCR in 8 patients. In all patients who experienced adenoviral infections, HADV antigen was detectable in the stool before the onset of a systemic infection. One patient died from herpes simplex virus (HSV) infection. Analysis of ADV infection showed that 90% of infections were during the first three months posttransplant. Analysis of the ADV subtype revealed infection with subtypes 2, 5, 1, 6, 31, and 4 at decreasing frequency. All infections strictly occurred during the first six months post-SCT. After this time span, infectious episodes became rare and were not life-threatening. Moreover, an analysis of different time periods showed that the incidence of severe viral infections was markedly reduced from 18% (1995–2001) to 8% within the last two years (2002–2004), in conjunction with the intensification of preventive/pre-emptive therapeutic strategies and the surveillance of virus loads.[37] In haplo-SCT with CD3-depleted stem cells (plus CD20 depletion *in vivo*) and reduced intensity conditioning, viral loads (ADV, CMV, EBV) in peripheral blood were significantly lower than in a CD34[+]-selected control group.[38] None out of 22 patients had died of viremia, probably due to the better recovery of thymus-dependent T cells and to a stronger NK-cell-mediated first line defense. Similar results have been obtained in an interim analysis of our ongoing study with T and B cell (CD3/CD19)–depleted stem cells, since no lethal viral infection occurred in 38 patients.[39]

In a large cohort of adult HSCT recipients an overall mortality rate of 26% was observed, with a higher mortality rate among patients with pneumonia (73%) and disseminated disease (61%).[34] Risk factors for dissemination included presence of graft-vs-host disease (GvHD), receipt of concurrent immunosuppressive therapy,[34] and delayed reconstitution of lymphocytes.[7,9,33] Mortality of disseminated disease has been closely associated with increasing and high levels of ADV DNA ($\leq$104 DNA copies/ml) in peripheral blood, with a median time of three weeks between the first detection of ADV DNA in blood and the onset of symptoms.[4,40,41]

Recently, lymphocyte reconstitution and an increase in lymphocyte counts during the first weeks after infection have been shown to play a crucial role in clearance of ADV viremia and survival of the host.[7,9] In our previous work we were able to detect ADV-specific T cells in children after HSCT and could demonstrate that ADV-specific T cells are protective against ADV disease after matched or mismatched (haploidentical) HSCT.[8,37] 93% of patients who cleared a documented ADV infection had ADV specific T cells, whereas patients with ADV-associated mortality developed no specific T cells at all. The mean frequency of such ADV-specific T cells until day 200 posttransplant was 0.56% and thus similar to that of healthy donors (0.38%).

It is now appreciated that T cell reconstitution is required for the control of ADV infections and that drug therapy might limit, but not clear, the infection. In a recent prospective survey of a large pediatric cohort of HSCT patients, a significantly lower mortality from disseminated ADV infection was reported.[42] This was attributed to a combination of regular

216

prospective monitoring for early disseminated ADV infection by peripheral blood PCR, with prompt pre-emptive cidofovir treatment and withdrawal of immunosuppression.

Diagnosis and Surveillance of Adenovirus Infection After Haploidentical Transplantation

In recent years ADV-DNA detection by polymerase chain reaction (PCR) has developed as a fast method with high sensitivity and specificity. This method improved in the detection of ADV-DNA from almost all serotypes in body fluids and tissue, using hexon-specific primers of the conserved region within the hexon gene.[43,44] Viral infection can now be defined as the detection of ADV-DNA or antigen. ADV disease is usually defined as the detection of viral antigen and/or DNA together with appropriate symptoms in the absence of any other recognizable cause. For assessment of the time course and severity of infection, viral quantification (ADV-DNA copies) in clinical samples has been established for ADV. Consensus primer pairs detected hexon sequences of all 51 different serotypes from multiple sites, including blood, serum, eye swabs, and feces.[4,45–47] Although detection of ADV-DNA has become a useful diagnostic tool and the standard of care in diagnostic and surveillance strategies post-HSCT, it has to be kept in mind that detection of viral DNA is not necessarily detection of viral replication or acute infection. Especially in stool samples, ADV-DNA could be found for months and even years after initial infection without evidence of acute reinfection.[17] Therefore, in the future, rt-PCR detection of viral m-RNA would be a more specific and fast diagnostic method for detection of viral replication, which has already been evaluated in infectivity culture assays.[48]

Intensive surveillance of viral infections has become an essential part especially in the management of haploidentical transplantation, in order to detect early those patients at risk for systemic infection and a need for fast therapeutic intervention. Since an increased risk of ADV infection can be correlated with the lack of endogenous T cell immunity, surveillance should include weekly immunological monitoring of total lymphocytes,

CD3[+], CD4[+], CD8[+], CD19[+], and CD56[+] lymphocytes, by flow cytometry until T cell recovery. In the case of infection the virus-specific T cell response should be evaluated in peripheral blood, if possible.[7–9,42] The surveillance strategy may differ between children and adults and among

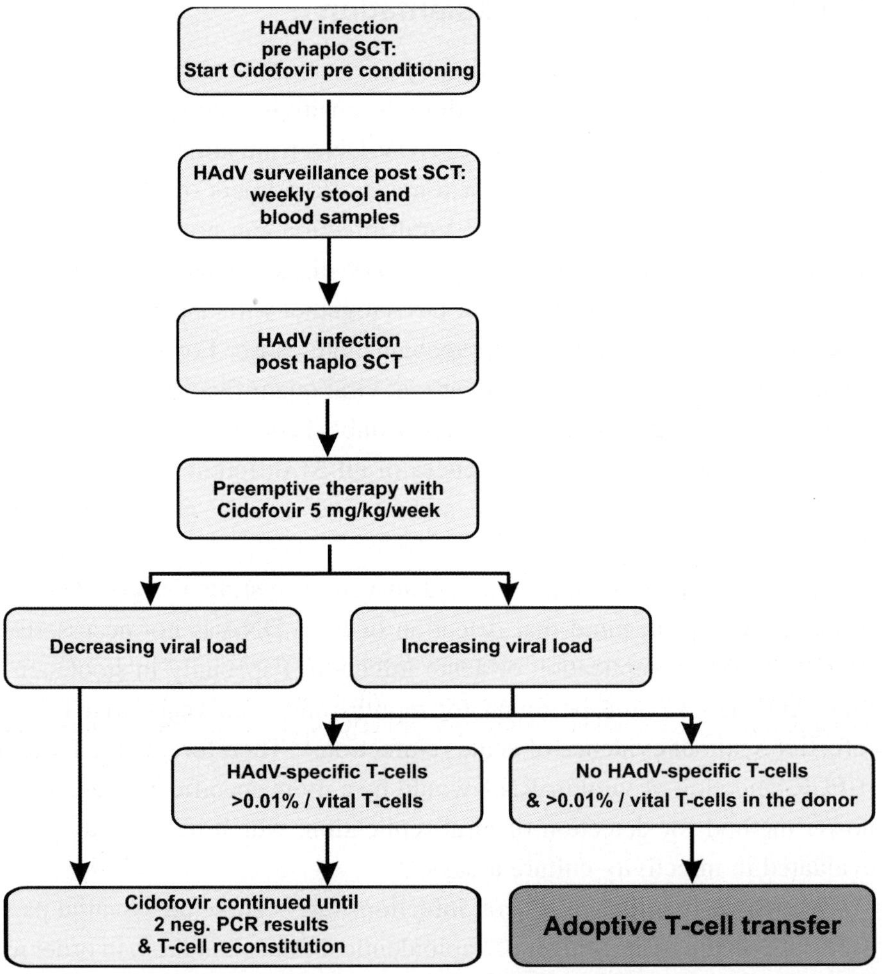

Fig. 1. Clinical decision algorithm for the management of adenovirus infection in haploidentical stem cell transplant recipients at the University Children's Hospital Tübingen. The approach to adenoviral infections post-haplo-SCT is based on different levels of evidence. No randomized controlled clinical trials have been performed to date

different transplant regimens. In haplo-SCT in children we recommend an intense approach with screening in peripheral blood and stool by PCR at weekly intervals beginning immediately prior to transplant until day +100 after transplantation, which has been shown to be superior to symptomatic testing[49] (Fig. 1). Urine and throat swabs can be investigated in the case of clinical symptoms. After day +100, surveillance should be carried out according to the recovery of T cells (absolute CD4 count >100/µl?) or in the case of an existing infection or clinically suspected viral infection.

Clinical Symptoms of Adenovirus Infection Posttransplant

Clinical symptoms post-HSCT have been described as three major localized manifestations and a number of severe complications of systemic infection; gastrointestinal symptoms of enteritis with diarrhea of variable severity are the most frequent manifestation in children,[42] which is often a source of diagnostic confusion with other causes of diarrhea. ADV

Fig. 1. (*Continued*)   Nevertheless, prospective data are available on the use of intensive surveillance and pre-emptive treatment with cidofovir. All other recommendations are based on retrospective data or even on an expert recommendation level. The prevention of life-threatening ADV infection post-HSCT starts with a diagnostic workup before the onset of the conditioning regimen, to begin treatment with cidofovir of patients with ADV-DNA in blood and stool before the induction of aplasia and hence reduce the risk of an endogenous ADV reactivation. Weekly surveillance by PCR of stool and blood and pre-emptive therapy with cidofovir are the mainstay of the current approach to adenoviral infections post-HSCT. Surveillance and pre-emptive therapy should be prolonged in patients at risk, lacking normal T cell reconstitution. Cidofovir treatment should be continued until two negative PCR results and until a sufficient T cell reconstitution. Since a sufficient host T cell response is essential for clearing the virus, all patients with an ADV infection post-haplo-SCT should be examined for virus-specific T cells in peripheral blood. The presence or absence of ADV-specific T cells allows a risk assessment of the viral infection. Adoptive immunotherapy with isolated specific T cells as a new treatment option should be considered in HSCT recipients with systemic ADV infection and high/increasing viral load under antiviral chemotherapy (as defined by the persistence or increase of ADV-DNA in peripheral blood and/or stool after two weeks of antiviral chemotherapy) and absent ADV-specific T cells.

Table 2. Clinical Presentations of Adenovirus Infections Post-Stem-Cell-Transplantation

Symptoms	Adults (%) (Ref. 30)	Children (%) (Ref. 59)
Asymptomatic	10	25
Fever	–	21
Enteritis	10	53
Pneumonitis	19	11
Cystitis	9	12

infections can involve the upper and the lower respiratory tract, and these infections are together the most frequent manifestation in adults.[30] While upper respiratory infection is often moderate, pneumonia can be fatal in the majority of cases in transplant recipients.[6,10,50] Involvement of the urothel is usually manifested as hemorrhagic cystitis. The most severe form of renal involvement by adenoviruses is acute renal failure due to necrotizing tubulointerstitial nephritis and obstructive uropathy, which could be fatal[51] (Table 2).

In cases of systemic infection a number of severe, life-threatening manifestations have been reported. Patients usually have high fever and elevated CRP levels up to 10 mg/dl. Finally, disseminated disease may manifest itself as multiorgan failure with CNS involvement, retinitis, heart failure, hepatitis, renal failure.[35] Hepatitis is a serious and often terminal complication of ADV infections.[52,53] In our own experience, continuously high fever for several days, associated with positive PCR results in the blood, were the only symptoms in some patients.

Pharmacologic Treatment of Adenovirus Infections Post-HSCT

For patients with insufficient T cell recovery, cidofovir seems to be the only antiviral drug at present that could be successfully used in treatment of ADV infections posttransplant. Cidofovir has been shown to reduce viral load in patients with viremia.[54,55] Clinical response has been documented in several studies[56–58] with a schedule of 5 mg/kg body weight/week given intravenously as induction therapy for the first 2–3 doses. After these doses, treatment could be changed to alternative-week dosing for the remainder of the therapy. Toxicities are mainly nephrotoxic side effects, which have been reported to be between 40% and 0%.[56,59] Children seem to tolerate cidofovir better than adult patients. Probenecid and extra prehydration should be given to all patients to reduce nephrotoxic side effects. Two recent reports have shown viral clearance under mean cidofovir treatment over 60 days.[55,59] Since immune reconstitution has not been included in these studies, the question whether the immune response or cidofovir has led to viral clearance is still not answered.

In patients with reduced renal clearance, lower doses (1–3 mg/ kg/week) or divided doses of 1 mg/kg 3 times weekly[60,61] have been reported. Although a considerable proportion of the patients in these studies still developed signs of nephrotoxicity (19–25%), the authors felt that this dose was better-tolerated, as treatment did not have to be stopped in any patient. An issue is the emergence of viral resistance (ADV, CMV, HSV) under subinhibitory concentrations of cidofovir. Resistance of adenovirus to cidofovir *in vitro* was first described in 2002.[62] Changes in the DNA-polymerase were found to be the mechanism underlying resistance induced in ADV type 5 following growth of the virus in subinhibitory concentrations of cidofovir.

Weekly surveillance of blood and stool, in combination with preemptive cidofovir treatment, as a first detection of ADV in any kind of specimen posttransplant has been attributed to marked reduction in ADV-related complications and survival.[42,59] In haploidentical transplantation, we additionally recommend evaluating ADV-DNA in blood and stool in advance of the conditioning regimen in order to treat those patients with asymptomatic carrier status prior to transplant (Fig. 1).

Ribavirin, a guanosine analog, has shown *in vitro* antiviral activity against ADV, with selective susceptibility of species C viruses.[63,64] There are some case reports of successful ribavirin treatment of ADV pneumonitis or cystitis,[65–67] but all larger series of patients with systemic infection post-HSCT have shown neither a clinical effect of ribavirin nor a reduction of the viral load.[34,57,68,69] Therefore, ribavirin cannot be recommended at present for the treatment of ADV infection post-HSCT until controlled clinical trials have addressed this question. However, the *in vitro* activity against species C ADV and the reactivation pattern of ADV infection post-HSCT support the rationale for a prophylactic use of ribavirin.

Adoptive T Cell Transfer in Adenovirus Infections Post-HSCT

T cell reconstitution is required for the control of ADV infections in HSCT recipients, and drug therapy seems to limit, but not cure, the infection.[7–9,70] This has led to efforts to reconstitute T cells in order to provide physiological protection against infection. Induction of a virus-specific T cell response in the patient by direct infusion of T cells is intended in a procedure known as adoptive transfer. So far, cellular immunotherapy has been directed almost exclusively against two herpes viruses, CMV and Epstein–Barr virus (EBV).[71–73] As a proof of principle for the use of T cell therapy in cases of ADV infection, successful reduction of viral replication was reported in seven of nine cases of unselected donor lymphocyte infusions (DLIs) for ADV infection post-HSCT.[7,31,57,74,75] However, unselected DLIs are associated with a high risk of GvHD and are not feasible in the haploidentical setting. Thus, an urgent clinical demand for donor lymphocyte preparations with enriched ADV-specific T cells and reduced alloreactivity has been expressed.[76] We have previously described a protocol using the antigen-specific IFN-γ secretion of T cells after *ex vivo* stimulation with viral antigen, to isolate a combination of CD4$^+$ and CD8$^+$ ADV-reactive T cells.[77] With this method, a more than 100-fold enrichment of specific T cells was achieved (preselection—0.6% IFN-secreting CD3$^+$ cells; postselection—85% IFN-secreting cells, means). Generated T cells showed specific killing of ADV-infectd B-LCL, and the alloreactive potential in mixed lymphocyte cultures was significantly reduced when compared to unmanipulated PBMCs (45-fold reduction in thymidine uptake). This approach offers several advantages, since the method is easy, fast, and can be readily standardized with various malignant and infectious antigens for antigen-specific cellular immunotherapy approaches. Moreover, there is a broad antigen specificity of the poly-clonal, specific T cell graft to several possible antigenic parts of the virus. The disadvantage of this approach is the limited availability of GMP grade antigens for T cell stimulation. Alternative approaches to the isolation of antigen-specific T cells are time-intensive *in vitro* culturing and MHC-peptide multimers. MHC-peptide multimers offer a theoretically higher specificity than the IFN-γ capture assay, but are limited by a narrowed antigenic spectrum and pure CD8$^+$ T cell populations.

In our first report on ADV-specific adoptive T cell therapy, feasibility and safety have been shown for the *ex vivo* isolation and infusion of IFN-γ-secreting T cells.[70] Virus-specific donor T cells were isolated and infused into nine children with systemic HAdV infection after unrelated and mismatched related SCT. Isolation was based on IFN-γ secretion after short *in vitro* stimulation with viral antigen, resulting in a combination of CD4$^+$ and CD8$^+$ T cells. 1.2–50 × 103/kg T cells were infused for adop-tive transfer. Isolated cells showed high specificity and markedly reduced alloreactivity *in vitro*. Adoptive transfer of HAdV-specific immunity was successful in five of six evaluable patients, documented by a dose-independent and sustained *in vivo* expansion of HAdV-specific T cells, associated with a durable clearance/decrease of viral copies. T cell infusion was well tolerated in all nine patients except for one case with GvHD°II of the skin. Thus, the induction of a specific T cell response through adoptive transfer was feasible and effective. When performed early in the course of infection, adoptive T cell transfer may protect against HAdV-related complications.[70,78,79]

In our ongoing multicenter trial we have transferred ADV-specific T cells from haploidentical donors in nine patients up to now. All patients had an increasing virus load despite cidofovir treatment, as measured by quanti-tative PCR in peripheral blood. A median cell number of 1500 cells / kg body weight was infused between day 18 and day 120 posttransplant, without any side effects. The majority of patients responded to this treatment. A clinical decision algorithm for the management of ADV infection and for the use of adoptive T cell therapy at our institution is shown in Fig. 1.

Conclusion

Pediatric patients have a relevant risk of adenovirus infection in the early posttransplant phase. The occurrence of lethal viral infections is associated with an incomplete reconstitution of T cells, in particular with the absence of virus-specific T cell subsets. Thus, further efforts are necessary to improve delayed T cell recovery after haploidentical transplantation. The use of high stem cell doses, new graft manipulation procedures and intensity-reduced conditioning regimens have contributed to speeding up immune reconstitution in this setting. Intensive surveillance of viral infections has become an essential component, in order to detect early those patients at risk for systemic disease with a need for pre-emptive antiviral therapy. Since a sufficient host T cell response is essential for clearing the virus, diagnostic procedures for detection of virus-specific T cells should be included in the management of haplo-SCT. Finally, adoptive immunotherapy is a new treatment option which appears to be feasible even in patients with mismatched donors.

Acknowledgments

We thank the nurses and physicians working in the pediatric stem cell transplant program for their dedication and their excellent care of the children, as well as the staff of the stem cell laboratory of the University Children's Hospital Tübingen. Last but not least, we are grateful to the Wilhelm-Sander-Stiftung, the Deutsche Forschungsgemeinschaft (SFB 685), and the Fortuen Program (University of Tuebingen) for their financial contributions through grants to P. L. and T. F.

References

1. Handgretinger R, Lang P, Schumm M *et al.* (2001) Immunological aspects of haploidentical stem cell transplantation in children. *Ann NY Acad Sci* **938**: 340–357.

2. Lang P, Handgretinger R, Niethammer D *et al.* (2003) Transplantation of highly purified CD34$^+$ progenitor cells from unrelated donors in pediatric leukemia. *Blood* **101**: 1630–1636.

3. Mohty M, Jacot W, Faucher C *et al.* (2003) Infectious complications following allogeneic HLA-identical sibling transplantation with antithymocyte globulin-based reduced intensity preparative regimen. *Leukemia* **17**: 2168–2177.

4. Lion T, Baumgartinger R, Watzinger F *et al.* (2003) Molecular monitoring of adenovirus in peripheral blood after allogeneic bone marrow transplantation permits early diagnosis of disseminated disease. *Blood* **102**: 1114–1120.

5. Walls T, Shankar AG, Shingadia D. (2003) Adenovirus: An increasingly important pathogen in paediatric bone marrow transplant patients. *Lancet Infect Dis* **3**: 79–86.

6. Flomenberg P, Babbitt J, Drobyski WR *et al.* (1994) Increasing incidence of adenovirus disease in bone marrow transplant recipients. *J Infect Dis* **169**: 775–781.

7. Chakrabarti S, Mautner V, Osman H *et al.* (2002) Adenovirus infections following allogeneic stem cell transplantation: Incidence and outcome in relation to graft manipulation, immunosuppression, and immune recovery. *Blood* **100**: 1619–1627.

8. Feuchtinger T, Lucke J, Hamprecht K *et al.* (2005) Detection of adenovirus-specific T cells in children with adenovirus infection after allogeneic stem cell transplantation. *Br J Haematol* **128**: 503–509.

9. Heemskerk B, Lankester AC, van Vreeswijk T *et al.* (2005) Immune reconstitution and clearance of human adenovirus viremia in pediatric stem-cell recipients. *J Infect Dis* **191**: 520–530.

10. Shields AF, Hackman RC, Fife KH *et al.* (1985) Adenovirus infections in patients undergoing bone-marrow transplantation. *N Engl J Med* **312**: 529–533.

11. Davison AJ, Benko M, Harrach B. (2003) Genetic content and evolution of adenoviruses. *J Gen Virol* **84**: 2895–2908.

12. Bergelson JM, Cunningham JA, Droguett G *et al.* (1997) Isolation of a common receptor for Coxsackie B viruses and adenoviruses 2 and 5. *Science* **275**: 1320–1323.

13. Gaggar A, Shayakhmetov DM, Lieber A. (2003) CD46 is a cellular receptor for group B adenoviruses. *Nat Med* **9**: 1408–1412.

14. Arnberg N, Edlund K, Kidd AH, Wadell G. (2000) Adenovirus type 37 uses sialic acid as a cellular receptor. *J Virol* **74**: 42–48.

15. Schmitz H, Wigand R, Heinrich W. (1983) Worldwide epidemiology of human adenovirus infections. *Am J Epidemiol* **117**: 455–466.

16. Sester M, Sester U, Salvador SA *et al.* (2002) Age-related decrease in adenovirus-specific T cell responses. *J Infect Dis* **185**: 1379–1387.

17. Fox JP, Brandt CD, Wassermann FE *et al.* (1969) The virus watch program: A continuing surveillance of viral infections in metropolitan New York families. VI. Observations of adenovirus infections: Virus excretion patterns, antibody response, efficiency of surveillance, patterns of infections, and relation to illness. *Am J Epidemiol* **89**: 25–50.

18. Garnett CT, Erdman D, Xu W, Gooding LR. (2002) Prevalence and quantitation of species C adenovirus DNA in human mucosal lymphocytes. *J Virol* **76**: 10608–10616.

19. Lang P, Griesinger A, Hamprecht K *et al.* (2004) Antiviral activity against CMV-infected fibroblasts in pediatric patients transplanted with CD34(+)-selected allografts from alternative donors. *Hum Immunol* **65**: 423–431.

20. Molinier-Frenkel V, Gahery-Segard H, Mehtali M *et al.* (2000) Immune response to recombinant adenovirus in humans: Capsid components from viral input are targets for vector-specific cytotoxic T lymphocytes. *J Virol* **74**: 7678–7682.

21. Smith CA, Woodruff LS, Kitchingman GR, Rooney CM. (1996) Adenovirus-pulsed dendritic cells stimulate human virus-specific T cell responses *in vitro*. *J Virol* **70**: 6733–6740.

22. Smith CA, Woodruff LS, Rooney C, Kitchingman GR. (1998) Extensive cross-reactivity of adenovirus-specific cytotoxic T cells. *Hum Gene Ther* **9**: 1419–1427.

23. Heemskerk B, Veltrop-Duits LA, van Vreeswijk T *et al.* (2003) Extensive cross-reactivity of CD4$^+$ adenovirus-specific T cells: Implications for immunotherapy and gene therapy. *J Virol* **77**: 6562–6566.

24. Molinier-Frenkel V, Lengagne R, Gaden F *et al.* (2002) Adenovirus hexon protein is a potent adjuvant for activation of a cellular immune response. *J Virol* **76**: 127–135.

25. Rux JJ, Kuser PR, Burnett RM. (2003) Structural and phylogenetic analysis of adenovirus hexons by use of high-resolution X-ray crystallographic, molecular modeling, and sequence-based methods. *J Virol* **77**: 9553–9566.

26. Olive M, Eisenlohr L, Flomenberg N *et al.* (2002) The adenovirus capsid protein hexon contains a highly conserved human CD4$^+$ T cell epitope. *Hum Gene Ther* **13**: 1167–1178.

27. Tang J, Olive M, Champagne K *et al.* (2004) Adenovirus hexon T cell epitope is recognized by most adults and is restricted by HLA DP4, the most common class II allele. *Gene Ther* **11**: 1408–1415.

28. Leen AM, Sili U, Vanin EF *et al.* (2004) Conserved CTL epitopes on the adenovirus hexon protein expand subgroup cross-reactive and subgroup-specific CD8$^+$ T cells. *Blood* **104**: 2432–2440.

29. Leen AM, Christin A, Khalil M *et al.* (2008) Identification of hexon-specific CD4 and CD8 T cell epitopes for vaccine and immunotherapy. *J Virol* **82**: 546–554.

30. Runde V, Ross S, Trenschel R *et al.* (2001) Adenoviral infection after allogeneic stem cell transplantation (SCT): Report on 130 patients from a single SCT unit involved in a prospective multicenter surveillance study. *Bone Marrow Transplant* **28**: 51–57.

31. Howard DS, Phillips II GL, Reece DE *et al.* (1999) Adenovirus infections in hematopoietic stem cell transplant recipients. *Clin Infect Dis* **29**: 1494–1501.

32. Baldwin A, Kingman H, Darville M *et al.* (2000) Outcome and clinical course of 100 patients with adenovirus infection following bone marrow transplantation. *Bone Marrow Transplant* **26**: 1333–1338.

33. van Tol MJ, Kroes AC, Schinkel J *et al.* (2005) Adenovirus infection in paediatric stem cell transplant recipients: Increased risk in young children with a delayed immune recovery. *Bone Marrow Transplant* **36**: 39–50.

34. La Rosa AM, Champlin RE, Mirza N *et al.* (2001) Adenovirus infections in adult recipients of blood and marrow transplants. *Clin Infect Dis* **32**: 871–876.

35. Hale GA, Heslop HE, Krance RA *et al.* (1999) Adenovirus infection after pediatric bone marrow transplantation. *Bone Marrow Transplant* **23**: 277–282.

36. Myers GD, Krance RA, Weiss H *et al.* (2005) Adenovirus infection rates in pediatric recipients of alternate donor allogeneic bone marrow transplants receiving either antithymocyte globulin (ATG) or alemtuzumab (Campath). *Bone Marrow Transplant* **36**: 1001–1008.

37. Feuchtinger T, Richard C, Pfeiffer M *et al.* (2005) Adenoviral infections after transplantation of positive selected stem cells from haploidentical donors in children: An update. *Klin Padiatr* **217**: 339–344.

38. Chen X, Hale GA, Barfield R *et al.* (2006) Rapid immune reconstitution after a reduced-intensity conditioning regimen and a CD3-depleted haploidentical stem cell graft for paediatric refractory haematological malignancies. *Br J Haematol* **135**: 524–532.

39. Handgretinger R, Chen X, Pfeiffer M *et al.* (2007) Feasibility and outcome of reduced-intensity conditioning in haploidentical transplantation. *Ann NY Acad Sci* **1106**: 279–289.

40. Echavarria M, Forman M, van Tol MJ *et al.* (2001) Prediction of severe disseminated adenovirus infection by serum PCR. *Lancet* **358**: 384–385.

41. Schilham MW, Claas EC, van Zaane W *et al.* (2002) High levels of adenovirus DNA in serum correlate with fatal outcome of adenovirus infection in children after allogeneic stem-cell transplantation. *Clin Infect Dis* **35**: 526–532.

42. Kampmann B, Cubitt D, Walls T *et al.* (2005) Improved outcome for children with disseminated adenoviral infection following allogeneic stem cell transplantation. *Br J Haematol* **130**: 595–603.

43. Allard A, Girones R, Juto P, Wadell G. (1990) Polymerase chain reaction for detection of adenoviruses in stool samples. *J Clin Microbiol* **28**: 2659–2667.

44. Pring-Akerblom P, Adrian T, Kostler T. (1997) PCR-based detection and typing of human adenoviruses in clinical samples. *Res Virol* **148**: 225–231.

45. Heim A, Ebnet C, Harste G, Pring-Akerblom P. (2003) Rapid and quantitative detection of human adenovirus DNA by real-time PCR. *J Med Virol* **70**: 228–239.

46. Lankester AC, van Tol MJ, Claas EC *et al.* (2002) Quantification of adenovirus DNA in plasma for management of infection in stem cell graft recipients. *Clin Infect Dis* **34**: 864–867.

47. Ebner K, Suda M, Watzinger F, Lion T. (2005) Molecular detection and quantitative analysis of the entire spectrum of human adenoviruses by a two-reaction real-time PCR assay. *J Clin Microbiol* **43**: 3049–3053.

48. Ko G, Cromeans TL, Sobsey MD. (2003) Detection of infectious adenovirus in cell culture by mRNA reverse transcription-PCR. *Appl Environ Microbiol* **69**: 7377–7384.

49. Walls T, Hawrami K, Ushiro-Lumb I *et al.* (2005) Adenovirus infection after pediatric bone marrow transplantation: Is treatment always necessary? *Clin Infect Dis* **40**: 1244–1249.

50. Hierholzer JC. (1992) Adenoviruses in the immunocompromised host. *Clin Microbiol Rev* **5**: 262–274.

51. Mori K, Yoshihara T, Nishimura Y *et al.* (2003) Acute renal failure due to adenovirus-associated obstructive uropathy and necrotizing tubulointerstitial nephritis in a bone marrow transplant recipient. *Bone Marrow Transplant* **31**: 1173–1176.

52. Chakrabarti S, Collingham KE, Fegan CD, Milligan DW. (1999) Fulminant adenovirus hepatitis following unrelated bone marrow transplantation: Failure of intravenous ribavirin therapy. *Bone Marrow Transplant* **23**: 1209–1211.

53. Johnson PR, Yin JA, Morris DJ *et al.* (1990) Fulminant hepatic necrosis caused by adenovirus type 5 following bone marrow transplantation. *Bone Marrow Transplant* **5**: 345–347.

54. Leruez-Ville M, Minard V, Lacaille F *et al.* (2004) Real-time blood plasma polymerase chain reaction for management of disseminated adenovirus infection. *Clin Infect Dis* **38**: 45–52.

55. Muller WJ, Levin MJ, Shin YK *et al.* (2005) Clinical and *in vitro* evaluation of cidofovir for treatment of adenovirus infection in pediatric hematopoietic stem cell transplant recipients. *Clin Infect Dis* **41**: 1812–1816.

56. Ljungman P, Ribaud P, Eyrich M *et al.* (2003) Cidofovir for adenovirus infections after allogeneic hematopoietic stem cell transplantation: A survey by the Infectious Diseases Working Party of the European Group for blood and Marrow Transplantation. *Bone Marrow Transplant* **31**: 481–486.

57. Bordigoni P, Carret AS, Venard V *et al.* (2001) Treatment of adenovirus infections in patients undergoing allogeneic hematopoietic stem cell transplantation. *Clin Infect Dis* **32**: 1290–1297.

58. Legrand F, Berrebi D, Houhou N *et al.* (2001) Early diagnosis of adenovirus infection and treatment with cidofovir after bone marrow transplantation in children. *Bone Marrow Transplant* **27**: 621–626.

59. Yusuf U, Hale GA, Carr J *et al.* (2006) Cidofovir for the treatment of adenoviral infection in pediatric hematopoietic stem cell transplant patients. *Transplantation* **81**: 1398–1404.

60. Hoffman JA, Shah AJ, Ross LA, Kapoor N. (2001) Adenoviral infections and a prospective trial of cidofovir in pediatric hematopoietic stem cell transplantation. *Biol Blood Marrow Transplant* **7**: 388–394.

61. Nagafuji K, Aoki K, Henzan H *et al.* (2004) Cidofovir for treating adenoviral hemorrhagic cystitis in hematopoietic stem cell transplant recipients. *Bone Marrow Transplant* **34**: 909–914.

62. Kinchington PR, Raullo-Cruz T, Vergnes JP *et al.* (2002) Sequence changes in the human adenovirus type 5 DNA polymerase associated with resistance to the broad spectrum antiviral cidofovir. *Antiviral Res* **56**: 73–84.

63. Morfin F, Dupuis-Girod S, Mundweiler S *et al.* (2005) *In vitro* susceptibility of adenovirus to antiviral drugs is species-dependent. *Antivir Ther* **10**: 225–229.

64. Stock R, Harste G, Madisch I, Heim A. (2006) A rapid quantitative PCR-based assay for testing antiviral agents against human adenoviruses demonstrates type specific differences in ribavirin activity. *Antiviral Res.*

65. Liles WC, Cushing H, Holt S *et al.* (1993) Severe adenoviral nephritis following bone marrow transplantation: Successful treatment with intravenous ribavirin. *Bone Marrow Transplant* **12**: 409–412.

66. Jurado M, Navarro JM, Hernandez J *et al.* (1995) Adenovirus-associated haemorrhagic cystitis after bone marrow transplantation successfully treated with intravenous ribavirin. *Bone Marrow Transplant* **15**: 651–652.

67. Miyamura K, Hamaguchi M, Taji H *et al.* (2000) Successful ribavirin therapy for severe adenovirus hemorrhagic cystitis after allogeneic marrow transplant from close HLA donors rather than distant donors. *Bone Marrow Transplant* **25**: 545–548.

68. Gavin PJ, Katz BZ. (2002) Intravenous ribavirin treatment for severe adenovirus disease in immunocompromised children. *Pediatrics* **110**: e9.

69. Lankester AC, Heemskerk B, Claas EC *et al.* (2004) Effect of ribavirin on the plasma viral DNA load in patients with disseminating adenovirus infection. *Clin Infect Dis* **38**: 1521–1525.

70. Feuchtinger T, Matthes-Martin S, Richard C *et al.* (2006) Safe adoptive transfer of virus-specific T cell immunity for the treatment of systemic adenovirus infection after allogeneic stem cell transplantation. *Br J Haematol* **134**: 64–76.

71. Rooney CM, Smith CA, Ng CY *et al.* (1998) Infusion of cytotoxic T cells for the prevention and treatment of Epstein–Barr virus-induced lymphoma in allogeneic transplant recipients. *Blood* **92**: 1549–1555.

72. Walter EA, Greenberg PD, Gilbert MJ *et al.* (1995) Reconstitution of cellular immunity against cytomegalovirus in recipients of allogeneic bone marrow by transfer of T cell clones from the donor. *N Engl J Med* **333**: 1038–1044.

73. Einsele H, Roosnek E, Rufer N *et al.* (2002) Infusion of cytomegalovirus (CMV)–specific T cells for the treatment of CMV

infection not responding to antiviral chemotherapy. *Blood* **99**: 3916–3922.

74. Chakrabarti S, Collingham KE, Fegan CD *et al.* (2000) Adenovirus infections following haematopoietic cell transplantation: Is there a role for adoptive immunotherapy? *Bone Marrow Transplant* **26**: 305–307.

75. Hromas R, Cornetta K, Srour E *et al.* (1994) Donor leukocyte infusion as therapy of life-threatening adenoviral infections after T cell-depleted bone marrow transplantation. *Blood* **84**: 1689–1690.

76. Moss P, Rickinson A. (2005) Cellular immunotherapy for viral infection after HSC transplantation. *Nat Rev Immunol* **5**: 9–20.

77. Feuchtinger T, Lang P, Hamprecht K *et al.* (2004) Isolation and expansion of human adenovirus specific CD4$^+$ and CD8$^+$ T cells according to IFN-gamma secretion for adjuvant immunotherapy. *Exp Hematol* **32**: 282–289.

78. Feuchtinger T, Richard C, Joachim S *et al.* (2008) Clinical grade generation of hexon-specific T Cells for adoptive T cell transfer as a treatment of adenovirus infection after allogeneic stem cell transplantation. *J Immunother* **31**: 199–206.

79. Leen AM, Myers GD, Sili U *et al.* (2006) Monoculture-derived T lymphocytes specific for multiple viruses expand and produce clinically relevant effects in immunocompromised individuals. *Nat Med* **12**: 1160–1166.

Chapter 11

Regulatory T Cell Therapy for Immunomodulation After Allogeneic Hematopoietic Cell Transplantation

Robert Zeiser and Robert S. Negrin[†]*

Introduction

While the existence of a suppressive T cell population was the subject of significant controversy for several decades, recent advances in the functional and molecular characterization of immunomodulatory cell populations have firmly established their existence and their critical role in the balance of the immune response. CD4[+]CD25[+] regulatory T cells (Treg) are a subset of immunomodulatory cells that play a fundamental role in controlling immune responses under physiological and pathological conditions.[67] Treg are characterized by the transcription factor forkhead box P3 (FoxP3), the regulator gene for their development in mice and humans.[4,39,54] Expression of FoxP3 is required for regulatory T cell development and appears to control a genetic program specifying a suppressor cell fate. In the setting of allogeneic hematopoietic cell transplantation (aHCT), early studies in which Treg were depleted from the bone marrow graft demonstrated a more aggressive course of GvHD,[81] indicating that

*Corresponding author. E-mail: robert.zeiser@uniklinik-freiburg.de.
[†]Department of Hematology and Oncology, Albert Ludwig University Freiburg, Freiburg, Germany.
[‡]Division of Blood and Marrow Transplantation, Department of Medicine, Stanford University School of Medicine, Stanford, CA 94305, USA. E-mail: negrs@stanford.edu.

physiological numbers of endogenous Treg counterbalance alloimmunity post-aHCT. A comparable observation was recently made in the human system-where the Treg frequency in the transplant and the incidence of GvHD were negatively correlated.[64] Besides studies on the physiological Treg frequencies, adoptive transfer studies have shown that Treg down-modulate GvHD across minor[42] and major[36,78] histocompatibility barriers. This biological activity was compatible with other preclinical animal models, indicating that adoptive Treg transfer can prevent autoimmune diseases[77] and allograft rejection,[41] by restoring immune tolerance to self antigens or alloantigens. The present chapter will focus on the role of Treg as regulators of GvHD as a major complication after aHCT in preclinical models and currently pursued approaches to translating these findings into clinical practice.

Evidence for Immunomodulation by Endogenous Regulatory T Cells in the Murine BMT Models

Early studies in which Treg were depleted from the bone marrow graft demonstrated a more aggressive course of GvHD.[81] These data indicate that alloimmune responses after aHCT are regulated by endogenous Treg contained in the donor graft. The observation that depletion of the CD25-positive cells was efficient in reducing the suppressive effects of Treg, despite bystander depletion of activated conventional CD4 T cells, is indicative of a central role of Treg as suppressor cells. These results were confirmed by others and extended to adoptive transfer studies demonstrating that the addition of Treg to the graft prevents GvHD in lethally irradiated mice.[18,24,36,42,78,83] Adoptive transfer studies were performed with either freshly isolated[36] or *ex vivo*-activated Treg.[78] In contrast to observations in the experimental models of autoimmunity, the transfer of Treg enriched for alloantigen specificity showed only moderately improved suppressor activity compared to the transfer of polyclonal Treg populations.[83] One could speculate that the different outcome in the experimental models of autoimmunity in comparison with aHCT may be due to the lymphopenic environment that supports the expansion of transferred Treg in BMT recipients, and that this may account for the difference observed in mice with autoimmunity receiving syngeneic Treg. In favor of this hypothesis was the demonstration that Treg expand robustly after murine BMT and that injecting the Treg prior to conventional T cells allows Treg expansion and the transfer of lower Treg cell numbers when conventional T cells are given at later time points after transplantation.[59] As human aHCT is performed across minor MHC barriers, it was important to demonstrate that Treg also suppress GvHD which results following HCT in the murine minor mismatch model.[42] Also, host type Treg that survive irradiation were shown to reduce chronic GvHD which develops following haploidentical or minor mismatch transplantation.[2]

Possible Mechanisms of Regulatory T Cell Control of GvHD

Although multiple effects of Treg on various immune cells have been described, the exact mechanism of suppression is not yet clarified. It is likely that protection from a complex immune reaction such as GvHD needs regulation at several levels. The pathophysiology of acute GvHD has been shown to be a three-step process in which the innate and adaptive immune systems interact. The initiation of aGvHD takes place during conditioning in the absence of donor cells when chemotherapy with or without radiotherapy administered for conditioning causes local tissue injury resulting in the production of cytokines, chemokines, adhesion molecules, costimulatory molecules and MHC antigens, indicating to the immune system that a systemic injury has occurred.[27] The most common inflammatory cytokines that are secreted by activated host cells are tumor necrosis factor (TNF) and interleukin (IL) 1.[91] Multiple inflammatory cytokines produced during this phase signal for the expression of adhesion molecules,[11] and are recognized as "danger signals"[53] which consequently lead to the activation of host dendritic cells (DCs) and recognition of host MHCs by alloreactive donor T cells. A first level on which Treg may interfere with immune activation is the reduction of costimulatory molecule expression on antigen-presenting cells (APCs). This finding is compatible with previous reports indicating that Treg downregulate CD80 and CD86 molecule expression on DCs in a cell–cell contact-dependent manner[10] and that Treg interfere with DC maturation.[56] In support of this hypothesis, it was shown that Treg migrate to and proliferate in draining lymph nodes

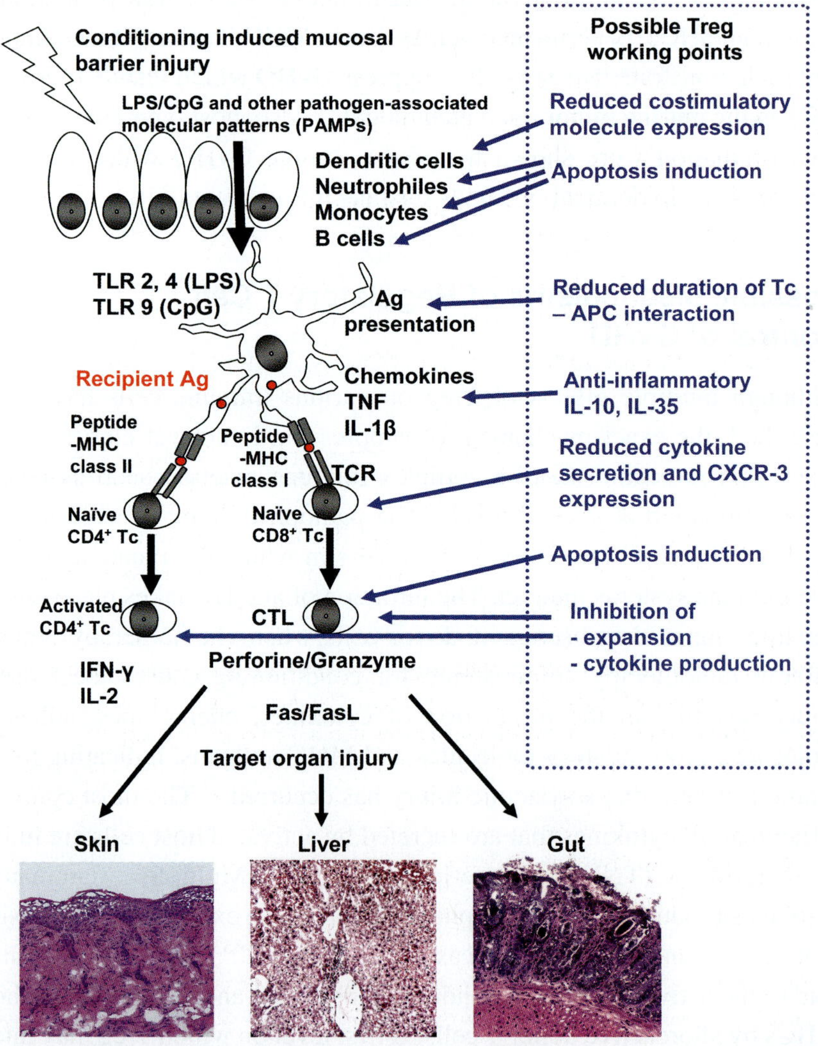

Fig. 1. Possible impact of Treg in protection from GvHD. Prior to aHCT, the conditioning regimen leads to damage of host tissues, particularly intestinal mucosae.

after BMT[59] which are the sites of donor T cell priming by host APCs. In addition, protection from GvHD by adoptively transferred Treg is dependent on CD62L expression,[25,79] which also suggests that migration of Treg to nodal sites where APCs are located is critical. Treg may also impact other APCs such as B cells in the draining lymph nodes, as it was shown that Treg are capable of killing B cells via granzyme B release.[31] Regarding the interaction between host APCs and donor T effector cells, Treg may impair it by reducing the stable contact between the two cell types, as was shown by two-photon microscopy in a model of autoimmune diabetes.[77] Treg have also been shown to influence monocyte and macrophage function by reducing their activation state[76] and inhibiting LPS-induced survival of these cells in a process depending on the Fas–FasL pathway.[85] These effects in concert with inhibition of neutrophil activity and promotion of neutrophil apoptosis[49] may disturb the antigen presentation process in the early phase of GvHD development (Fig. 1).

Fig. 1. (***Continued***) Consecutively, microbial products, such as lipopolysaccharide, and CpG motives as pathogen-associated molecular patterns (PAMPs) from pathogens located in the intestines access the bloodstream. Antigen-presenting cells that encounter PAMPs are activated via Toll-like receptors (TLRs), which leads to maturation and the secretion of proinflammatory cytokines, such as interleukin 1 (IL-1) and tumor necrosis factor (TNF). In response, activated macrophages produce chemokines that activate neutrophils, which further enhances inflammation. The release of these proinflammatory cytokines increases the expression of MHCs and adhesion molecules on host cells, enhancing their antigen-presenting capacity toward donor T cells which produce interferon γ (IFN-γ) with a positive feedback loop on the expression of MHCs and adhesion molecules, chemokines on APCs. Also, host-specific cytotoxic CD8$^+$ and CD4$^+$ T cells migrate to the target organs, where they mediate tissue injury that leads to multiorgan failure mediated mainly by the CD95–CD95 ligand and the perforin–granzyme pathways. It is likely that Treg interfere at different levels to control GvHD: (1) *Maturation and Ag presentation of APCs*: Treg can interfere with the maturation and expression of costimulatory molecule and MHC class II.[10,56] They can kill B cells as APCs via granzyme B release.[31] They can reduce the stable contact between APCs and effector T cells.[77] Finally, Treg can affect the function and survival of monocytes, macrophages[76,85] and neutrophils.[49] (2) *Effects on effector T cells*: Inhibition of proliferation,[24,83] cytokine production[9] and migration;[68] apoptosis induction in effector T cells after BMT[95] and other models.[62] (3) *Effects on the local cytokine milieu*: Treg require IL-10 for suppression of GvHD,[36] and IL-35[19] is critical for Treg-mediated suppression in other models.

Treg have also been shown to inhibit effector T cells at different levels, including proliferation,[24] cytokine production[9] and migration.[68] The hypothesis that Treg impact effector T cell migration is supported by data indicating that they reduce the expression of adhesion molecules and chemokine receptors by effector T cells,[68] an effect that may also account for the reduced numbers of conventional T cells in GvHD target organs when Treg are adoptively transferred too. In addition, recent data indicate that Treg can induce apoptosis of effector T cells after BMT[95] and in other models by cytokine deprivation.[62] Besides cell-contact-mediated effects on the donor T cells, soluble factors such as IL-10[36] or IL-35[19] may be critical for Treg-mediated suppression of alloresponses.

In summary, the effects of Treg on the immune response are likely to occur at multiple levels, which may explain their effectiveness in a disease as aggressive as GvHD. The described effects are summarized in Fig. 1.

Impact of Regulatory T Cells on Antitumor Immunity

Importantly, Treg were not only capable of suppressing GvHD but also facilitated engraftment[33] and allowed for graft-vs-tumor activity.[24,42,83] Therefore, they hold promise of being applied as prophylaxis or treatment of GvHD after aHCT for hematological malignancies. One explanation for this selective suppression of GvHD might be the observation that Treg inhibit proliferation but not activation of alloreactive T cells.[24]

Treg are highly effective in suppressing immune responses at different levels, and in the autologous setting they were shown to counteract antitumor immunity.[21] Also, increased numbers of Treg within the tumor tissue, tumor-infiltrating lymphocyte populations and in the peripheral blood of tumor patients have been shown in several tumor types, including gastric and esophageal cancer, hepatocellular carcinoma, B cell non-Hodgkin lymphoma, Hodgkin lymphoma, lung and ovarian cancer, pancreas and breast adenocarcinoma.[40,52,61,89,92]

However, the situation following aHCT is fundamentally different from the syngeneic situation as elimination of tumor cells is not solely based on tumor-specific antigens but also on alloreactivity. In the minor mismatch model it was shown that CD8[+] T cell-mediated GvL effects against the myeloid leukemia cell line MMCBA6 are preserved in the presence of Treg.[42] This finding was complemented by data from the major mismatch model demonstrating that GvL effects were conserved against two different lymphoma models — one transferred after lethal irradiation and one nine days prior to irradiation to mimic minimal residual disease.[24] The observed rejection of A20 cells was confirmed by others;[83] however, this group also found that the mastocytoma cell line P815 which was injected subcutaneously was not rejected in the presence of Treg. These data indicate that multiple variables, including the tumor type, the location and the ratio of Treg/T effector cells, may play a critical role in GvL effects in the setting of adoptive Treg transfer.

One way to think of the impact of Treg on GvHD and GvL is to consider that both involve the activation of alloreactive T cells. In the setting of GvHD significant proliferation and infiltration of GvHD target tissues is required, which ultimately results in tissue damage and the clinical syndrome of GvHD. In the setting where there is a high precursor frequency for the tumor (i.e. allogeneic settings, especially across major histompatibility barriers), GvL is preserved even in the setting of reduced alloreactive T cell proliferation since there are sufficient numbers of alloreactive T cells present even without proliferation once these cells are activated. Killing then proceeds through a perforin-mediated mechanism. In contrast, in the setting where antitumor T cells are in low numbers and significant proliferation is required (i.e. syngeneic transplantation and vaccination), suppression of T cell proliferation by Treg can negatively impact antitumor activity.

Differential Susceptibility of Regulatory T Cells to Immunosuppressive Agents

Calcineurin Inhibitors: Cyclosporine A and Tacrolimus (FK506)

The calcineurin inhibitors cyclosporine A and tacrolimus (FK506) are frequently utilized in human aHCT. A typical feature of Treg[74] is their dependence on IL-2 for survival and function as compared to CD4[+]CD25[−] T cells.[28,58,82] In that context it was shown that a critical requirement for Treg function and expansion is calcineurin-dependent IL-2 production, and that its inhibition by the calcineurin inhibitor cyclosporine A (CSA) impacts human and murine Treg.[16,17,94] In light of the finding that the interaction between NFATc and FoxP3 is required for the suppressive effects of Treg,[35,90] interference with NFAT by CSA may also contribute to the observed effects of CSA on Treg biology. Mechanistically, it was demonstrated that CSA affects Treg development, expansion and GvHD suppressor function.[16,87,94] In a murine skin graft model, CSA interfered with the *de novo* conversion of T_{conv} into alloantigen-specific Treg.[30] *In vitro* studies on human cells suggested that CSA affects the highly suppressive subpopulation of human CD27[+] Treg.[17] Clinical data indicated that CSA treatment of patients undergoing renal allograft transplantation reduced Treg frequencies as compared to other immunosuppressive regimens.[60,66,72]

Impact of Rapamycin on Treg and Effector T Cells

Rapamycin (RAPA) inhibits protein kinase activity of mTOR/raptor complex 1 and is clinically used to prevent allograft rejection. The initial step during the biological action of RAPA is the binding to the intracellular immunophilin FK506-binding protein (FKBP12), which resembles calcineurin inhibitors.[1] In contrast to calcineurin inhibitors, RAPA does not inhibit TCR-induced calcineurin activity but the RAPA-FKBP12 complex inhibits the serine/threonine protein kinase mTOR, the activation of which is required for protein synthesis and cell cycle progression. Therefore, RAPA blocks signaling in response to cytokines/growth factors, whereas calcineurin inhibitors exert their inhibitory effects by blocking TCR-induced activation.[1] Recent data indicate that mTOR blockade enhances lasting induction of Treg, irrespective of the initial antigen dose used to activate the antigen-specific T cells in a murine skin allograft model.[43] *In vitro* studies demonstrated that RAPA enables *in vitro* expansion of functionally suppressive Treg of murine[6] or human[7,75,84] origin. *In vivo* the presence of RAPA allowed the expansion and effector function of Treg in a GvHD model[93] and the combination of RAPA and IL-10 induced tolerance in a diabetes model.[7] Furthermore, a synergistic effect between Treg and RAPA has been demonstrated in a model of bone marrow graft rejection[73] and GvHD.[93] Mechanistically, different groups have suggested that the beneficial effect of RAPA is through selective Treg expansion,[6] conversion of CD4 T cells into Treg[84] and improved survival of Treg as compared to T_{conv}.[75] Treg as a subset of T cells are unusual, since engagement of the IL-2R fails to activate downstream targets of the PI-3K signaling pathway, including Akt, mTOR or p70[s6kinase].[8,93] This observation has important therapeutic implications for aHCT, since the immunosuppressive drug RAPA targets the mTOR pathway. RAPA was shown to be useful for the expansion of Treg *in vitro*[6,7,84] and preserves the *in vivo* suppressive effects of Treg.[94] These altered IL-2R PI-3 kinase downstream events may account for the hypoproliferative response of Treg to IL-2 and are mediated through the inhibitory effect of PTEN (phosphatase and tensin homolog deleted on chromosome 10).[86] Recent studies indicate that a blockade of the AKT-mTOR axis directly induces FoxP3 expression[34] and that the PI3K/Akt/mTOR signaling network regulates FoxP3 expression.[69]

Mycophenolate Mofetil

Mycophenolate mofetil (MMF) is a prodrug of mycophenolic acid (MPA), an inhibitor of inosine monophosphate dehydrogenase, and suppresses proliferation of antigen-stimulated T cells. Preclinical studies have demonstrated that MMF contributes to the generation of Treg and enhances their activity.[32] However, in these studies MMF was combined with $1\alpha,25$-dihydroxyvitamin D_3 in a diabetes model. Thus, there was no direct evidence that the expansion of $CD4^+CD25^+$ cells was due to either MMF or $1\alpha,25$-dihydroxyvitamin D_3.[32] Recent *in vitro* studies of murine Treg indicate that MMF does not interfere with the expansion and suppressor function of Treg in the presence of alloantigen stimulation.[50] In human renal allograft recipients, the use of MMF and calcineurin inhibitor sparing was associated with increased Treg frequencies.[14]

Impact of Glucocorticosteroids on Treg

Since dexamethasone (DEX) induces cell death in T cells, this drug could have unfavorable effects on Treg. However, Treg were shown to express higher levels of the glucocorticoid receptor and Bcl-2, which coincided with an increased resistance to DEX-mediated cell death as compared to CD4[+]CD25[−] T cells.[13] The first direct evidence that steroids affect Treg came from the observation that the female sex hormone, estrogen, up-regulates FoxP3 expression in mice both *in vitro* and *in vivo*.[63] In agreement with this concept, the steroid fluticasone propionate increased Treg-mediated suppression of allergen-stimulated T effector cells through an IL-10-dependent mechanism,[22] and inhaled or systemic glucocorticoids have been found to induce FoxP3 and IL-10 expression and generation of Treg[44] and glucocorticoid-amplified IL-2-dependent expansion of Treg in a model of EAE.[12] Further evidence that steroid treatment is compatible with intact Treg functions comes from studies on myasthenia gravis patients showing that the number of Treg in the blood is significantly lower in untreated myasthenia gravis patients than in age-matched healthy subjects, whereas it is normal or elevated in patients receiving prednisone.[26] Similar results were reported for the synthetic corticosteroid, dexamethasone, which induced FoxP3 expression in short- and long-term T cell cultures, while preserving the suppressive capacity of Treg.[44] In the murine system, the administration of DEX to BALB/c mice enhances the proportion of Treg and the ratio of Treg/CD4[+]CD25[−] cells the lymphoid organs, especially the thymus. Furthermore, IL-2 selectively protected Treg from DEX-induced cell death, while IL-7 and IL-15 did not exert such preferential protective effects.[13]

Anti-IL-2 Receptor Antibodies

Ás the monoclonal antibodies basiliximab and daclizumab are therapeutic agents directed against the α-chain of the IL-2 receptor (CD25), an unfavorable effect on Treg could be expected. In line with this notion, one study showed inhibition of FoxP3 mRNA induction by CD25 mAb daclizumab in allostimulated peripheral blood mononuclear cells[3] and another study showed downregulation of FoxP3 protein expression.[46] However, in direct coincubations of Treg and T_{eff}, CD25 mAb did not interfere in the suppressive activities of CD4$^+$CD25$^+$ Treg.[29] But it was shown in the murine model that particular CD25 mAb reduced the percentage of FoxP3$^+$ T cells within the CD4 fraction *in vivo*,[20] or reduced their suppressive activity.[45] Based on these reports, the anti-CD25 mAb may negatively impact Treg, which could lead to suboptimal function.

FTY720

The sphingosine-1-phosphate analog FTY720 has shown promising immunomodulatory properties based on its pronounced effects on lymphoid migration. One could speculate that FTY720 may interfere with Treg function since it abrogates S1P/S1P$_1$-dependent egression of lymphoid cells from lymphoid organs and in light of the fact that Treg express S1P, which appears to be required for optimal suppression of effector T cell activities.[88] In contrast, it has been shown that FTY720 does not block the sequestration of Treg and, importantly, increases their functional activity in a murine model of suppression of OVA-induced airway inflammation.[70] In a murine colitis model, FTY720 treatment induced a prominent upregulation of regulatory cytokines and transcription factors including IL-10, TGFβ, FoxP3 and CTLA-4. Supporting the hypothesis that FTY720 directly affects functional activity of Treg, a significant increase of CD25 and FoxP3 expression in isolated lamina propria CD4$^+$ T cells of FTY720-treated mice was found. Functional studies employing an *in vivo* blockade of CTLA-4 or IL-10R demonstrated that the impact of FTY720 on Treg induction could be antagonized. These data indicate that in addition to its well-established effects on migration, FTY720 leads to a specific downregulation of proinflammatory signals while simultaneously inducing functional activity of Treg. Furthermore, data from a different mouse model indicate that FTY720 does not impair Treg-mediated suppression of GvHD.[80]

The Role of Regulatory T Cells in Clinical Allogeneic Hematopoietic Cell Transplantation

A number of studies have attempted to evaluate the role of human Treg in aHCT by correlating Treg numbers either in the graft or in the recipient with the occurrence of acute or chronic GvHD. Miura *et al.* were the first to show a significant reduction of FoxP3 mRNA levels in peripheral blood lymphocytes (PBLs) from patients with GvHD compared with those without GvHD.[57] While some studies described a positive correlation between high numbers of circulating Treg and a reduced risk of GvHD,[57,64,96] others reported the opposite.[15,55] The opposing findings may be explained in part by the different methods used to determine Treg, as one study on chronic GvHD utilized CD25 as a surrogate maker for Treg.[15] Also, the heterogeneous patient populations, differences in the underlying diseases, different immunosuppressive regimens and the use of leukapheresis as compared to bone marrow cells for analysis may contribute to the different findings. Apart from these limitations, the peripheral blood is unlikely to be the critical anatomical site in which Treg that exert immune regulation are located. Based on the trafficking studies in murine models, secondary lymphoid organs or inflamed GvHD target tissues are highly infiltrated by Treg and are likely to be the sites of function.[59] In one clinical study reduced Treg numbers in the intestinal mucosa correlated with the presence of acute and chronic GvHD,[65] which is compatible with the hypothesis that Treg exert their suppressive effects at this location.

Isolation and Expansion Strategies for Human Regulatory T Cells

Isolation and Expansion

Human Treg can be isolated from apheresis products by using a magnetic cell separation protocol performed under conditions of good manufacturing practice.[38] However, the relative paucity of the Treg cell population is a major limitation on the potential clinical application as Treg represent approximately 5–10% of CD4[+] cells in the peripheral blood.[23] To overcome this limitation, different expansion strategies have been evaluated and it was shown that the expansion of human CD4[+]CD25[+] T cells using feeder cells can be successfully performed.[47] Expansion of highly purified human CD4[+]CD25[high] T cells *in vitro* through the use of artificial APCs for repeated stimulation with cross-linked CD3 and CD28 antibodies in the presence of high-dose IL-2 within 3–4 weeks resulted in an up-to-40,000-fold expansion.[37] Expanded CD4[+]CD25[high] T cells were polyclonal (as demonstrated by TCR Vβ analysis), maintained their phenotype and exceeded the suppressive activity of freshly isolated CD4[+]CD25[high] T cells.[37] One concern is that in murine models only the CD62L[+] subfraction of CD4[+]CD25[high] Treg suppressed GvHD whereas both CD62L[+] and CD62L[−] Treg suppressed the MLR *in vitro*.[25] These data indicated that homing to secondary lymphoid organs is likely to be critically important for Treg function. Following *in vitro* expansion the homing properties of the cells could be attenuated. However, expanded Treg maintained expression of relevant lymph-node-homing receptors, such as CD62L and CC-chemokine receptor 7 (CCR7).[37] Expansion of Treg under stimulatory cell culture conditions could also favor the expansion of effector T cell populations, which can contaminate the purified Treg population and abrogate their effects. In contrast to the murine setting, in humans, even the CD4[+]CD25[high] T cell subset contains 30–45% of *in vivo* recently activated CD25[+] T cells, which could outgrow Treg after prolonged culturing *in vitro*.[48] This concern may be overcome by using additional markers to reisolate Treg from expansion cultures, such as the negative Treg marker IL-7R (CD127),[51,71] or by the addition of mTOR inhibitors to the culture.[6]

Clinical Trials

As the major question is whether Treg display comparable efficacy in the clinical setting as shown for the murine experiments, clinical trials have been designed to test Treg function postallografting. In the first clinical trial patients with high risk of cancer relapse or molecular relapse after allogeneic HCT receive a pre-emptive donor lymphocyte infusion (DLI) after immunosuppression with cyclosporin A has been discontinued (Matthias Edinger, personal communication). Eight to ten weeks after immunosuppressive treatment is withdrawn, patients receive between 1×10^6 and 5×10^6 freshly isolated donor Treg cells per kg of body weight, followed by DLI of equal T cell numbers. Data derived from this trial may provide essential insight into the safety and feasibility of adoptive transfer of unmanipulated Treg in humans. A second trial, designed by B. Blazar and C. June (University of Minnesota, USA), will evaluate the effects of Treg expanded with beads coated with CD3- and CD28-specific antibodies and high-dose IL-2. The Treg are expanded from umbilical cord blood and will given at the time point of aHCT. A third trial, at Stanford University, will use purified human Treg isolated by magnetic bead and high speed cell sorting with purification of CD4$^+$CD25^{high}CD127^{low} cells.

Summary and Conclusions

In light of the multiple observations from preclinical models, Treg represent a promising therapeutic approach to be applied in clinical aHCT. The adoptive transfer of Treg may have several advantages in comparison with conventional immunosuppressive therapy. A major benefit could be the potential to induce long-term immunotolerance as compared to short-term immunosuppression. Another advantage over currently applied immunosuppressive regimens may be the antigen specificity of the regulatory T cell compartment, which could avoid generalized immune paralysis. However, to take advantage of Treg as a cellular therapy multiple barriers need to be overcome. To study Treg in large-scale clinical trials more information on the expansion methods with regard to efficiency and safety is needed. Also, the patient population that may benefit most from Treg transfer and the application of Treg in the pre-emptive or the therapeutic setting for GvHD protection needs to be determined. These data may become available with patient recruitment of the ongoing early phase clinical trials. Information from the rodent models may help to estimate Treg effects on antiviral and antitumor immunity, the ideal time point for their adoptive transfer after aHCT and the impact of immunosuppressive drugs on Treg.

References

1. Abraham R, Wiederrecht GJ. (1995) Immunopharmacology of rapamycin. *Annu Rev Immunol* **14**: 483–510.
2. Anderson BE, McNiff J, Matte C *et al.* (2004) Recipient CD4$^+$ T cells that survive irradiation regulate chronic graft-vs-host disease. *Blood* **104**: 1565–1573.
3. Baan C, van der Mast BJ, Klepper M *et al.* (2005) Differential effect of calcineurin inhibitors, anti-CD25 antibodies and rapamycin on the induction of FoxP3 in human T cells. *Transplantation* **80**: 110–117.
4. Baecher-Allan CBJ, Freeman GJ, Hafler DA. (2001) CD4$^+$CD25 high regulatory cells in human peripheral blood. *J Immunol* **167**: 1245–1253.
5. Battaglia M, Stabilini A, Migliavacca B *et al.* (2006) Rapamycin promotes expansion of functional CD4$^+$CD25$^+$FoxP3$^+$ regulatory T cells of both healthy subjects and type 1 diabetic patients. *J Immunol* **177**: 8338–8347.
6. Battaglia M, Stabilini A, Roncarolo MG. (2005) Rapamycin selectively expands CD4$^+$CD25$^+$FoxP3$^+$ regulatory T cells. *Blood* **105**: 4743–4748.
7. Battaglia M, Stabilini A, Draghici E *et al.* (2006) Rapamycin and interleukin-10 treatment induces T regulatory type 1 cells that mediate antigen-specific transplantation tolerance. *Diabetes* **55**: 40–49.
8. Bensinger S, Walsh PT, Zhang J *et al.* (2004) Distinct IL-2 receptor signaling pattern in CD4$^+$CD25$^+$ regulatory T cells. *J Immunol* **172**: 5287–5296.
9. Bergerot I, Arreaza GA, Cameron MJ *et al.* (1999) Insulin B-chain reactive CD4$^+$ regulatory T cells induced by oral insulin treatment protect from type 1 diabetes by blocking the cytokine secretion and pancreatic infiltration of diabetogenic effector T cells. *Diabetes* **48**: 1720–1729.

10. Cederbom L, Hall H, Ivars F. (2004) CD4$^+$CD25$^+$ regulatory T cells down-regulate co-stimulatory molecules on antigen-presenting cells. *Eur J Immunol* **30**: 1538–1543.

11. Chang RJ, Lee SH. (1986) Effects of interferon-gamma and tumor necrosis factor-alpha on the expression of an Ia antigen on a murine macrophage cell line. *J Immunol* **173**: 2853–2856.

12. Chen X, Oppenheim JJ, Winkler-Pickett RT *et al.* (2006) Glucocorticoid amplifies IL-2-dependent expansion of functional FoxP3(+)CD4(+)CD25(+) T regulatory cells *in vivo* and enhances their capacity to suppress EAE. *Eur J Immunol* **36**: 2139–2143.

13. Chen X, Murakami T, Oppenheim JJ, Howard OM. (2004) Differential response of murine CD4$^+$CD25$^+$ and CD4$^+$CD25$^-$ T cells to dexamethasone-induced cell death. *Eur J Immunol* **34**: 859–869.

14. Cicinnati VR, Yu Z, Klein CG *et al.* (2007) Clinical trial: Switch to combined mycophenolate mofetil and minimal dose calcineurin inhibitor in stable liver transplant patients — assessment of renal and allograft function, cardiovascular risk factors and immune monitoring. *Aliment Pharmacol Ther* **26**: 1195–1208.

15. Clark F, Gregg R, Piper K *et al.* (2004) Chronic graft-versus-host disease is associated with increased numbers of peripheral blood CD4$^+$CD25 high regulatory T cells. *Blood* **103**: 2410–2416.

16. Coenen J, Koenen, HJ, van Rijssen E *et al.* (2007) Rapamycin, not cyclosporine, permits thymic generation and peripheral preservation of CD4(+)CD25(+)FoxP3(+) T cells. *Bone Marrow Transplant*, Mar. 12 epub.

17. Coenen JJA, Koenen HJM, van Rijssen E *et al.* (2006) Rapamycin, and not cyclosporin A, preserves the highly suppressive CD27$^+$ subset of human CD4$^+$CD25$^+$ regulatory T cells. *Blood* **107**: 1018–1023.

18. Cohen JL, Trenado A, Vasey D *et al.* (2002) Immunoregulatory T cells: New therapeutics for graft-versus-host disease. *J Exp Med* **196**: 401–406.

19. Collison LW, Workman CJ, Kuo TT *et al.* (2007) The inhibitory cytokine IL-35 contributes to regulatory T cell function. *Nature* **450**: 566–569.

20. Couper KN, Blount DG, de Souza JB *et al.* (2007) Incomplete depletion and rapid regeneration of FoxP3$^+$ regulatory T cells following anti-CD25 treatment in malaria-infected mice. *J Immunol* **178**: 4136–4141.

21. Curiel T, Coukos G, Zou L *et al.* (2004) Specific recruitment of regulatory T cells in ovarian carcinoma fosters immune privilege and predicts reduced survival. *Nat Med* **10**: 942–949.

22. Dao Nguyen X, Robinson DS. (2004) Fluticasone propionate increases CD4CD25 T regulatory cell suppression of allergen-stimulated CD4CD25 T cells by an IL-10-dependent mechanism. *J Allergy Clin Immunol* **114**: 296–301.

23. Dieckmann DPH, Berchtold S, Berger T, Schuler G. (2001) *Ex vivo* isolation and characterization of CD4(+)CD25(+) T cells with regulatory properties from human blood. *J Exp Med* **193**: 1303–1311.

24. Edinger M, Hoffmann P, Ermann J *et al.* (2003) CD4$^+$CD25$^+$ regulatory T cells preserve graft-vs-tumor activity while inhibiting graft-vs-host disease after bone marrow transplantation. *Nat Med* **9**: 1144–1149.

25. Ermann J, Hoffmann P, Edinger M *et al.* (2005) Only the CD62L$^+$ subpopulation of CD4$^+$CD25$^+$ regulatory T cells protects from lethal acute GvHD. *Blood* **105**: 2220–2226.

26. Fattorossi A, Battaglia A, Buzzonetti A *et al.* (2005) Circulating and thymic CD4 CD25 T regulatory cells in myasthenia gravis: Effect of immunosuppressive treatment. *Immunology* **116**: 134–141.

27. Ferrara JL, Cooke KR, Teshima T. (2003) The pathophysiology of acute graft-versus-host disease. *Int J Hematol* **78**: 181–187.

28. Furtado G, de Lafaille MAC, Kutchukhidze N, Lafaille JJ. (2002) Interleukin-2 signaling is required for CD4$^+$ regulatory T-cell function. *J Exp Med* **196**: 851–857.

29. Game DS, Hernandez-Fuentes MP, Lechler RI. (2005) Everolimus and basiliximab permit suppression by human CD4$^+$CD25$^+$ cells *in vitro*. *Am J Transplant* **5**: 454–459.

30. Gao W, Lu Y, El Essawy B *et al.* (2007) Contrasting effects of cyclosporine and rapamycin in *de novo* generation of alloantigen-specific regulatory T cells. *Am J Transplant* **7**: 1722–1732.

31. Gondek D, Lu LF, Quezada SA *et al.* (2005) Cutting edge: Contact-mediated suppression by CD4+CD25+ regulatory cells involves a granzyme B-dependent, perforin-independent mechanism. *J Immunol* **174**: 1783–1786.

32. Gregori S, Casorati M, Amuchastegui S *et al.* (2001) Regulatory T cells induced by 1 alpha, 25-dihydroxyvitamin D3 and mycophenolate mofetil treatment mediate transplantation tolerance. *J Immunol* **167**: 1945–1953.

33. Hanash AM, Levy RB. (2005) Donor CD4+CD25+ T cells promote engraftment and tolerance following MHC-mismatched hematopoietic cell transplantation. *Blood* **105**: 1828–1836.

34. Haxhinasto S, Mathis D, Benoist C. (2008) The AKT-mTOR axis regulates *de novo* differentiation of CD4+FoxP3+ cells. *J Exp Med* **205**: 565–574.

35. Ho L, Crabtree G. (2006) A Foxy tango with NFAT. *Nat Immunol* **7**: 906–908.

36. Hoffmann P, Ermann J, Edinger M *et al.* (2002) Donor-type CD4(+)CD25(+) regulatory T cells suppress lethal acute graft-versus-host disease after allogeneic bone marrow transplantation. *J Exp Med* **196**: 389–399.

37. Hoffmann P, ER, Kunz-Schughart LA, Andreesen R, Edinger M. (2004) Large scale *in vitro* expansion of polyclonal human CD4+CD25 high regulatory T cells. *Blood* **104**: 895–903.

38. Hoffmann P *et al.* (2006) Isolation of CD4+CD25+ regulatory T cells for clinical trials. *Biol Blood Marrow Transplant* **12**: 267–274.

39. Hori S, Nomura T, Sakaguchi S. (2003) Control of regulatory T cell development by the transcription factor FoxP3. *Science* **299**: 1057–1061.

40. Ichihara F, Kono K, Takahashi A *et al.* (2003) Increased populations of regulatory T cells in peripheral blood and tumor-infiltrating lymphocytes in patients with gastric and esophageal cancers. *Clin Cancer Res* **9**: 4404–4408.

41. Joffre O, Santolaria T, Calise D *et al.* (2007) Prevention of acute and chronic allograft rejection with CD4+CD25+FoxP3+ regulatory T lymphocytes. *Nat Med* **14**: 88–92.

42. Jones S, Murphy GF, Korngold R. (2003) Post-hematopoietic cell transplantation control of graft-versus-host disease by donor CD425 T cells to allow an effective graft-versus-leukemia response. *Biol Blood Marrow Transplant* **9**: 243–256.

43. Kang J, Huddleston SJ, Fraser JM, Khoruts A. (2008) *De novo* induction of antigen-specific CD4$^+$CD25$^+$FoxP3$^+$ regulatory T cells *in vivo* following systemic antigen administration accompanied by blockade of mTOR. *J Leukoc Biol*, epub ahead of print: PMID 18270248.

44. Karagiannidis C, Akdis M, Holopainen P *et al.* (2004) Glucocorticoids upregulate FoxP3 expression and regulatory T cells in asthma. *J Allergy Clin Immunol* **114**: 1425–1433.

45. Kohm AP, McMahon JS, Podojil JR *et al.* (2006) Cutting edge: Anti-CD25 monoclonal antibody injection results in the functional inactivation, not depletion, of CD4$^+$CD25$^+$ T regulatory cells. *J Immunol* **176**: 3301–3312.

46. Kreijveld E, Koenen HJ, Klasen IS *et al.* (2007) Following anti-CD25 treatment, a functional CD4$^+$CD25$^+$ regulatory T-cell pool is present in renal transplant recipients. *Am J Transplant* **7**: 249–254.

47. Levings M, Sangvegorio R, Roncarolo M. (2001) Human CD25$^+$CD4$^+$ T regulatory cells suppress naive and memory T cell pro-liferation and can be expanded *in vitro* without loss of function. *J Exp Med* **193**: 1295–1301.

48. Levings MK *et al.* (2002) Human CD25$^+$CD4$^+$ T suppressor cell clones produce transforming growth factor, but not interleukin 10, and are distinct from type 1 T regulatory cells. *J Exp Med* **196**: 1335–1346.

49. Lewkowicz P, Lewkowicz N, Sasiak A, Tchorzewski H. (2006) Lipopolysaccharide-activated CD4$^+$CD25$^+$ T regulatory cells inhibit neutrophil function and promote their apoptosis and death. *J Immunol* **177**: 7155–7163.

50. Lim DG, Joe IY, Park YH *et al.* (2007) Effect of immunosuppressants on the expansion and function of naturally occurring regulatory T cells. *Transplant Immunol* **18**: 94–100.

51. Liu W, Putnam AL, Xu-Yu Z *et al.* (2006) CD127 expression inversely correlates with FoxP3 and suppressive function of human CD4$^+$ T reg cells. *J Exp Med* **203**: 1701–1711.

52. Marshall NA, Christie LE *et al.* (2004) Immunosuppressive regulatory T cells are abundant in the reactive lymphocytes of Hodgkin lymphoma. *Blood* **103**(5): 1755–1762.

53. Matzinger P. (2002) The danger model: A renewed sense of self. *Science* **296**: 301–305.

54. McHugh R, Whitters MJ, Piccirillo CA *et al.* (2002) CD4$^+$CD25$^+$ immunoregulatory T cells: Gene expression analysis reveals a functional role for the glucocorticoid-induced TNF receptor. *Immunity* **16**: 311–323.

55. Meignin V *et al.* (2005) Numbers of FoxP3-expressing CD4$^+$CD25 high T cells do not correlate with the establishment of long-term tolerance after allogeneic stem cell transplantation. *Exp Hematol* **33**: 894–900.

56. Misra N, Bayry J, Lacroix-Desmazes S *et al.* (2004) Cutting edge: Human CD4$^+$CD25$^+$ T cells restrain the maturation and antigen-presenting function of dendritic cells. *J Immunol* **172**: 4676–4680.

57. Miura Y, Thoburn CJ, Bright EC *et al.* (2004) Association of FoxP3 regulatory gene expression with graft-versus-host disease. *Blood* **104**: 2187–2193.

58. Nelson BH. (2004) IL-2, regulatory T cells, and tolerance. *J Immunol* **172**: 3983–3988.

59. Nguyen V, Zeiser R, Dasilva DL *et al.* (2006) *In vivo* dynamics of regulatory T cell trafficking and survival predict effective strategies to control graft-versus-host disease following allogeneic transplantation. *Blood* **109**: 2649–2656.

60. Noris M, Casiraghi F, Todeschini M *et al.* (2007) Regulatory T cells and T cell depletion: Role of immunosuppressive drugs. *J Am Soc Nephrol* **18**: 1007–1018.

61. Ormandy LA, Hillemann T, Wedemeyer H *et al.* (2005) Increased populations of regulatory T cells in peripheral blood of patients with hepatocellular carcinoma. *Cancer Res* **65**(6): 2457–2464.

62. Pandiyan P, Zheng L, Ishihara S *et al.* (2007) CD4$^+$CD25$^+$FoxP3$^+$ regulatory T cells induce cytokine deprivation–mediated apoptosis of effector CD4$^+$ T cells. *Nat Immunol* **8**: 1353–1362.

63. Polanczyk MJ, Carson BD, Subramanian S *et al.* (2004) Cutting edge: Estrogen drives expansion of the CD4$^+$CD25$^+$ regulatory T cell compartment. *J Immunol* **173**: 2227–2234.

64. Rezvani K, Mielke S, Ahmadzadeh M *et al.* (2006) High donor FoxP3-positive regulatory T cell (Treg) content is associated with a low risk of GvHD following HLA-matched allogeneic SCT. *Blood* **108**: 1291–1297.

65. Rieger K *et al.* (2006) Mucosal FoxP3$^+$ regulatory T cells are numerically deficient in acute and chronic GvHD. *Blood* **107**: 1717–1723.

66. Ruggenenti P, Perico N, Gotti E *et al.* (2007) Sirolimus versus cyclosporine therapy increases circulating regulatory T cells, but does not protect renal transplant patients given alemtuzumab induction from chronic allograft injury. *Transplantation* **84**: 956–964.

67. Sakaguchi S, Sakaguchi N, Asano M *et al.* (1995) Immunological self-tolerance maintained by activated T cells expressing IL-2 receptor alpha-chains (CD25). *J Immunol* **155**: 1151–1164.

68. Sarween N *et al.* (2004) CD4$^+$CD25$^+$ cells controlling a pathogenic CD4 response inhibit cytokine differentiation, CXCR-3 expression, and tissue invasion. *J Immunol* **173**: 2942–2951.

69. Sauer S, Bruno L, Hertweck A. (2008) T cell receptor signaling controls FoxP3 expression via PI3K, Akt, and mTOR. *Proc Natl Acad Sci USA* **105**: 7797–7802.

70. Sawicka E, Dubois G, Jarai G *et al.* (2005) The sphingosine 1-phosphate receptor agonist FTY720 differentially affects the sequestration of CD4$^+$/CD25$^+$ T-regulatory cells and enhances their functional activity. *J Immunol* **175**: 7973–7980.

71. Seddiki N, Santner-Nanan B, Martinson J *et al.* (2006) Expression of interleukin (IL)-2 and IL-7 receptors discriminates between human regulatory and activated T cells. *J Exp Med* **203**: 1693–1700.

72. Segundo D, Ruiz JC, Izquierdo M *et al.* (2006) Calcineurin inhibitors, but not rapamycin, reduce percentages of CD4$^+$CD25$^+$FoxP3$^+$ regulatory T cells in renal transplant recipients. *Transplantation* **82**: 550–557.

73. Steiner D, Brunicki N, Bachar-Lustig E *et al.* (2006) Overcoming T cell–mediated rejection of bone marrow allografts by T-regulatory cells: Synergism with veto cells and rapamycin. *Exp Hematol* **34**: 802–808.

74. Stephens LA, Mottet C, Mason D, Powrie F. (2001) Human CD4(+)CD25(+) thymocytes and peripheral T cells have immune suppressive activity *in vitro*. *Eur J Immunol* **31**: 1247–1254.

75. Strauss L, Whiteside TL, Knights A *et al.* (2007) Selective survival of naturally occurring human CD4$^+$CD25$^+$FoxP3$^+$ regulatory T cells cultured with rapamycin. *J Immunol* **178**: 320–329.

76. Taams LS *et al.* (2005) Modulation of monocyte/macrophage function by human CD4$^+$CD25$^+$ regulatory T cells. *Hum Immunol* **66**: 222–230.

77. Tang Q, Adams JY, Tooley AJ *et al.* (2005) Visualizing regulatory T cell control of autoimmune responses in nonobese diabetic mice. *Nat Immunol* **7**: 83–92.

78. Taylor P, Lees CJ, Blazar BR. (2002) The infusion of *ex vivo* activated and expanded CD4(+)CD25(+) immune regulatory cells inhibits graft-versus-host disease lethality. *Blood* **99**: 3493–3499.

79. Taylor P, Panoskaltsis-Mortari A, Swedin JM *et al.* (2004) L-selectin(hi) but not the L-selectin(lo) CD4$^+$25$^+$ T-regulatory cells are potent inhibitors of GvHD and BM graft rejection. *Blood* **104**: 3804–3812.

80. Taylor PA, Ehrhardt MJ, Lees CJ *et al.* (2007) Insights into the mechanism of FTY720 and compatibility with regulatory T cells for the inhibition of graft-versus-host disease (GvHD) *Blood* **110**: 3480–3488.

81. Taylor PA, Noelle RJ, Blazar BR. (2001) CD4(+)CD25(+) immune regulatory cells are required for induction of tolerance to alloantigen via costimulatory blockade. *J Exp Med* **193**: 1311–1318.

82. Thornton A, Donovan EE, Piccirillo CA, Shevach EM. (2004) Cutting edge: IL-2 is critically required for the *in vitro* activation of CD4$^+$CD25$^+$ T cell suppressor function. *J Immunol* **172**: 6519–6523.

83. Trenado A, Charlotte F, Fisson S *et al.* (2003) Recipient-type specific CD4$^+$CD25$^+$ regulatory T cells favor immune reconstitution and control graft-versus-host disease while maintaining graft-versus-leukemia. *J Clin Invest* **112**: 1688–1696.

84. Valmori D, Tosello V, Souleimanian NE *et al.* (2006) Rapamycin-mediated enrichment of T cells with regulatory activity in stimulated CD4 T cell cultures is not due to the selective expansion of naturally occurring regulatory T cells but to the induction of regulatory functions in conventional CD4 T cells. *J Immunol* **177**: 944–949.

85. Venet F *et al.* (2006) Human CD4$^+$CD25$^+$ regulatory T lymphocytes inhibit lipopolysaccharide-induced monocyte survival through a Fas/Fas ligand-dependent mechanism. *J Immunol* **177**: 6540–6547.

86. Walsh P, Buckler JL, Zhang J *et al.* (2006) PTEN inhibits IL-2 receptor-mediated expansion of CD4 CD25 Treg. *J Clin Invest* **116**: 2521–2531.

87. Wang H, Zhao L, Sun Z *et al.* (2006) A potential side effect of cyclosporin A: Inhibition of CD4(+)CD25(+) regulatory T cells in mice. *Tranplantation* **82**: 1484–1492.

88. Wang W, Graeler MH, Goetzl EJ. (2004) Physiological sphingosine 1-phosphate requirement for optimal activity of mouse CD4$^+$ regulatory T cells. *FASEB J* **18**: 1043–1045.

89. Woo E, Chu CS, Goletz TJ *et al.* (2001) Regulatory CD4(+)CD25(+) T cells in tumors from patients with early-stage non-small cell lung cancer and late-stage ovarian cancer. *Cancer Research* **61**: 4766–6772.

90. Wu Y, Borde M, Heissmeyer V *et al.* (2006) FoxP3 controls regulatory T cell function through cooperation with NFAT. *Cell* **126**: 375–387.

91. Xun CQ, TJ, Jennings CD, Brown SA, Widmer MB. (1994) Effect of total body irradiation, busulfan-cyclophosphamide, or cyclophosphamide conditioning on inflammatory cytokine release and

development of acute and chronic graft-versus-host disease in H-2-incompatible transplanted SCID mice. *Blood* **83**: 2360–2367.

92. Yang ZZ, Novak AJ *et al.* (2006) Attenuation of CD8(+) T cell function by CD4(+)CD25(+) regulatory T cells in B-cell non-Hodgkin's lymphoma. *Cancer Res* **66**(20): 10145–10152.

93. Zeiser R, Leveson-Gower DB, Zambricki EA *et al.* (2008) Differential impact of mTOR inhibition on $CD4^+CD25^+FoxP3^+$ regulatory T cells as compared to conventional $CD4^+$ T cells. *Blood* **111**: 453–462.

94. Zeiser R, Nguyen VH, Beilhack A *et al.* (2006) Inhibition of $CD4^+CD25^+$ regulatory T cell function by calcineurin dependent interleukin-2 production. *Blood* **108**: 390–399.

95. Zeiser R, Nguyen VH, Hou JZ *et al.* (2007) Early CD30 signaling is critical for adoptively transferred $CD4^+CD25^+$ regulatory T cells in prevention of acute graft versus host disease. *Blood* **109**: 2225–2233.

96. Zorn E, Nelson EA, Mohseni M *et al.* (2006) IL-2 regulates FoxP3 expression in human $CD4^+CD25^+$ regulatory T cells through a STAT dependent mechanism and induces the expansion of these cells *in vivo. Blood* **108**: 1571–1579.

Chapter 12

Pathogen-induced Immune Regulation in Transplantation

*Luigina Romani**

Rodent models of transplantation have demonstrated that it is possible to induce specific immunological tolerance of donor antigens and indefinite graft survival in the absence of any continued nonspecific immunosuppression, through the exploitation of mechanisms that normally maintain immune homeostasis and tolerance to self-antigens. Regulatory T cells are important mediators of peripheral tolerance, and deficiency of this population is associated with autoimmune inflammation and onset of acute lethal graft-vs-host disease in transplantation. The interplay between regulatory T cells and antigen-responsive T cells for tolerance induction is modulated by tolerogenic dendritic cells. Indoleamine 2,3-dioxygenase, a rate-limiting enzyme in the tryptophan catabolism, is one recognized mediator of tolerance induction by dendritic cells. Evidence indicates that mechanisms that regulate both T cell and dendritic cell activity to a model pathogen and moreover a common cause of morbidity in hematopoietic transplantation, *Aspergillus fumigatus*, could be successfully exploited to elicit antimicrobial immunity and concomitant tolerance via acquired local immune privilege.

Introduction

Current treatment strategies in organ transplantation, as well as allergy and autoimmunity treatment, nonspecifically block immune reactions, leading to a wide range of adverse effects. Broad immunosuppression

*Microbiology Section, Department of Experimental Medicine and Biochemical Sciences, University of Perugia, Via del Giochetto, 06122 Perugia, Italy. Tel. and Fax: 039-075-585-7411. E-mail: lromani@unipg.it.

predisposes patients to disorders of immune surveillance and response, resulting in an increased incidence and severity of infections, often with uncommon nosocomial bacteria, fungi or viruses, and neoplasms. To minimize these adverse effects, research is focusing on antigen-specific suppression of the immune response. Rodent models of transplantation have demonstrated that it is possible to induce specific immunological tolerance of donor antigens and indefinite graft survival in the absence of any continued nonspecific immunosuppression, through the exploitation of mechanisms that normally maintain immune homeostasis and tolerance to self-antigens. If this situation could be achieved clinically, it would avoid many of the longer term complications of organ grafting, such as the increased risk of infection and cancer and the nephrotoxicity of many immunosuppressive agents.

Like natural tolerance, transplantation tolerance is achieved through control of T cell reactivity by central and peripheral mechanisms of tolerance. Significant enthusiasm has emerged for manipulating regulatory T cells (T_{reg}) either *ex vivo* or *in vivo* for the generation of dominant immune tolerance without chronic immunosuppression.[18,24,62] The fact that T cells with regulatory capacity constitute 5–10% of human CD4[+] peripheral blood T cells,[45] decrease in the initial phase of graft-vs-host disease (GvHD) after allogeneic stem cell transplantation (HSCT)[35,69] but can be actively induced directly via immunosuppressive medication or indirectly as a result of endogenous anti-inflammatory mechanisms,[59] suggests that a breakdown of regulation is an important factor in immune disorders, such as those associated with defective induction of transplantation tolerance.

The interplay between T_{reg} and antigen-responsive T cells is modulated by dendritic cells (DCs). DCs not only play a key role in the induction of immune responses, but also serve as potential targets and therapeutic agents for protection against infectious diseases and the long-term improvement of transplant outcome.[39,63,66] Several clinical studies indicated that plasmacytoid (p)DC may contribute to the T cell repertoire reconstitution, facilitate engraftment[15] and prevent GvHD[5] in hematopoietic stem cell transplantation (HSCT). As DC function is impaired during the immediate period posttransplant,[51] the administration of donor DCs may have beneficial effects on immune recovery in early HSCT. Interestingly, donor DCs present in the G-CSF-mobilized peripheral blood stem cell transplant are preferentially tolerogenic DCs that might have been responsible for decreased GvHD after posttransplant administration of G-CSF.[50] The potential use of tolerogenic DCs as negative cellular vaccines to induce experimental transplantation tolerance has been suggested.[2,23,25,29,39,67]

In addition to the many speculations on how DCs induce tolerance, various molecular mediators have been linked to the mediation of suppression by DCs.[42] One molecule is the indoleamine 2,3-dioxygenase (IDO), a rate-limiting enzyme in the tryptophan catabolism that controls the rejection of the fetus during pregnancy.[34,49] Ultimately, the mechanism used by the immune system for suppressing autoreactive responses could conceivably be used for therapeutic purposes in transplantation.

In this review we shall consider the interplay between T_{reg}, DC and IDO and the resulting protective mechanisms that are coordinated to induce antimicrobial immunity and maintain the tolerant state. We will discuss how mechanisms that regulate both T cell and antigen-presenting cell activity to a model pathogen and moreover a common cause of morbidity in HSCT, *Aspergillus fumigatus*, could be successfully exploited to elicit antimicrobial immunity and concomitant tolerance via acquired local immune privilege.

Fungi and Immunity: An Intriguing Relationship

Fungal infections have historically been and remain important causes of transplant-related morbidity in HSCT. However, several studies have reported the predominance of aspergillosis cases occurring in the postengraftment rather than the neutropenic period in allogeneic HSCT recipients.[20,31] Clinically, severe fungal infections occur in patients with immune reconstitution syndrome (IRS), an entity characterized by local and systemic reactions that have both beneficial and deleterious effects on infection.[61] Intriguingly, IRS responses are also found in immunocompetent individuals and after rapid resolution of immunosuppression, indicating that inflammatory responses can result in quiescent or latent infections manifesting as opportunistic mycoses. These considerations indicate that host immunity is crucial in eradicating infection, but immunological recovery can also be detrimental and may contribute toward worsening disease in opportunistic and nonopportunistic infections. Therefore, proper manipulation of deregulated innate and adaptive responses could offer strategies to control or prevent exacerbations in those diseases.[56] Recent observations highlight a truly bipolar nature of the inflammatory process in infection, at least by specific fungi, such as *Candida* or *Aspergillus* spp.[56,58]

Largely viewed as proinflammatory, innate responses combine with adaptive immunity to generate the most effective form of antifungal resistance, and T cells feed back onto a tenuous balance of diverse effects of inflammation on infection. Some degree of inflammation is required for protection — particularly in mucosal tissues — during the transitional response occurring temporally between the rapid innate and slower adaptive response. However, progressive inflammation may worsen disease and ultimately may prevent pathogen eradication. IDO, tryptophan catabolites ("kynurenines") and T_{reg} have all been shown to help tame overzealous and exaggerated inflammatory responses. In this context, IL-23 and the Th17 pathway, which downregulate tryptophan catabolism, may instead favor pathology and serve to accommodate the seemingly paradoxical association of chronic inflammation with fungal persistence (Fig. 1). As a matter of fact, IL-23/IL-17 antagonistic strategies, including the administration of synthetic kynurenines, could represent a means of harnessing progressive or potentially harmful inflammation.[56,58] This condition is crucially exemplified in CGD mice in which an intrinsic, genetically determined failure to control inflammation to sterile fungal components determines the animals' inability to resolve an actual infection with *A. fumigatus*.[55] It is of interest that the IL-23/Th17 pathway has recently been considered to have a role in transplantation immunity and tolerance.[1,11]

A main implication of these findings is that, at least in specific clinical settings, it is an exaggerated inflammatory response that likely

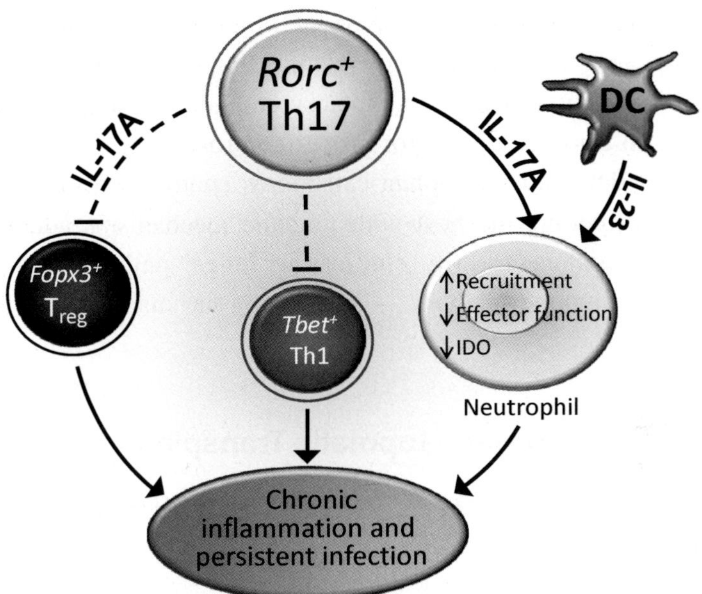

Fig. 1. The contribution of the IL-23/Th17 pathway to pathogen persistence, chronic inflammation and antifungal immunity. IL-23 and IL-17A, produced by Th17 cells, contribute to neutrophil mobilization, impairment of antifungal effector activities and activation of an inflammatory program by opposing IFN-γ-dependent activation of immunosuppressive IDO. Fungal persistence and inflammation in this setting may further be promoted by the concomitant antagonistic activity of the Th17 pathway on Th1 or T_{reg} cell activation. Thus, in its ability to inhibit Th1 or T_{reg} activation, the Th17-dependent pathway could be responsible for failure to resolve infection in the face of ongoing inflammation. This implies that failure to downregulate microbe-induced expression of IL-23/IL-17 could be an important link between infection and chronic inflammation. T_{reg} — regulatory T cells; DC — dendritic cells. See Ref. 58 for further details.

compromises a patient's ability to eradicate infection, and not an "intrinsic" susceptibility to infection that determines a state of chronic or intractable disease. The above findings may serve to accommodate fungi within the host immune system and at the same time explain why, despite the fact that human beings are constantly exposed to fungi, fungal diseases are relatively rare. Should a degree of coexistence have occurred between fungi and their mammalian hosts, this would implicate the possible, underestimated contribution of fungi to the plasticity of the immune system. Recent evidence would support the belief that the continued integration of proinflammatory and anti-inflammatory stimuli in response to fungi is critical for proper control of infection and T cell homeostasis. IDO and tryptophan catabolites contribute to this delicate balance, by providing the host with immune mechanisms adequate for protection without necessarily eliminating fungal pathogens — which would impair immune memory — or causing an unacceptable level of tissue damage.[56,58]

Dendritic Cells in Hematopoietic Transplantation

Dendritic Cells Provide Antifungal Immune Resistance

Fungus-pulsed DCs activated adaptive Th cell responses upon adoptive transfer into immunocompetent mice.[6,8,53] The ability of fungus-pulsed DCs to prime for Th1 and Th2 cell activation upon adoptive transfer *in vivo* correlated with the occurrence of resistance or susceptibility to infections. The infusion of fungus-pulsed DCs also accelerated myeloid and functional Th1 cells, producing IFN-γ recovery in mice with allogeneic HSCT.[53]

Different categories of DCs have been described in both experimental and human settings.[12] Type I IFN-producing pDCs not only mediate Th1 and Th2 type responses but also participate in the induction and maintenance of tolerance, by promoting the development of T_{reg} with suppressive activity.[12] Expansion of pDCs is contingent upon the haematopoietic growth factor FLT3L and not GM-CSF/IL-4, known to expand conventional, myeloid DCs (GM-DCs).[44] On comparative analysis of murine and human DC subsets for Th priming against *A. fumigatus*, FL-DCs but not GM-DCs conferred resistance to *Aspergillus* infection in experimental HSCT. A paradoxical effect was observed with GM-DCs, which although capable of efficiently controlling the fungal growth, were nevertheless associated with inflammatory toxicity.[53] Thus, instructive immunotherapy with fungus-pulsed DCs may generate both protective and nonprotective antifungal responses, a finding emphasizing the importance of DC plasticity and functional specialization in response to fungi.[54]

At a time when vaccination of stem cell transplant recipients is highly recommended,[30] developing new strategies to expand and modulate the functions of distinct DC subsets associated with specific regulation of host immunity may provide novel immune-based therapies in HSCT.[66] Within the instructive model of DC-mediated regulation of the Th repertoire, it is conceivable that an improved understanding of the pathogen/DC interaction will allow the potential use of pathogen- or TLR-conditioned DCs for the induction of patient-tailored T_{reg} with indirect antidonor allospecificity.

Dendritic Cells Induce Protective Tolerance

The infusion of the DC populations along with donor T cells further unmasked the potential for immunotoxicity versus protection in HSCT of each DC subset. The infusion of GM-DCs greatly accelerated the induction of GvHD by T cells, whereas FL-DCs not only failed to do so but actually totally prevented it.[53] FL-DCs, in contrast, were able to control both inflammation in infection and GvHD. The protection conferred by FL-DCs was associated with the concomitant activation of IFN-γ^+Th1 cells and FOXP3$^+$IL-10$^+$CD25$^+$T$_{reg}$. It has been demonstrated that a division of labor occurs between functionally distinct T_{reg} that are coordinately activated by a CD28/B7-dependent costimulatory pathway after exposure of mice to *Aspergillus* resting conidia.[37] Inflammation is controlled by the expansion, activation and recruitment of CD4$^+$CD25$^+$ T_{reg} suppressing neutrophils through the combined actions of IL-10 and CTLA-4. Late in infection, and similarly in allergy, tolerogenic T_{reg} which produce IL-10 and TGF-β inhibit Th2 cells and prevent allergy to the fungus. Thus, the capacity of T_{reg} to inhibit aspects of innate and adaptive immunity is central to their regulatory activity in fungal infections.[53]

Together, our results suggest that FL-DCs are fully competent at inducing antifungal resistance and protective tolerance upon adoptive transfer in HSCT recipients through the combined action of immunizing and tolerizing DCs. In contrast, GM-DCs are endowed with immunotoxicity, which may include the promotion of inflammation and GvHD.

Antifungal T_{reg} Concomitantly Suppress Inflammation and Alloreactivity

Allogeneic, but not *Aspergillus*-specific, proliferation was induced by the infusion of GM-DCs. In contrast, alloreactivity decreased but pathogen-specific reactivity recovered upon the infusion of FL-DCs. As comparable responses to mitogen were observed, the above results suggest that T_{reg} directly impacted on both allogeneic and pathogen-specific Th1 reactivity. This was indeed the case as purified $CD4^+CD25^+$ T cells efficiently blocked *Aspergillus*- or alloantigen-specific proliferation and IFN-γ production by the corresponding effector $CD4^+CD25^-$ T cells.[53] In agreement with the notion that lung T_{reg} are endowed with potent anti-inflammatory activity in pulmonary aspergillosis,[37] lung $CD4^+CD25^+$ T cells, induced by FL-DCs, potently inhibited the antifungal effector and inflammatory activities of neutrophils, such as TNF-α and oxidant production. Thus, the ability of *Aspergillus*-induced T_{reg} to inhibit alloreactivity while sparing responsiveness to mitogens suggests that pathogen-induced T_{reg} may be associated with minimal bystander suppression. From a mechanistic perspective, this implies that the function of T_{reg} in transplantation can be controlled by the specificity of the T cell receptor expressed on T_{reg}[2] and is in line with the observation of a positive effect on posttransplant immunity of antigen exposure at the time of transplantation.[40]

Several studies have addressed the effects that infections have on transplantation tolerance, and the overall view is that both prior and concurrent exposure to pathogens can prevent tolerance induction. However, much less attention has been paid to the effect that pathogen-directed tolerance based on active T cell regulation might have on tolerance to donor antigens. Because of the cross-reactivity in the T cell repertoire between antimicrobial, environmental and transplantation antigens,[32,47] the above results raise the intriguing possibility that pathogen-conditioned DCs could be potential reagents for promoting donor-specific transplantation through the induction of CD4$^+$CD25$^+$ T$_{reg}$ with indirect antidonor allospecificity. Strategies to generate human CD4$^+$CD25$^+$ T cell lines with indirect allospecificity for therapeutic use for the induction of donor-specific transplantation tolerance have recently been described.[25]

IDO Contributes to Protective Tolerance

IDO is an interferon-gamma-inducible intracellular enzyme which catalyzes the catabolism of tryptophan.[34,49] Work has demonstrated a complex and crucial role for IDO in immunoregulation during infection, pregnancy, autoimmunity, transplantation and neoplasia.[34,49] The effects of IDO activity are tryptophan deficiency, excess tryptophan breakdown products (kynurenines) and consumption of reactive oxygen species. Tryptophan deficiency and kynurenine excess have immunodulatory effects, including suppression of lymphocyte responses particularly by sensitizing them to apoptosis, which is of potential interest in transplantation. Transplantation tolerance essentially involves two critical processes: (i) deletion of alloreactive T cells and (ii) development of anergy and regulatory activity of alloreactive T cells. After allogeneic cell transplantation a state of immune activation, driven by recognition of major or minor histocompatibility antigens, will invariably emerge in the recipient, even in the HLA-matched donor. In addition, some immune activation will result from tissue damage in the recipient caused by HSCT or the conditioning regimens. This state of immune activation will include the secretion of proinflammatory cytokines, including IFN-γ, by innate cells or activated T cells. Because of the intimate association of IFN-γ and induction of IDO, it is likely that IDO by its immunoregulatory effects may actively participate in downregulating allogeneic immune responses in transplantation.

In several transplant models, increased IDO activity in transplanted cells has been demonstrated to have antirejection properties both *in vitro* and *in vivo*.[21,42] Evidence for IDO activity being involved in human transplantation immunology has also been demonstrated.[9,22] The state of immunosuppression after HSCT involved an enhanced tryptophan metabolism mediated by activated monocytes that were able to suppress T cell proliferation. A striking finding was that after HSCT monocytes were highly sensitive to upregulate IDO activity upon exposure to even low doses of IFN-γ. Thus, IDO-competent cells might become sensitive to upregulate IDO activity upon exposure to inflammatory cytokines such that conversion into suppressor cells rather than stimulatory cells is facilitated. As a previous study, although small-scale, showed that lack of IDO activity in recipients of HSCT was associated with high-grade GvHD,[64] this indicates that systemic IDO activity, rather than being associated with general immunosuppression after transplantation, contributes to tolerance induction and prevention of GvHD or rejection. Overall, the available data suggest a potentially dominant role of IDO governing alloreactivity through a mechanistic pathway possibly involving IDO induction by reverse signaling through costimulatory receptors.[7] This concept is compatible with viewing IDO as a negative feedback mechanism in which activated T cells that express CTLA-4 interact with CD80/86 expressed by DCs. In turn, the capacity of IDO-competent DCs to induce T_{reg} suggests a positive loop through which peripheral tolerance is likely maintained.[19]

IDO plays many roles in fungal infections (Fig. 2), the most relevant being the induction of $CD4^+CD25^+$ T_{reg} via FL-DCs.[36,37] Murine pDCs have been credited with a unique ability to express IDO function and with a general and important role in regulating T cell homeostasis.[43,46] Tolerogenic IDO^+DCs proved to be pivotal in the generation of dominant regulation that ultimately controlled inflammation, pathogen immunity and tolerance in transplant recipients, eventually leading to prevention of GvHD and reduction of the aspergillosis incidence.[38] Thus, antifungal resistance within a regulatory environment is achievable by adoptive cellular therapy of *Aspergillus*-pulsed IDO^+DCs exerting IDO-dependent homeostatic control over the proliferation and survival of peripheral T cells, and can promote Ag-specific tolerance. These data would indicate that the exploitation of IDO activity in an intelligent manner may be a way to achieve the magical goal of transplantation immunology,

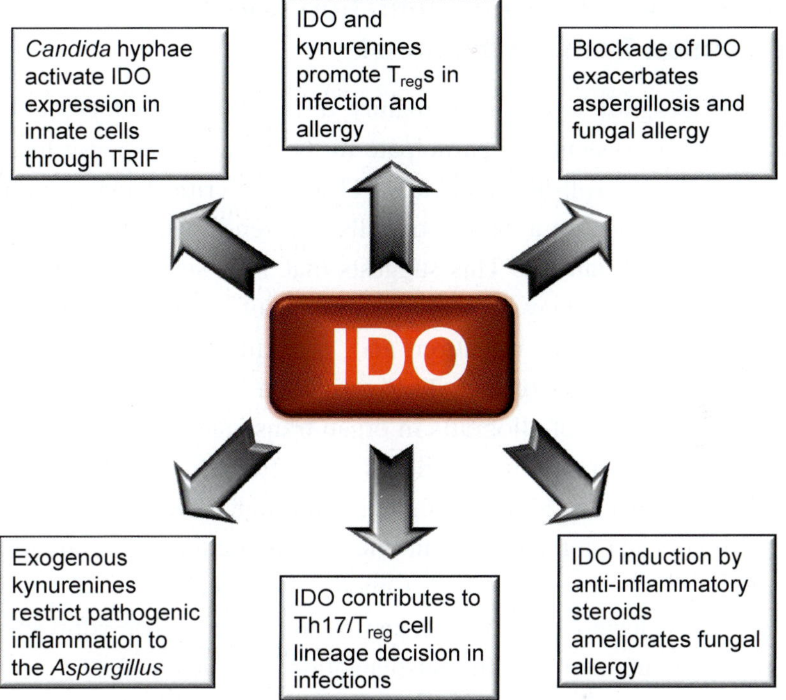

Fig. 2. The multifaceted activity of IDO in fungal infections. See Ref. 56 for further details.

which is to tolerize against alloantigens while preserving immunity against pathogens.[42]

It is intriguing that fungi have exploited IDO manipulation as a means of inducing or subverting the tolerogenic program of pDCs.[57] Regulation of IDO activity in pDCs occurred in a morphotype-dependent manner and, interestingly, in an opposite manner for *Candida* and *Aspergillus*. IDO activity was promoted by *Candida* hyphae and by *Aspergillus* resting conidia, and inhibited by *Aspergillus* swollen conidia or hyphae. The implication is that *Candida* hyphae, by promoting tolerance, contribute to commensalism and eventually to immunoevasion while swollen *Aspergillus* conidia promote host inflammatory response by subverting tolerance.

Exploiting TLR for Transplantation Tolerance: The Lesson from Thymosin α1

Although allograft rejection is mainly a T cell-mediated process, the innate immune system can participate in the immune response to organ transplantation.[28] Toll-like receptors (TLRs) are critical innate immune receptors expressed on a variety of cells that sense pathogens as well as injury-associated damage. This suggests that TLR signaling participates in inflammation that may occur in the absence of overt infection and promotes acute allograft rejection and prevention of transplantation tolerance.[3] As a matter of fact, TLR activation is involved in the innate immune recognition of allografts in organ transplantation.[17] Strategies to prevent innate immunity-mediated rejection have already been described.[27] However, although signaling through TLRs, and recruitment of the MyD88 adaptor, can prevent tolerance induction and promote graft rejection,[10] TLR signaling also promotes the induction of T_{reg}.[26] This implies that selected TLR ligands can be useful candidate adjuvants for T_{reg} induction/maintenance in transplantation. Thymosin α1 (Tα1), a naturally occurring thymic peptide,[16] promoted maturation of and cytokine production by human and murine DCs by signaling through TLR9.[52] By tipping the balance between IL-12- and IL-10-producing DCs, Tα1 acted as an endogenous immune regulator capable of inducing protective immunity to *Aspergillus*. As TLR9 stimulation may lead to IDO activation[14,33] and can promote pDC-mediated generation of $CD4^+CD25^+$ T_{reg} cells,[41] it was conceivable that Tα1 could affect the tolerogenic program of DCs. This was indeed the case as Tα1 induced IDO expression and kynurenin production by murine GM-DCs and greatly increased that of FL-DCs, an effect that was ablated in the absence of TLR9 or type I IFNR signaling.[53] As with murine DC cultures, Tα1 promoted the mobilization of $CD123^+$ pDCs while decreasing that of $CD1a^+$ DCs in GM-CSF+IL-4 cultures of peripheral $CD14^+$ cells from healthy donors.[53] In terms of functional activity, Tα1 converted inflammatory IL-12-producing GM-DCs into tolerogenic pDCs which, as with FL-DCs, produced higher levels of IL-10 and primed for IL-10-producing $CD4^+$ T cells *in vitro*. These data indicate that Tα1, by taming inflammatory DCs, may meet the requirement for

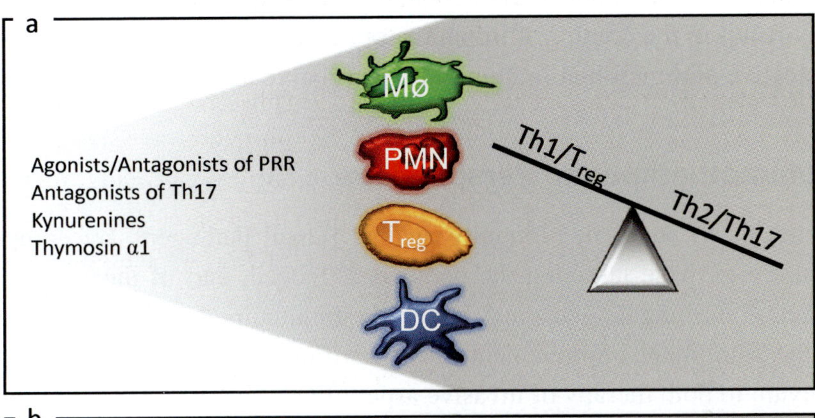

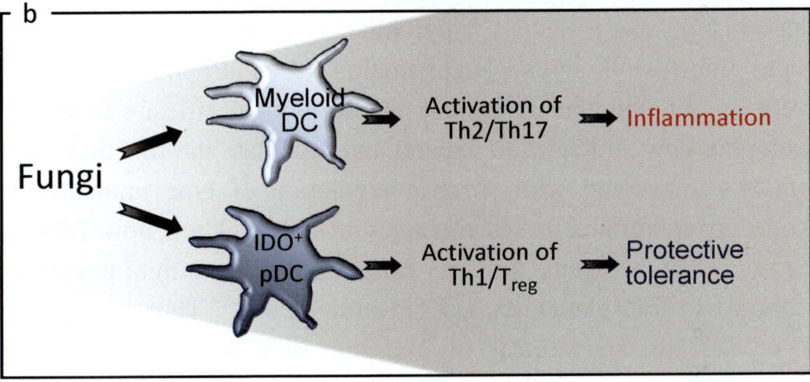

Fig. 3. Possible immunotherapeutic strategies in HSCT. Shown are (a) the possible utility of selective maneuvers that target innate immune pathways in the balance between inflammatory and tolerogenic response to fungi, and (a) the exploitation of fungus-pulsed DC subsets for active and negative vaccination in hematopoietic transplantation (see text and Refs. 52, 53 and 58 for further details).

successful antifungal $Th1/T_{reg}$ cell priming devoid of alloreactivity in haematopoietic transplantation. By activating the IDO-dependent tolerogenic program in DCs via TLR9 and type I IFNR signaling, Tα1 acted as a fine regulator of peripheral inflammation via tolerance induction through T_{reg} cell induction. Although Tα1 activates innate cells, including DCs, to an antimicrobial[52] and antitumor state,[60] the attenuation of the immunogenic/inflammatory activity of myeloid DCs by Tα1 through IDO induction qualifies Tα1 as a unique immunoregulatory molecule capable of fine-tuning and controlling the quality of the immune response, which may result in the control of inflammatory response and the restoration of protective antimicrobial immunity in the relative absence of GvHD.

Immunotherapeutic Perspectives

Strategies to augment immunity against fungal pathogens are complementary to those targeting the pathogens. Indeed, part of the antifungal effect of antifungal agents may occur via immunomodulation. In addition to the significant improvement in the antifungal armamentarium that is relevant to both therapy of invasive aspergillosis and prevention of fungal disease in high-risk patients,[13,68] cytokine/anticytokine therapy[4] and granulocyte transfusion and/or augmentation of neutrophil number[48] are current immunotherapeutic options whose clinical efficacy is not clear. Developing new strategies to expand and modulate the functions of distinct DCs associated with specific regulation of host immunity may provide novel immune-based therapies in HSCT. Until now DCs have been used only in vaccine trials for cancer, where the aim of treatment is, in contrast to transplantation, immunostimulation.[63] Thus, one potential risk of DC-based treatment in transplantation is immunostimulation versus tolerance, depending on the route of administration and DC reversibility to the inflammatory state. An alternative strategy to the use of positive or negative vaccination with DCs generated *in vitro* is the targeting of DCs *in vivo* by biologic or pharmacologic agents. Strategies that lead to recipient DC depletion and/or modulation are currently being tested in HSCT.[65] Tα1, which is approved in 30 countries for treatment of some viral infections and as an immune adjuvant,[16] appears to be a suitable candidate for modulating DC functioning for active and negative vaccination in transplantation. Finally, the therapeutic adoption of IDO-mediated immunoregulation appears attractive for use in transplantation. As a systemic enhancement of IDO activity by pharmacologic IDO induction would carry the risk of inducing general immunosuppression and IDO activity itself is modulated by the microenvironment and factors that cannot be controlled for *in vivo*, these considerations argue against a therapeutic approach of systemic IDO induction as a means of facilitating the generation of tolerance. The enrichment of IDO activity at targeted sites, as with IDO-competent DCs, is an attractive option.

Acknowledgements

We thank Dr. Cristina Massi Benedetti for digital art and editing. The original studies conducted in the author's laboratory were supported by the Specific Targeted Research Project "SYBARIS" (FP7-Health-2009-single-stage, contract number 242220), by the Italian Projects PRIN 2007KLCKP8_004 (to LR) and by the Project 2006.020.0291 from Fondazione Cassa di Risparmio di Perugia.

References

1. Afzali B, Lombardi G, Lechler RI, Lord GM. (2007) The role of T helper 17 (Th17) and regulatory T cells (T_{reg}) in human organ transplantation and autoimmune disease. *Clin Exp Immunol* **148**: 32–46.

2. Albert MH, Anasetti C, Yu XZ. (2006) T regulatory cells as an immunotherapy for transplantation. *Expert Opin Biol Ther* **6**: 315–324.

3. Alegre ML, Leemans J, Le Moine A *et al.* (2008) The multiple facets of toll-like receptors in transplantation biology. *Transplantation* **86**: 1–9.

4. Antachopoulos C, Roilides E. (2005) Cytokines and fungal infections. *Br J Haematol* **129**: 583–596.

5. Arpinati M, Chirumbolo G, Urbini B *et al.* (2003) Role of plasmacytoid dendritic cells in immunity and tolerance after allogeneic hematopoietic stem cell transplantation. *Transpl Immunol* **11**: 345–356.

6. Bacci A, Montagnoli C, Perruccio K *et al.* (2002) Dendritic cells pulsed with fungal RNA induce protective immunity to *Candida albicans* in hematopoietic transplantation. *J Immunol* **168**: 2904–2913.

7. Belladonna ML, Puccetti P, Orabona C *et al.* (2007) Immunosuppression via tryptophan catabolism: The role of kynurenine pathway enzymes. *Transplantation* **84**: S17–S20.

8. Bozza S, Gaziano R, Lipford GB *et al.* (2002) Vaccination of mice against invasive aspergillosis with recombinant *Aspergillus* proteins and CpG oligodeoxynucleotides as adjuvants. *Microbes Infect* **4**: 1281–1290.

9. Brandacher G, Margreiter R, Fuchs D. (2008) Clinical relevance of indoleamine 2,3-dioxygenase for alloimmunity and transplantation. *Curr Opin Organ Transplant* **13**: 10–15.

10. Chen L, Wang T, Zhou P *et al.* (2006) TLR engagement prevents transplantation tolerance. *Am J Transplant* **6**: 2282–2291.

11. Chen Y, Wood KJ. (2007) Interleukin-23 and TH17 cells in transplantation immunity: Does 23+17 equal rejection? *Transplantation* **84**: 1071–1074.

12. Colonna M, Trinchieri G, Liu YJ. (2004) Plasmacytoid dendritic cells in immunity. *Nat Immunol* **5**: 1219–1226.

13. Cornely OA, Maertens J, Winston DJ *et al.* (2007) Posaconazole vs. fluconazole or itraconazole prophylaxis in patients with neutropenia. *N Engl J Med* **356**: 348–359.

14. Fallarino F, Puccetti P. (2005) Toll-like receptor 9-mediated induction of the immunosuppressive pathway of tryptophan catabolism. *Eur J Immunol* **36**: 8–11.

15. Fugier-Vivier IJ, Rezzoug F, Huang Y *et al.* (2005) Plasmacytoid precursor dendritic cells facilitate allogeneic hematopoietic stem cell engraftment. *J Exp Med* **201**: 373–383.

16. Goldstein AL, Badamchian M. (2004) Thymosins: Chemistry and biological properties in health and disease. *Expert Opin Biol Ther* **4**: 559–573.

17. Goldstein DR. (2006) Toll-like receptors and acute allograft rejection. *Transpl Immunol* **17**: 11–15.

18. Golshayan D, Buhler L, Lechler RI, Pascual M. (2007) From current immunosuppressive strategies to clinical tolerance of allografts. *Transpl Int* **20**: 12–24.

19. Grohmann U, Orabona C, Fallarino F *et al.* (2002) CTLA-4-Ig regulates tryptophan catabolism *in vivo*. *Nat Immunol* **3**: 1097–1101.

20. Grow WB, Moreb JS, Roque D *et al.* (2002) Late onset of invasive *Aspergillus* infection in bone marrow transplant patients at a university hospital. *Bone Marrow Transplant* **29**: 15–19.

21. Hainz U, Jurgens B, Heitger A. (2007) The role of indoleamine 2,3-dioxygenase in transplantation. *Transpl Int* **20**: 118–127.

22. Hainz U, Obexer P, Winkler C *et al.* (2005) Monocyte-mediated T-cell suppression and augmented monocyte tryptophan catabolism after human hematopoietic stem-cell transplantation. *Blood* **105**: 4127–4134.

23. Horibe EK, Sacks J, Unadkat J *et al.* (2008) Rapamycin-conditioned, alloantigen-pulsed dendritic cells promote indefinite survival of vascularized skin allografts in association with T regulatory cell expansion. *Transpl Immunol* **18**: 307–318.

24. Jiang S, Herrera O, Lechler RI. (2004) New spectrum of allorecognition pathways: Implications for graft rejection and transplantation tolerance. *Curr Opin Immunol* **16**: 550–557.

25. Jiang S, Lombardi G. (2006) New trends in immunosuppression and immunotherapy. *Int Immunopharmacol* **6**: 1874–1878.

26. Kabelitz D, Wesch D, Oberg HH. (2006) Regulation of regulatory T cells: Role of dendritic cells and toll-like receptors. *Crit Rev Immunol* **26**: 291–306.

27. Land WG. (2007) Innate immunity-mediated allograft rejection and strategies to prevent it. *Transplant Proc* **39**: 667–672.

28. LaRosa DF, Rahman AH, Turka LA. (2007) The innate immune system in allograft rejection and tolerance. *J Immunol* **178**: 7503–7509.

29. Lechler R, Ng WF, Steinman RM. (2001) Dendritic cells in transplantation — friend or foe? *Immunity* **14**: 357–368.

30. Ljungman P, Engelhard D, de la Camara R *et al.* (2005) Vaccination of stem cell transplant recipients: Recommendations of the Infectious Diseases Working Party of the EBMT. *Bone Marrow Transplant* **35**: 737–746.

31. Marr KA, Carter RA, Boeckh M *et al.* (2002) Invasive aspergillosis in allogeneic stem cell transplant recipients: Changes in epidemiology and risk factors. *Blood* **100**: 4358–4366.

32. Mason D. (1998) A very high level of crossreactivity is an essential feature of the T-cell receptor. *Immunol Today* **19**: 395–404.

33. Mellor AL, Baban B, Chandler PR *et al.* (2005) Cutting edge: CpG oligonucleotides induce splenic CD19$^+$ dendritic cells to acquire potent indoleamine 2,3-dioxygenase-dependent T cell regulatory functions via IFN type 1 signaling. *J Immunol* **175**: 5601–5605.

34. Mellor AL, Munn DH. (2008) Creating immune privilege: Active local suppression that benefits friends, but protects foes. *Nat Rev Immunol* **8**: 74–80.

35. Miura Y, Thoburn CJ, Bright EC *et al.* (2004) Association of FoxP3 regulatory gene expression with graft-versus-host disease. *Blood* **104**: 2187–2193.

36. Montagnoli C, Bacci A, Bozza S *et al.* (2002) B7/CD28-dependent CD4$^+$CD25$^+$ regulatory T cells are essential components of the memory-protective immunity to *Candida albicans*. *J Immunol* **169**: 6298–6308.

37. Montagnoli C, Fallarino F, Gaziano R *et al.* (2006) Immunity and tolerance to *Aspergillus* involve functionally distinct regulatory T cells and tryptophan catabolism. *J Immunol* **176**: 1712–1723.

38. Montagnoli C, Perruccio K, Bozza S *et al.* (2008) Provision of antifungal immunity and concomitant alloantigen tolerization by conditioned dendritic cells in experimental hematopoietic transplantation. *Blood Cells Mol Dis* **40**: 55–62.

39. Morelli AE, Thomson AW. (2007) Tolerogenic dendritic cells and the quest for transplant tolerance. *Nat Rev Immunol* **7**: 610–621.

40. Mori S, Kocak U, Shaw JL, Mullen CA. (2005) Augmentation of post-transplant immunity: Antigen encounter at the time of hematopoietic stem cell transplantation enhances antigen-specific donor T-cell responses in the post-transplant repertoire. *Bone Marrow Transplant* **35**: 793–801.

41. Moseman EA, Liang X, Dawson AJ *et al.* (2004) Human plasmacytoid dendritic cells activated by CpG oligodeoxynucleotides induce the generation of CD4$^+$CD25$^+$ regulatory T cells. *J Immunol* **173**: 4433–4442.

42. Mulley WR, Nikolic-Paterson DJ. (2008) Indoleamine 2,3-dioxyge-nase in transplantation. *Nephrology (Carlton)* **13**: 204–211.

43. Munn DH, Sharma MD, Lee JR *et al.* (2002) Potential regulatory func-tion of human dendritic cells expressing indoleamine 2,3-dioxygenase. *Science* **297**: 1867–1870.

44. Naik SH, Proietto AI, Wilson NS *et al.* (2005) Cutting edge: Generation of splenic CD8$^+$ and CD8$^-$ dendritic cell equivalents in Fms-like tyrosine kinase 3 ligand bone marrow cultures. *J Immunol* **174**: 6592–6597.

45. Ng WF, Duggan PJ, Ponchel F *et al.* (2001) Human CD4(+)CD25(+) cells: A naturally occurring population of regulatory T cells. *Blood* **98**: 2736–2744.

46. Orabona C, Puccetti P, Vacca C *et al.* (2006) Toward the identifica-tion of a tolerogenic signature in IDO-competent dendritic cells. *Blood* **107**: 2846–2854.

47. Pantenburg B, Heinzel F, Das L *et al.* (2002) T cells primed by Leishmania major infection cross-react with alloantigens and alter the course of allograft rejection. *J Immunol* **169**: 3686–3693.

48. Price TH. (2007) Granulocyte transfusion: Current status. *Semin Hematol* **44**: 15–23.

49. Puccetti P, Grohmann U. (2007) IDO and regulatory T cells: A role for reverse signalling and non-canonical NF-kappaB activation. *Nat Rev Immunol* **7**: 817–823.

50. Reddy V, Hill GR, Pan L *et al.* (2000) G-CSF modulates cytokine profile of dendritic cells and decreases acute graft-versus-host disease through effects on the donor rather than the recipient. *Transplantation* **69**: 691–693.

51. Reddy V, Iturraspe JA, Tzolas AC *et al.* (2004) Low dendritic cell count after allogeneic hematopoietic stem cell transplantation predicts relapse, death, and acute graft-versus-host disease. *Blood* **103**: 4330–4335.

52. Romani L, Bistoni F, Gaziano R *et al.* (2004) Thymosin alpha 1 acti-vates dendritic cells for antifungal Th1 resistance through toll-like receptor signaling. *Blood* **103**: 4232–4239.

53. Romani L, Bistoni F, Perruccio K *et al.* (2006) Thymosin alpha 1 activates dendritic cell tryptophan catabolism and establishes a regulatory environment for balance of inflammation and tolerance. *Blood* **108**: 2265–2274.

54. Romani L, Bistoni F, Puccetti P. (2002) Fungi, dendritic cells and receptors: A host perspective of fungal virulence. *Trends Microbiol* **10**: 508–514.

55. Romani L, Fallarino F, De Luca A *et al.* (2008) Defective tryptophan catabolism underlies inflammation in mouse chronic granulomatous disease. *Nature* **451**: 211–215.

56. Romani L, Puccetti P. (2007) Controlling pathogenic inflammation to fungi. *Expert Rev Anti Infect Ther* **5**: 1007–1017.

57. Romani L, Puccetti P. (2006) Protective tolerance to fungi: The role of IL-10 and tryptophan catabolism. *Trends Microbiol* **14**: 183–189.

58. Romani L, Zelante T, De Luca A *et al.* (2008) IL-17 and therapeutic kynurenines in pathogenic inflammation to fungi. *J Immunol* **180**: 5157–5162.

59. Schneider M, Munder M, Karakhanova S *et al.* (2006) The initial phase of graft-versus-host disease is associated with a decrease of $CD4^+CD25^+$ regulatory T cells in the peripheral blood of patients after allogeneic stem cell transplantation. *Clin Lab Haematol* **28**: 382–390.

60. Shrivastava P, Singh SM, Singh N. (2005) Antitumor activation of peritoneal macrophages by thymosin alpha-1. *Cancer Invest* **23**: 316–322.

61. Singh N, Perfect JR. (2007) Immune reconstitution syndrome associated with opportunistic mycoses. *Lancet Infect Dis* **7**: 395–401.

62. Soiffer R. (2008) Immune modulation and chronic graft-versus-host disease. *Bone Marrow Transplant* **42**(Suppl 1): S66–S69.

63. Solari MG, Thomson AW. (2008) Human dendritic cells and transplant outcome. *Transplantation* **85**: 1513–1522.

64. Steckel NK, Kuhn U, Beelen DW, Elmaagacli AH. (2003) Indoleamine 2,3-dioxygenase expression in patients with acute

graft-versus-host disease after allogeneic stem cell transplantation and in pregnant women: Association with the induction of allogeneic immune tolerance? *Scand J Immunol* **57**: 185–191.

65. Steinman RM, Banchereau J. (2007) Taking dendritic cells into medicine. *Nature* **449**: 419–426.

66. Steinman RM, Hawiger D, Nussenzweig MC. (2003) Tolerogenic dendritic cells. *Annu Rev Immunol* **21**: 685–711.

67. Turnquist HR, Thomson AW. (2008) Taming the lions: Manipulating dendritic cells for use as negative cellular vaccines in organ transplantation. *Curr Opin Organ Transplant* **13**: 350–357.

68. Ullmann AJ, Lipton JH, Vesole DH *et al.* (2007) Posaconazole or fluconazole for prophylaxis in severe graft-versus-host disease. *N Engl J Med* **356**: 335–347.

69. Zorn E, Kim HT, Lee SJ *et al.* (2005) Reduced frequency of FOXP3$^+$ CD4$^+$CD25$^+$ regulatory T cells in patients with chronic graft-versus-host disease. *Blood* **106**: 2903–2911.

Chapter 13

Immune Reconstitution After Haploidentical Hematopoietic Stem Cell Transplantation

*Ami Shah, Neena Kapoor, Hisham Abdel-Azim and Robertson Parkman**

Introduction

The development of a competent immune system following hematopoietic stem cell transplantation (HSCT) is necessary in order to control posttransplant infections as well as reducing the likelihood of neoplastic relapse.[1–5] Immune reconstitution is a particular problem following haploidentical HSCT, for the reasons that will be presented. The recipient immune system following HSCT is a combination of the recipient pre-existing immune system and the newly transplanted donor cells, including both hematopoietic stem cells (HSCs) and the infused donor T and B lymphocytes. A variety of factors can impact the development of a competent immune system, including the transplant conditioning regimen, T cell depletion (TCD), the HSC source, recipient age/thymic function and graft-vs-host disease (GvHD).

*Corresponding author. Division of Research Immunology/Bone Marrow Transplantation, Children's Hospital Los Angeles, The Saban Research Institute, 4650 Sunset Boulevard, Mail Stop 62, Los Angeles, CA 90027, USA. Tel.: 323-361-2196 Fax: 323-906-8193 E-mail: rparkman@chla.usc.edu.

Factors in the Development of Immune Competence

Conditioning Regimen

Traditionally, HSCT recipients received a conditioning regimen that eliminated all recipient HSCs, T lymphocytes, and the majority of B lymphocytes. Following HSCT, all elements of the recipient immune system became donor-derived. The donor HSC innoculum contained both mature antigen-specific and naïve T and B lymphocytes as well as pluripotent HSCs which, through a recapitulation of immune ontogeny, can develop into new T and B lymphocytes of donor origin. Thus, both passively acquired and new T and B lymphocytes contribute to post-HSCT immune function.

The introduction of reduced intensity conditioning (RIC) regimens has resulted in the initial persistence of the recipient immune system, though in most recipients the T lymphocytes are almost exclusively of donor origin by 100 days following transplantation.[6] If sustained donor T lymphocyte chimerism is not established following an RIC HSCT, it is likely that the residual recipient T lymphocytes will reject the donor HSCs and the recipient will undergo autologous hematopoietic and immune recovery or develop aplasia.

T Cell Depletion

Based upon animal experiments, it has been clear for more than 30 years that mature donor T lymphocytes initiate acute GvHD.[7] The use of related HSC donors with significant histocompatibility differences from the recipient was initially possible only when the mature donor T lymphocytes were removed from the HSC product.[8] T lymphocyte depletion (TCD) prior to HSCT has been critical to the development of haploidentical transplantation for adult recipients.[9] The reduction of donor T lymphocytes to less than 1×10^4 functional or 3×10^4 immunophenotypic T lymphocytes/ml has resulted in successful donor HSC engraftment without significant acute GvHD if conditioning regimens with adequate anti-immune and anti-HSC properties are used. TCD has also been used in histocompatible HSCT to reduce acute GvHD.[10] The use of a TCD HSC product means, however, that there will be no contribution to the post-HSCT immune system by the mature naïve and antigen-specific T lymphocytes usually present in the HSC innoculum. All recipient immune function will have to be derived from the newly engrafted donor HSCs.

HSC Source

Initially, bone marrow was the only HSC source of allogeneic HSCTs. When bone marrow is obtained by multiple iliac crest aspirates, a significant amount of peripheral blood is also collected, resulting in an HSC product that contains mature donor T lymphocytes. If bone marrow, however, is obtained by the physical removal of bone marrow after the surgical uncovering of the iliac crest, no significant contamination with peripheral blood occurs. The clinical consequence of these differences in obtaining bone marrow is that no significant acute GvHD occurs if surgically obtained bone marrow is used while, if bone marrow is aspirated, significant acute GvHD may occur. Unless recipients are infected or vaccinated, donor-derived antigen-specific T lymphocytes cannot be detected in the peripheral blood of allogeneic recipients of bone marrow.

Because of delays in myeloid engraftment, studies were undertaken using hematopoietic growth factors to mobilize HSCs and progenitors to the peripheral blood. Following GCSF administration, circulating HSCs and progenitors can be collected by leukapheresis. The administration of the peripheral blood cells (PBCs) results in more rapid hematopoietic engraftment with a reduction in neutropenia and earlier platelet transfusion independence.[11] In addition to accelerated hematopoietic engraftment, ten fold more donor T lymphocytes are infused with PBCs than with bone marrow. In both related and unrelated transplants the incidence of chronic GvHD is twice as great in recipients who receive PBCs than bone marrow.[12] Following PBC transplantation, it has been possible to demonstrate the presence of antigen-specific donor T lymphocytes in the recipient peripheral blood.[13] However, no decrease in the incidence of post-HSCT infection complications has been demonstrated.

Cord blood as an HSC source is characterized by the fact that the donor T lymphocytes present in the cord blood are relatively immuno-incompetent and have no antigen-specific function. The lack of transfer of antigen-specific T lymphocytes has resulted in an increased frequency of viral infections following cord blood transplantation but also a decreased incidence of acute GvHD.[14,15] Therefore, degrees of donor–recipient histoincompatibility, which would not have been possible without TCD of other HSC sources, can be tolerated. Four out of six HLA matched donor–recipient combinations are routinely successfully transplanted.

Recipient Age

Although mature T and B lymphocytes can be transferred with the HSC innoculum and may contribute to antigen-specific T and B lymphocyte function early after HSCT, long-term immunocompetence after HSCT is dependent upon the engraftment of donor HSCs and a recapitulation of normal lymphoid ontogeny with the development of both T and B lymphocytes. Central to the production of new T lymphocytes and normal T lymphocyte function is adequate thymopoiesis. Thymic function peaks in the first/second decade of life, and subsequently there is a continuing decrease in the capacity of the thymus to generate new T lymphocytes. The decrease in thymic function can be followed morphologically by CAT scans of the thymus gland or by immunophenotypic analysis for recent thymic emigrants [CD4, CD45RA; CD4, CD31; and TCR excision circle (TREC) analysis].[16–18] All of these analyses are concordant and demonstrate decreased thymic function with increasing age although adequate thymic function is present in normal-aged adults to sustain a broad antigen repertoire as measured by T cell receptor (TCR) usage well into the eighth decade. Antineoplastic drugs have a negative effect on the thymic function, as does total body irradiation (TBI), used in many HSCT conditioning regimens. The impact of these agents during conventional therapy and the conditioning regimen can lead to decreased thymic function and an inability to generate new T lymphocytes, resulting in a prolonged lymphopenia and restricted TCR heterogeneity.

GvHD

Almost all transplant recipients have a graft-versus-host reaction (GvHR) and many have clinical GvHD, depending upon their degree of donor–recipient histoincompatibility. One of the major target organs for GvHD is the thymus.[19] Both animal and human experiments have shown that the presence of chronic GvHD results in defects in thymopoiesis with severe reductions in the number of recent thymic emigrants.[20] Thus, recipients with chronic GvHD may have a protracted inability to produce new T lymphocytes and, therefore, have severe defects in posttransplant immunocompetence.

Immune Reconstitution

Following HSCT the evolution of the recipient immune system can be evaluated either immunophenotypically or functionally. The immunophenotypic assays are easier to perform. In the absence of immunophenotypic T or B lymphocytes, adequate immune reconstitution will not exist. Once adequate numbers of immunophenotypic T and B lymphocytes are present, the determination of their function, especially antigen-specific function, is necessary in order to fully characterize recipient immunocompetence.

Immunophenotypic Analysis of T Lymphocytes

The simplest clinical setting in which to immunophenotypically analyze the posttransplant immune system is following the infusion of autologous HSCs after myeloablative conditioning. In this clinical setting there will be no GvHD, and the recipient's pre-existing immune system will have been eliminated. The transplantation of either whole or TCD PBCs results in lymphopenia early after HSCT; natural killer (NK) cells are the earliest lymphoid population to be identified, and by three months both CD4 and CD8 T lymphocytes can be detected.[21,22] By one year after transplantation, the CD4 counts have stabilized. In adult recipients there is no correlation between the recipient age and the recovery of CD4 T lymphocyte counts. However, in pediatric patients there is a correlation with younger patients having a more rapid recovery of CD4 counts than older pediatric patients, suggesting that more residual thymic function was present in younger patients.[23] In adult patients, the study of thymopoiesis by TREC analysis has shown that individuals with higher TREC numbers have a broader TCR repertoire, indicating that with greater recipient thymopoiesis, more T lymphocytes are produced with a broader antigeneic repertoire.[18]

When histocompatible bone marrow is used as an HSC source, there are delays in the recovery of both CD4 and CD8 T lymphocytes as compared to autologous HSCs.[24,25] CD8 T lymphocyte counts normalize sooner than CD4 T lymphocytes due to the homeostatic expansion of CD8 T lymphocytes, which occurs after HSCT, whereas the increase in the number of CD4 T lymphocytes requires thymopoiesis. When histocompatible PBCs are utilized, there is more rapid normalization both of CD4 and of CD8 T lymphocyte counts, presumably due to the fact that 1–2 logs more T lymphocytes are infused with PBCs as compared to bone marrow.[13]

Following unrelated HSCT, the immunophenotypic recovery of T lymphocytes in the recipients of either unrelated bone marrow or PBCs is more variable than following autologous or related HSCT. Children can develop normal numbers of CD4 T lymphocytes by one year after unrelated HSCT, while in adult recipients delays in the normalization of CD4 T lymphocyte counts can last for two or three years after HSCT, primarily to defects in thymopoiesis.[26]

When TCD products are used, immunophenotypic T lymphocytes are not detectable during the first three months after transplantation, at which time, in young children receiving bone marrow for severe combined immune deficiency, immunophenotypic T lymphocytes can first be identified.[27] The presence of immunophenotypic T lymphocytes correlates with the initial presence of TREC and other markers of recent thymic emigrants. However, when TCD HSC products are infused into adult recipients, recent thymic emigrants may not be detectable until 9 or 12 months after transplantation, indicating that significant defects in thymopoiesis exist and predicting that the recipients may be at increased risk of opportunistic infections and potentially neoplastic relapse.[26] Following cord blood transplantation, early delays in the recovery of both CD4 and CD8 T lymphocytes are seen; the rise in CD8 T lymphocytes is more rapid than for CD4 T lymphocytes, suggesting that homeostatic expansion for CD8 T lymphocytes occurs sooner than thymopoiesis. In the absence of significant GvHD, the immunophenotypic recovery of T lymphocytes is normal by 12 months after cord blood transplantation.[2]

In the specific case of haploidentical transplantation, which is routinely TCD and which occurs in older individuals with a history of prior chemotherapy, prolonged deficits in the recovery of immunophenotypic T lymphocytes are routinely seen as there is no passive transfer of T lymphocytes with the HSC product. The detrimental effects of prior chemoradiotherapy on an aging thymus further result in a marked inability of the recipient thymus to produce new T lymphocytes. Thus, many adult haploidentical transplant recipients have a limited number of CD4 T lymphocytes even one year after transplantation. These results are to be distinguished from those for pediatric recipients, particularly children with severe combined immune deficiency, in whom the transplantation of TCD bone marrow results in the appearance of immunophenotypic T lymphocytes by 90–100 days after HSCT, with normal proliferative responses by six months and the ability to respond to vaccinations by one year after transplantation.

Immunophenotypic Analysis of B Lymphocytes

B lymphocytes recover to normal immunophenotypic levels by 1–2 months after HSCT, and recovery is unaffected by recipient age or TCD.[28] Analysis of variable heavy chain (VH) gene usage in circulating B lymphocytes early after transplantation shows VH usage similar to that seen in fetal B lymphocytes, indicating that a recapitulation of normal B lymphocyte ontogeny occurs after HSCT.[29] Defects in mucosal IgA production exist for the first six months after transplantation but are normalizing by year except in patients with significant chronic GvHD.[30] Patients without chronic GvHD normalize their serum IgG levels by 8–9 months, their IgM levels by 9–12 months, and their IgA by 2–3 years.[31]

Antigen-Specific Immunity Following HSCT

Antigen-Specific T Lymphocyte Function

The presence of normal numbers of immunophenotypic T and B lymphocytes following HSCT is not adequate for demonstrating that HSCT recipients have normal immunocompetence. In order to maintain protection against opportunistic infections, HSCT recipients need to have antigen-specific T and B lymphocyte immunity, and particularly the ability to respond to neoantigens. Recipients of HSC products (PBCs) that contain a significant number of antigen-specific T lymphocytes may have detectable antigen-specific T lymphocytes early following transplantation. Although it has still not been definitely demonstrated, the presence of the donor-derived antigen-specific T lymphocytes may reduce the incidence of posttransplant infectious complications. The recipients of cord blood or TCD HSC products, which contain no antigen-specific T lymphocytes, will have no passive acquisition of antigen-specific T lymphocytes, and all of their antigen-specific T lymphocyte function would have to be generated by T lymphocytes that are derived from donor HSCs after differentiation through the recipient thymus. Recipients of allogeneic PBCs have antigen-specific T lymphocytes of donor origin early after HSCT, whereas it has not been possible to detect antigen-specific T lymphocytes in the peripheral blood of bone marrow recipients.[13] The difference may be explained in part by the fact that 1–2 logs more T lymphocytes are administered with PBCs than with bone marrow. Also, the routine use of methotrexate for GvHD prophylaxis to eliminate donor-derived T lymphocytes with specificity for recipient histocompatibility antigens may lead to the destruction of donor-derived antigen-specific T lymphocytes that are stimulated by viral and fungal antigens present in the recipient, resulting in the selective loss of those T lymphocytes that are most needed by the recipient for protection against opportunistic infections.

Few studies have been done in which HSC recipients have been challenged with neoantigens to determine their capacity to respond to primary antigen stimulation. Most studies of antigen-specific function have determined the presence of antigen-specific T lymphocytes by measuring their blastogeneic responses to recall antigens [cytomegalovirus (CMV), herpes simplex virus (HSV), varicella zoster virus (VZV)] as well as vaccination antigens such as the tetanus toxoid. Since most donors are immune to one if not all of these recall antigens, it is difficult to determine the origin of the antigen-specific T lymphocyte function following HSCT as both passively acquired donor T lymphocytes and recent thymic emigrants have the potential to respond to these antigens.

The clinical setting which has been most informative about the ability of HSC recipients to respond to a neoantigen has been the evaluation of the recipients of cord blood.[32] Since cord blood has no antigen-specific T lymphocytes, the development of an antigen-specific T lymphocyte response must have occurred in the recipient. However, it is not possible to state definitively whether the passively acquired naïve T lymphocytes contained in cord blood or newly generated T lymphocytes are the source of the antigen-specific function. The longitudinal evaluation of unrelated cord blood recipients has shown that antigen-specific T lymphocytes can be identified as early as one month after transplantation, a time at which no T lymphocytes derived from recipient thymopoiesis are yet present. The observation is the first definitive evidence that the passively acquired naïve T lymphocytes contained in the donor HSC innoculum can give rise to antigen-specific T lymphocytes. In the cord blood study viral reactivation was required to generate the antigeneic stimulus for the development of antigen-specific function, which means that, if there was a lack of viral reactivation, there was no antigenic stimulus to assess whether normal immunocompetence was present. Thus, the lack of antigen-specific function may be due to a lack of antigen stimulation rather than immunoincompetence. Definitive studies in which HSC recipients are sequentially immunized with a neoantigen are necessary in order to determine the kinetics of the ability of HSCT recipients to respond to primary antigeneic stimulation, and in order to determine the impact of variables such as GvHD, recipient age, and conditioning regimens on immune reconstitution.

Just as there is an immunophenotypic recapitulation of normal T lymphocyte ontogeny following transplantation, there is a functional recapitulation of T lymphocyte function. When immunophenotypic T lymphocytes are first present after HSCT and their function is analyzed with stimulation with either mitogens (phytohemagglutin) or specific antigens, the lack of blastogenesis by the T lymphocytes of some recipients can be corrected by the addition of exogenous IL-2, demonstrating that the recipients had T lymphocytes capable of expressing IL-2 receptors but T lymphocytes capable of producing IL-2 were not present.[33,34] Thus, IL-2 receptors expressing T lymphocytes appear earlier in ontogeny than IL-2 producing T lymphocytes. In addition, other defects in cytokine production, particularly γ-interferon, can be identified early following transplantation.[35] When cytoplasmic cytokines are evaluated following antigen stimulation of normal T lymphocytes, γ-interferon production by T lymphocytes is more frequent than IL-2 production. Early following HSCT, however, the frequency of γ-interferon-producing cells is less than that of IL-2-producing cells, which may explain why some recipients with antigen-specific T lymphocyte blastogenesis to herpes viruses, particularly VZV, still have recurrent clinical infections, presumably due to lack of a full range of protective antiviral mechanisms, including the production of γ-interferon and cytotoxic T lymphocytes (CTLs), which may not normalize until a year after HSCT.[36]

Antigen-Specific B Lymphocyte Function

Although following myeloablative conditioning all recipient T lymphocytes are eliminated, not all recipient antibody-producing cells are eliminated. Plasma cells are relatively resistant to the effect of the chemoradiotherapy given prior to HSCT, and recipient antibody production to infectious and vaccination antigens can be detected for up to one year after HSCT, at which time the recipient plasma cells have been replaced by antibody-producing cells of donor origin.[37–39]

By two years after HSCT the majority of recipients can respond to vaccination with protein or viral antigens unless they have significant chronic GvHD. An exception to the general ability of HSCT recipients to respond to vaccination/infection by antibody production is their inability to produce protective levels of antibody to bacterial polysaccharide antigens, which are necessary for protection against infection with respiratory bacteria. Histocompatible recipients with chronic GvHD and all recipients of unrelated PBCs and bone marrow are at increased risk of late bacterial infections.[4,40] Analysis of the ability of HSCT recipients to generate antibody to naturally occurring bacterial polysaccharides, such as polyribosophosphate (PRP), the capsular antigens of *Haemophilus influenzae* type b, reveals a recapitulation of normal antibody ontogeny.[41] In autologous and histocompatible recipients without chronic GvHD, the development of protection levels of anti-PRP antibody is first detected 18 months after HSCT, which corresponds to the time at which normal infants start to produce anti-PRP antibody. However, histocompatible recipients with chronic GvHD and almost all unrelated recipients have a permanent inability to make antipolysaccharide antibodies to wild type infections although they can respond, as normal newborn infants can, to conjugated polysaccharide vaccines. HSCT recipients with an inability to respond to wild type bacterial polysaccharides should be on replacement immunoglobulin therapy or prophylactic antibiotics.

Attempts to Improve Post-HSCT Immune Reconstitution

The sustained inability of HSCT recipients, especially adults receiving TCD HSC products, to generate new T lymphocytes necessary for the development of antigen-specific function and protection against infectious agents, has led to an evaluation of innovative approaches to enhancing post-HSCT immune reconstitution. These approaches can be characterized into two major areas: (1) improvement of recipient thymopoiesis to enhance the ability of the recipients to generate new T lymphocytes, and (2) attempts to adoptively transfer T lymphocytes that have the ability to generate antigen-specific immunity.

Cytokine Therapy

IL-7

Animal studies have shown that IL-7 is a central cytokine in both thymopoiesis and the homeostatic expansion of CD8 T lymphocytes following transplantation. Pretransplant conditioning, especially TBI, and chronic GvHD have a negative impact on the capacity of the thymic epithelial cells to produce IL-7. The posttransplant administration of IL-7 can reverse the defects in thymopoiesis, resulting in normalization of post-HSCT T lymphocyte recovery and generation of antigen-specific T lymphocyte function.[42,43] The first clinical trials with recombinant IL-7 after autologous HSCT have shown that IL-7 increases the numbers of peripheral blood CD4 and CD8 T lymphocytes with a broadening of the TCR diversity.[44] In contrast to the animal experiments which had demonstrated increased thymopoiesis following IL-7 administration, there was no increase in thymic size or the frequency of TREC. Therefore, in these preliminary human studies, most of the biological effects of IL-7 administration are on homeostatic expansion of the existing mature T lymphocytes rather than an improvement in thymic function.

Keratinocyte Growth Factor

A major cause of the thymic dysfunction seen after chemoradiotherapy is a decrease in thymic epithelial cells and the IL-7 production necessary for normal thymic function. Keratinocyte growth factor (KGF) is produced by mesenchymal cells and some thymocytes. In preclinical studies, the administration of KGF before chemotherapy or irradiation protects the thymus against chemoradiotherapy-induced damage with maintenance of relatively normal thymic function with normal peripheral T lymphocyte numbers and function.[45,46] In addition, some experiments have shown decreased GvHD, suggesting that KGF may have a protective effect on the targets of GvHD. KGF also has a protective effect on mucosal epithelial cells and has been approved for clinical administration for this indication. However, human studies have not yet demonstrated that the peritransplant administration of KGF results in maintenance of thymopoietic function or more rapid immune reconstitution.

Androgen Receptor Antagonists

A decade ago animal experiments made the unique observation that castration in aged male mice resulted in a rapid increase in thymic size and improved thymopoiesis.[47] Chemical castration through the administration of androgen receptor antagonists can produce the same biological effects. The mechanism by which the androgen receptor antagonists function is, however, not clear. Preliminary clinical studies have shown improved immunophenotypic recovery after HSCT in noncontrolled investigations.[48] However, definitive studies demonstrating improved antigen-specific function after the administration of androgen receptor antagonists are still needed.

Adoptive Cellular Therapy

Delayed Lymphocyte Infusions

The use of TCD HSC products is linked with an increased incidence of EBV-associated lymphoproliferative disease. Because the increased incidence was found primarily in HSCT recipients who received either *in vivo* or *in vitro* TCD HSCs, a logical clinical response was to infuse donor T lymphocytes so as to improve recipient anti-EBV immunity, i.e. delayed lymphocyte infusions (DLIs).[49] Initially, whole donor peripheral blood cells were infused. Clinical responses of the EBV lymphoproliferative disease to the DLIs were observed, usually starting 2–3 months after the infusion. The major complication of the DLIs was the development of acute GvHD in the majority of recipients, who had clinical responses even though a limited number of T lymphocytes was infused. These experiments, however, clearly demonstrated that the adoptive transfer of donor T lymphocytes was capable of contributing to post-HSCT antigen-specific function.

Antigen-Specific Donor Lymphocyte Infusions

The initial DLIs contained both antigen-specific and naïve T lymphocytes, some of which had the potential to respond to recipient histocompatibility antigens and, therefore, initiate GvHD. In an attempt to provide the benefits of the infusion of antigen-specific T lymphocytes without the associated risks of acute and chronic GvHD, T lymphocyte clones were established with specificity to CMV.[50] These clones were then pedigreed in proliferative assays to demonstrate that they were CMV-specific and that they did not have alloreactivity to recipient-restricted histocompatibility antigens. In prophylactic studies the infusion of the CMV clones eliminated the risk of CMV disease in seropositive recipients without clinical GvHD. These pioneering studies were followed by studies with T lymphocyte clones to *Aspergillus*. *Aspergillus*-specific T lymphocyte clones without alloreactivity were infused into recipients at high risk of pulmonary *Aspergillus* disease. There was markedly improved survival in the treated recipients, demonstrating that the adoptive transfer of donor-derived antigen-specific T lymphocytes could contribute to posttransplant immunocompetence with clinical benefit.

Alloreactive-Depleted Donor Lymphocyte Infusions

The initial studies with antigen-specific T lymphocyte clones demonstrated the benefit of adoptive cellular therapy. There are several limitations to the approach: (1) cost, since clones have to be derived from each donor and screened for specificity and alloreactivity; (2) protection is achieved only for the antigen/agent to which the clones were specific. In order to improve posttransplant immunity, especially to give cells in a prophylactic manner, it is necessary to infuse naïve donor T lymphocytes, which have the capacity *in vivo* to respond to neoantigens in the same manner that was seen after the transplantation of cord blood cells. Therefore, it has been necessary to develop strategies for removing the alloreactive T lymphocytes contained in the donor peripheral blood T lymphocytes while retaining the naïve and antigen-specific T lymphocytes. Studies have been completed in which the donor T lymphocytes were stimulated *in vitro* with recipient antigen-presenting cells and then the alloreactive donor T lymphocytes, identified by the expression of CD25, were removed by either columns or immunotoxins.[51,52] The administration of these alloreactive-depleted donor T lymphocytes has been clinically evaluated, with improvement in the recipient immunophenotypic T lymphocyte recovery and the detection of antigen-specific T lymphocyte responses.

Anergization

The administration of alloreactive-depleted donor T lymphocytes has been characterized by clinically acceptable levels of GvHD. Therefore, investigators have undertaken studies to determine if it is possible to anergize the donor T lymphocytes against the recipient histocompatibility antigens rather than physically removing them. Normal T lymphocyte activation requires the stimulation of naïve T lymphocytes through their TCR and costimulatory molecules (CD28, B7.1). The blockade of the costimulatory molecules results in the T lymphocytes being stimulated only through their TCR and the development of T lymphocyte anergy to the stimulating histocompatible antigens. Studies on haploidentical transplantation, in which the donor bone marrow was stimulated for 36 h with recipient cells in the presence of CTLA4-Ig antibody, resulted in donor HSC engraftment with no clinically significant GvHD.[53] Because of concerns about prolonged *in vivo* incubation of the HSC product, subsequent studies have evaluated the infusion on day 35 of donor peripheral blood T lymphocytes that have been stimulated with recipient cells in the presence of anti–B7.1 and B7.2 antibodies — a time at which donor HSC engraftment has been established.[54] These preliminary studies have demonstrated that the anergized T lymphocytes can be safely infused without clinically significant GvHD and the recipients have more rapid immunophenotypic T lymphocyte reconstitution. However, definitive studies to demonstrate that their antigen-specific T lymphocyte function is improved and that the recipients have a decreased incidence of clinical infections have yet to be done.

Haploidentical HSCT

Haploidentical HSCT has the advantage that almost all individuals have a potential HSC donor who is readily available without the delays associated with obtaining unrelated bone marrow or the limitations on size associated with the use of unrelated cord blood.[55] Traditionally, haploidentical HSCT has been done with TCD products, resulting in significant delays in immune reconstitution, especially in adult recipients who have had prior chemotherapy. The present HSCT protocols use TBI, which additionally damages the recipient thymus, resulting in a reduced capacity of the recipient thymus to support the development of a new immune system. Initially, GCSF was administered after haploidentical TCD transplantation to hasten myeloid engraftment. However, studies have demonstrated that the GCSF had a negative effect on immune reconstitution, and the routine post-HSCT administration of GCSF has been discontinued.[56]

To reduce the posttransplant complications seen after haploidentical transplantation, including infectious complications and/or neoplastic relapse, the defective immune reconstitution presently associated with haploidentical transplantation has to be improved. The two major strategies, which may be clinically integrated, would be first to improve recipient thymopoiesis by the administration of drugs such as KGF which protect the thymus from the deleterious effects of the chemoradiotherapy used in the preparatory regimen, and/or the administration of drugs such as IL-7 and androgen receptor antagonists to improve recipient thymopoiesis.

Secondly, recipients should receive anergized or alloreactive-depleted T lymphocytes to obtain a broad T lymphocyte repertoire of both antigen-specific and naïve T lymphocytes. It must be noted that, if only mature T lymphocytes are infused without the establishment of normal thymopoiesis, recipients would with time develop defects in their TCR repertoire, resulting in immunodeficiency. Therefore, the most effective approach to improving the immune reconstitution of haploidentical HSCT recipients would be (1) to infuse donor T lymphocytes incapable of alloreactivity following HSCT so as to generate a population of T lymphocytes capable responding to both infectious and neoplastic antigens early following transplantation, and (2) to use drugs capable of correcting/preventing thymic damage so that the donor HSCs can undergo normal thymic differentiation.

Acknowledgment

This study was supported by a grant from the National Institutes of Health and the National Cancer Institute to Robertson Parkman and Neena Kapoor (PO1 CA100265).

References

1. Storek J, Geddes M, Khan F *et al.* (2008) Reconstitution of the immune system after hematopoietic stem cell transplantation in humans. *Semin Immunopathol* **30**: 425–437.
2. Parkman R, Cohen G, Carter SL *et al.* (2006) Successful immune reconstitution decreases leukemic relapse and improves survival in recipients of unrelated cord blood transplantation. *Biol Blood Marrow Transplant* **12**: 919–927.
3. Witherspoon RP, Lum LG, Storb R. (1984) Immunologic reconstitution after human marrow grafting. *Semin Hematol* **21**: 2–10.

4. Ochs L, Shu XO, Miller J *et al.* (1995) Late infections after allogeneic bone marrow transplantation: Comparison of incidence in related and unrelated donor transplant recipients. *Blood* **86**: 3979–3986.

5. Storek J, Gooley T, Witherspoon RP *et al.* (1997) Infectious morbidity in long-term survivors of allogeneic marrow transplantation is associated with low CD4 T cell counts. *Am J Hematol* **54**: 131–138.

6. Bahceci E, Epperson D, Douek DC *et al.* (2003) Early reconstitution of the T-cell repertoire after non-myeloablative peripheral blood stem cell transplantation is from post-thymic T-cell expansion and is unaffected by graft-versus-host disease or mixed chimaerism. *Br J Haematol* **122**: 934–943.

7. Sprent J, Boehmer HV, Nabholz M. (1975) Association of immunity and tolerance to host H-2 determinants in irradiated F1 hybrid mice reconstituted with bone marrow cells from one parental strain. *J Exp Med* **142**(2): 321–331.

8. Reisner Y, Kapoor N, Kirkpatrick D *et al.* (1983) Transplantation for severe combined immunodeficiency with HLA-A, B, D, DR incompatible parental marrow cells fractionated by soybean agglutinin and sheep red blood cells. *Blood* **61**: 341–348.

9. Aversa F, Tabilio A, Verlardi *et al.* (1998) Treatment of high-risk acute leukemia with T cell-depleted stem cells from related donors with one fully mismatched HLA haplotype. *N Engl J Med* **339**: 1186–1193.

10. Jakubowski AA, Small TN, Young JW *et al.* (2007) T cell-depleted stem-cell transplantation for adults with hematologic malignancies: Sustained engraftment of HLA-matched related donor grafts without the use of antithymocyte globulin. *Blood* **110**: 4452–4459.

11. Storek J, Dawson MA, Stoere B *et al.* (2001) Immune reconstitution after allogeneic marrow transplantation compared with blood stem cell transplantation. *Blood* **97**: 3380–3389.

12. Schmitz N, Eapen M, Horowitz MM *et al.* (2006) Long-term outcome of patients given transplants of mobilized blood or bone marrow: A report from the International Bone Marrow Transplant Registry and the European Group for Blood and Marrow Transplantation. *Blood* **108**: 4288–4290.

13. Ottinger HD, Beelen DW, Scheulen B *et al.* (1996) Improved immune reconstitution after allotransplantation of peripheral blood stem cells instead of bone marrow. *Blood* **88**: 2775–2779.

14. Rocha V, Wagner JE Jr., Sobocinski KA *et al.* (2000) Graft-versus-host disease in children who have received a cord-blood or bone marrow transplant from an HLA-identical sibling. *N Engl J Med* **342**: 1846–1854.

15. Rocha V, Cornish J, Sievers EL *et al.* (2001) Comparison of outcomes of unrelated bone marrow and umbilical cord blood transplants in children with acute leukemia. *Blood* **97**: 2962–2970.

16. Weinberg KI, Annett GM, Kashyap A *et al.* (1995) The effect of thymic function on immunocompetence following bone marrow transplantation. *Biol Blood Marrow Transplant* **1**: 18–23.

17. Mackall CL, Fleisher TA, Brown MR *et al.* (1995) Age, thympoiesis, and $CD4^+$ T-lymphocyte regeneration after intensive chemotherapy. *N Engl J Med* **332**: 143–149.

18. Kouek DC, Vescio RA, Betts MR *et al.* (2000) Assessment of thymic output in adults after haematopoietic stem-cell transplantation and prediction of T cell reconstitution. *Lancet* **355**: 1875–1881.

19. Krenger W, Holländer GA. (2008) The immunopathology of thymic GvHD. *Semin Immunopathol* **30**: 439–456.

20. Weinberg K, Blazar BR, Wagner JE *et al.* (2001) Factors affecting thymic function after allogeneic hematopoietic stem cell transplantation. *Blood* **97**: 1458–1466.

21. Koehne G, Zeller W, Stockschlaeder M, Zander AR. (2007) Phenotype of lymphocyte subsets after autologous peripheral blood stem cell transplantation. *Bone Marrow Transplant* **19**: 149–156.

22. Singh RK, Varney ML, Leutzinger C *et al.* (2007) Immune reconstitution after autologous hematopoietic transplantation with Lin^-, $CD34^+$, Thy-1^{lo} selected or intact stem cell products. *Int Immunopharmacol* **7**: 1033–1043.

23. Mackall CL, Stein D, Fleisher TA *et al.* (2002) Prolonged CD4 depletion after sequential autologous peripheral blood progenitor cell infusions in children and young adults. *Blood* **96**: 754–762.

24. Linch DC, Knott LJ, Thomas RM *et al.* (1983) T cell regeneration after allogeneic and autologous bone marrow transplantation. *Br J Haematol* **53**: 451–458.

25. Atkinson K. (1990) Reconstitution of the haemopoietic and immune systems after marrow transplantation. *Bone Marrow Transplant* **5**: 2009–2026.

26. Small TN, Papadopoulos EB, Boulad F *et al.* (1999) Comparison of immune reconstitution after unrelated and related T cell-depleted bone marrow transplantation: Effect of patient age and donor leukocyte infusions. *Blood* **93**: 467–480.

27. O'Reilly RJ, Keever CA, Small TN, Brochstein J. (1989) The use of HLA-non-identical T cell-deplete marrow transplants for correction of severe combined immunodeficiency disease. *Immunodeficiency Rev* **1**: 273–309.

28. Ault KE, Antin JH, Ginsburg D *et al.* (1985) Phenotype of recovering lymphoid cell populations after marrow transplantation. *J Exp Med* **161**: 1483–1502.

29. Storek J, King L, Ferrara S *et al.* (1994) Abundance of a restricted fetal B cell repertoire in marrow transplant recipients. *Bone Marrow Transplant* **14**: 783–790.

30. Chaushu S, Chaushu G, Garfunkel AA *et al.* (1994) Salivary immunoglobulins in recipients of bone marrow grafts. 1. A longitudinal follow-up. *Bone Marrow Transplant* **14**: 871–876.

31. Noel Dr, Witherspoon RP, Storb R *et al.* (1978) Does graft-versus-host-disease influence the tempo of immunologic recovery after allogeneic human marrow transplantation? An observation on long-term survivors. *Blood* **51**: 1087–1105.

32. Cohen G, Carter SL, Weinberg KI *et al.* (2006) Antigen-specific T-lymphocyte function after cord blood transplantation. *Biol Blood Marrow Transplant* **12**: 1335–1342.

33. Roosnek EE, Brouwer MC, Vossen JM *et al.* (1987) The role of interleukin-2 in proliferative responses *in vitro* of T cells from patients after bone marrow transplantation. *Transplantation* **43**: 855–860.

34. Welte K, Kobanu N, More MAS *et al.* (1984) Defective interleukin-2 production in patients after bone marrow transplantation and *in vitro* restoration of defective T-lymphocyte proliferation by highly purified interleukin 2. *Blood* **64**: 380–385.

35. Levin MJ, Parkman R, Oxman MN *et al.* (1978) Proliferative and interferon responses following transplantation in man. *Inf Immun* **20**: 678–684.

36. Quinnan GV, Kirmani N, Rook AH *et al.* (1982) Cytotoxic cells in cytomegalovirus infection: HLA-restricted T-lymphocyte and non-T-lymphocyte cytotoxic responses correlate with recovery from cytomegalovirus infection in bone marrow transplant recipients. *N Engl J Med* **307**: 7–13.

37. Wahren B, Gahrton G, Linde A *et al.* (1984) Transfer and persistence of viral antibody-producing cells in bone marrow transplantation. *J Infec Dis* **150**: 358–365.

38. Shiobara S, Lum LG, Witherspoon RP, Storb R. (1985) Antigen-specific antibody responses of lymphocytes to tetanus toxoid after human marrow transplantation. *Transplantation* **41**: 587–592.

39. Lum LG, Munn NA, Schanfield MS, Storb R. (1986) The detection of specific antibody formation to recall antigens after human bone marrow transplantation. *Blood* **67**: 582–587.

40. Atkinson K, Storb R, Prentice RL *et al.* (1979) Analysis of late infections in 89 long-term survivors of bone marrow transplantation. *Blood* **53**: 720–731.

41. Kapoor N, Chan R, Weinberg KI *et al.* (1999) Defective anticarbohydrate antibody responses to naturally occurring bacteria following bone marrow transplantation. *Biol Blood Marrow Transplant* **5**: 46–50.

42. Bolotin E, Smogorzewska M, Smith S *et al.* (1996) Enhancement of thymopoiesis after bone marrow transplant by *in vivo* interleukin-7. *Blood* **88**: 1887–1894.

43. Mackall CL, Fry TJ, Bare C *et al.* (2001) IL-7 increases both thymic-dependent and thymic-independent T-cell regeneration after bone marrow transplantation. *Blood* **97**: 1491–1497.

44. Sportès C, Hakim FT, Memon SA *et al.* (2008) Administration of rhIL-7 in humans increases *in vivo* TCR repertoire diversity by preferential expansion of naïve T cell subsets. *J Exp Med* **205**: 1701–1714.

45. Rossi S, Blazar BR, Farrell CL *et al.* (2002) Keratinocyte growth factor preserves normal thymopoiesis and thymic microenvironment during experimental graft-versus-host disease. *Blood* **100**: 682–691.

46. Min D, Panoskaltsis-Morari A, Kuro OM *et al.* (2007) Sustained thymopoiesis and improvement in functional immunity induced exogenous KGF administration in murine models of aging. *Blood* **109**: 2529–2537.

47. Windmill KF, Lee VW. (1986) Effects of castration on the lymphocytes of the thymus, spleen and lymph nodes. *J Endocrinol* **110**: 417–422.

48. Sutherland JS, Spyroglou L, Muirhead JL *et al.* (2008) Enhanced immune system regeneration in humans following allogeneic or autologous hemopoietic stem cell transplantation by temporary sex steroid blockade. *Clin Cancer Res* **14**: 1138–1149.

49. Papadopoulos EB, Ladanyi M, Emanuel D *et al.* (1994) Infusions of donor leukocytes to treat Epstein–Barr virus-associated lymphoproliferative disorders after allogeneic bone marrow transplantation. *N Engl J Med* **330**: 1185–1191.

50. Perruccio K, Tosti A, Burchielli E *et al.* (2005) Transferring functional immune responses to pathogens after haploidentical hematopoietic transplantation. *Blood* **106**: 4397–4406.

51. Davies JK, Koh MB, Lowdell MW. (2004) Antiviral immunity and T-regulatory cell function are retained after selective alloreactive T cell depletion in both the HLA-identical and HLA-mismatched settings. *Biol Blood Marrow Transplant* **10**: 259–268.

52. Amrolia PJ, Muccioli-Casadei G, Hus H *et al.* (2006) Adoptive immunotherapy with allodepleted donor T-cells improves immune reconstitution after haploidentical stem cell transplantation. *Blood* **108**: 1797–1808.

53. Guinan EC, Boussiotis VA, Neuberg D *et al.* (1999) Transplantation of anergic histoincompatible bone marrow allografts. *N Engl J Med* **340**: 1704–1714.

54. Davies JK, Gribben JG, Brennan LL *et al.* (2008) Outcome of alloanergized haploidentical bone marrow transplantation after *ex vivo* costimulatory blockade: Results of 2 phase 1 studies. *Blood* **112**: 2232–2241.

55. Aversa F. (2008) Haploidentical haematopoietic stem cell transplantation for acute leukaemia in adults: Experience in Europe and the United States. *Bone Marrow Transplant* **41**: 473–481.

56. Volpi I, Perriccio K, Tosti A *et al.* (2001) Postgrafting administration of granulocyte colony-stimulating factor impairs functional immune recovery in recipients of human leukocyte antigen haplotype-mismatched hematopoietic transplants. *Blood* **97**: 2514–2521.

Chapter 14

The Role of the Thymus in Hematopoietic Stem Cell Transplantation

Werner Krenger[*,†] *and Georg A. Holländer*[*,‡]

Introduction

The present cytoreductive conditioning regimens in the context of hematopoietic stem cell transplantation (HSCT) cause deficits within the immune system. Either transient or protracted in nature, the post-HSCT immune deficiency can last for more than a year and is invariably associated with an increased risk of opportunistic infections, inflammation, reactivation of latent infections, disease relapse and the development of secondary malignancies. Hence, rebuilding innate and adaptive immunity is a critical issue for patients receiving HSCT (for recent reviews see Refs. 1–15). The process of posttransplant immune reconstitution depends on two — but not mutually exclusive — pathways which involve (1) the clonal expansion of donor graft- and residual host-derived mature hematopoietic cells in the host periphery, and (2) the *de novo* generation of lymphoid and myeloid lineage cells from the transferred hematopoietic stem cells (HSCs). Whereas the innate immune system (specifically epithelial barriers, phagocytes and natural killer cells) typically recovers

*Laboratory of Pediatric Immunology, Department of Biomedicine, University of Basel, Mattenstrasse 28, 4058 Basel, Switzerland. E-mails: [†]werner.krenger@unibas.ch, [‡]georg-a.hollaender@unibas.ch

within a few weeks posttransplant, the renewal of the adaptive immune system is subject to a complex and slow process which usually takes months (for B cells) to years (for T cells) to be accomplished, even under favorable conditions.[7,8,13,15]

Inadequate T cell reconstitution after HSCT is associated with infections by viruses, fungi and bacteria, and serves as a prognostic indicator for poor transplant outcome.[16–21] Knowledge regarding the size and quality of the T cell compartment in patients who have received lymphodepleting conditioning and HSCT will hence be paramount for establishing an optimal management of transplant-related immunodeficiency. It is now recognized that the speed of T cell reconstitution following HSCT is determined by multiple parameters: host factors such as age, gender, type of conditioning and underlying pathology; genetic differences between donor and host; stem cell source; post-HSCT events such as acute and chronic graft-versus-host disease (GvHD) and their respective therapies; relapse of malignancy; and infection by various microbial pathogens contribute to the kinetics of peripheral T cell recovery.[13] Early T cell immunity present in transplant recipients may be provided by residual, conditioning resistant host T cells or, alternatively, by passively transferred naïve or memory T cells of donor origin. However, as the oligoclonal expansion of these cell populations confers a limited degree of immune competence, new T cells need to be generated, which in turn necessitates an intact thymic function. The thymic generation of new T cells assures the long-term regeneration of a broad T cell antigen receptor (TCR) repertoire able to recognize a wide range of antigens. The cellular and molecular mechanisms operational in the maintenance of thymic function in healthy, diseased and aged individuals have therefore received considerable attention over the last few years. The gained insights reveal that thymus-dependent T cell reconstitution is limited by age-related thymic changes, pretransplant conditioning and, particularly, existing GvHD. This chapter discusses recent insight into how GvHD affects thymic function and how an understanding of the molecular and cellular mechanisms of this pathology may aid the design of new therapeutic approaches that boost thymic function after HSCT and thus T cell reconstitution.

Normal Postnatal Thymic T Cell Maturation and Export

The thymus is the primary site of T lymphopoiesis during fetal and early postnatal life.[22–26] Arranged in distinct phenotypic compartments, such as the subcapsular region, the cortex, the cortical–medullary junction and the medulla, the typical structural organization of the thymus displays several features that are highly conserved between different vertebrate species and may hence reflect their importance for thymic function.

The Thymic Lymphoid Compartment

Within the thymus, lymphoid cells develop in an ordered maturational progression from immature precursors to phenotypically and functionally mature T cells that express an appropriately selected TCR. As the thymus does not contain precursor stem cells with an unlimited self-renewal capacity, T cell progenitors need to be continuously recruited from the bone marrow via the blood to maintain permanent thymopoiesis. These precursors enter the thymus at the corticomedullary junction and bear a $CD3^-CD4^-CD8^-$ (triple negative, TN) phenotype. Once positioned within the thymic microenvironment, these cells are commonly termed "early thymic precursors" (ETPs) and develop in close physical and functional interaction with thymic epithelial cells (TECs) (see Refs. 27 and 28; discussed in more detail below). Maturation of the TN thymocytes occurs in the depth of the cortex and in the subcapsular region along several well-defined developmental stages, which are typically characterized by phenotypic changes and robust cell proliferation. Thymocytes that have concomitantly acquired a $CD4^+CD8^+$ (double positive, DP) phenotype represent the next sequential stage in intrathymic T cell development. As DP cells assemble and express a complete but randomly chosen TCR $\alpha\beta$/CD3 complex, they are subjected at this stage of development to a stringent selection that assures the utility of the chosen TCR specificity. It is the designated purpose of this process, known as positive thymic selection, to pick TCRs that display a sufficiently high affinity for the combination of self-peptides and self-MHC (p-MHC) complexes expressed by cortical (c) TECs. Thymocytes that bear a TCR with these specifications will receive a signal that prevents a default program of apoptosis and stimulates further differentiation of the cells. In contrast, DP thymocytes will undergo apoptosis if their TCR displays an affinity for p-MHC that is too small to elicit such a survival signal. Positively selected DP thymocytes that are restricted in their antigen recognition to MHC class I molecules will keep the expression of CD8 on their cell surface while downmodulating that of CD4, whereas DP thymocytes that express an MHC class II–restricted TCR will adopt upon further differentiation a $CD4^+CD8^-$ phenotype. These so-called single positive (SP) thymocytes accumulate in the medulla, where their TCR specificity is now monitored for reactivity to self-peptides presented by either medullary (m) TECs or dendritic cells (DCs) and possibly other bone-marrow-derived stromal cells. Known as negative thymic selection, this step in the maturation of T cells results in the clonal deletion of those thymocytes that express a TCR with a high affinity for the p-MHC complexes.[29] Positive and negative selection shape a repertoire of TCRs which endows the adaptive immune system with the capacity to respond to a seemingly unlimited array of foreign ("Nonself") antigens whilst remaining unresponsive to the host's own tissues ("Self"). This essential capacity is referred to as central (i.e. thymic) T cell tolerance induction. During the obligatory post-selection maturation in the medulla, which usually lasts in the mouse between 7–10 days, thymocytes acquire full functional competence and the ability to be exported to the periphery.[30]

T cells are continuously exported to peripheral lymphoid tissues by mechanisms that are only incompletely understood at present but that are seemingly independent of a feedback mechanism sensing the number of peripheral T cells.[31] Informative cell surface markers that accurately identify recent thymic emigrants (RTEs) among mature peripheral T cells are lacking for both mice and humans. Consequently, it has been difficult in practice to precisely estimate *in vivo* the thymic export of new T cells during the steady state and under conditions of disease. The expression of CD45 splice variants is commonly but not always correctly used as a marker to enumerate naïve (i.e. CD45RA$^+$) T cells. However, the number of T cells expressing CD45RA should not simply be taken as a measure for thymic output of naïve T cells, since these cells may expand peripherally without changing their phenotype and since CD45RO$^+$ T cells can revert to a CD45RA$^+$ phenotype despite their continued function as memory T cells.[32] Detection of other cell surface markers such as CD62L, CD27, CD31 or CD103 ($\alpha E\beta 7$ integrin) may also aid in the identification of human naïve T cells, but again, their cell surface expression is not exclusive for RTEs.[2,9,33–35] As a consequence, thymic T cell output has been quantified in more recent studies by measuring T cell receptor rearrangement excision circles (TRECs).[2,3,36–50] These extrachromosomal DNA circles are generated during DNA rearrangement steps to build either the TCR-β-chain from the TCRB locus or the TCR-α-chain from the TCRAD locus.[36,51,52] The TCRB locus is recombined in TN thymocytes and forms Dβ-JβTREC, whereas the TCRAD locus is rearranged in DP thymocytes and generates sjTREC. Since the TCRB recombination occurs prior to TN expansion and because episomal DNA circles cannot replicate with cell division, Dβ-JβTREC are progressively diluted among TN thymocytes as these cells proliferate and progress to adopt a DP phenotype. The sj/Dβ-JβTREC ratio thus provides a quantitative marker for the proliferation of thymocytes that have rearranged their TCRB locus.[52] As the magnitude of TN expansion is the key determinant of the number of RTEs exported,[53] it is the sj/DβJβ TREC ratio measured among peripheral T cells that serves as a suitable marker to quantify thymic output.[52]

New T cells are generated in the thymus throughout life but the size of this organ and in consequence the number of RTE changes as a function of age.[11] Thymic T cell output in humans is particularly high during the fetal and perinatal period, but thymopoietic function and consequently the exit of naïve T cells decrease swiftly following the first year of life and again shortly before and with puberty. Although structural and functional involution are hallmarks of the aging thymus and are already present at a relatively young age, phenotypically naïve TREC$^+$ cells can still be detected in the peripheral blood of octogenarians and even older individuals.[54–56] Physiological thymic involution affects both the lymphoid and the stromal compartments of the thymus, and is paralleled by an increase in perivascular space and adipose tissue.[57,58] Several endogenous and exogenous factors have been identified to promote thymic involution, among which sex steroids, insulin-like growth factor, glucocorticoids and inflammatory cytokines are those that have been investigated best (reviewed in Refs. 11, 59 and 60). The finding that age determines the kinetics by which lymphoid tissue is populated by RTEs has been made by studies detailing the rate at which the CD4$^+$ T cell compartment is rebuilt in complication-free recipients of an autologous HSCT. This process necessitates two and more years in adult transplant recipients, whereas normal CD4$^+$ T cell counts are recovered in children within a year of transplantation.[45] At an advanced stage in its structural remodeling (as typically observed in individuals at 50 and more years of age), the thymus remains permanently compromised in function as it does not substantially recover its size or thymopoietic activity following conditioning and HSCT.[60,61] In consequence, the delayed kinetics observed in the older transplant recipient has been linked to the enhanced susceptibility of older transplant recipients to suffer from immunodeficiency and/or autoimmunity.

The Thymic Stromal Compartment

In addition to autochthonous epithelial cells, the thymic stromal compartment also contains mesenchymal cells such as reticular fibroblasts and hematopoietic cells, including DCs and macrophages. Together, these cells form a complex microenvironment that is not only competent to attract bloodborne T cell precursors but also uniquely able to efficiently support the survival, expansion, differentiation and selection of thymocytes so that functionally and phenotypically mature T cells are generated. TECs constitute the most abundant component of the thymic stroma. Contrary to epithelia in all other tissues, the vast majority of TECs lack the typical cell polarity of epithelia and are not placed on a basal membrane but arranged via dendrite-like processes that form cell–cell contacts in a three-dimensional orientation to form a continuous network.[25,27,28]

The epithelium itself is phenotypically and functionally heterogeneous not only between the structurally distinct cortical and medullary compartments but also within these domains. While TEC subsets still await a refined characterization in the human, several cell surface and cytoplasmic molecules precisely distinguish in the mouse the separate TEC subpopulations. For example, the expression of the cytokeratins-5 (K5) and K18 in conjunction with the detection of a UEA-1 binding lectin and other not-yet-well-characterized cell surface glycoproteins allows one to identify cTECs and mTECs as well as subpopulations within these particular groups of thymic epithelia (murine major cortical TECs display a $K18^+K5^-UEA-1^-MTS10^-$ phenotype, the minor cortical TECs are $K18^+K5^+UEA-1^-MTS10^-$, major medullary TECs are characterized as $K5^+MTS10^+$ and minor medullary epithelial cells stain $K18^+UEA-1^+$ [22,62,63]). The microenvironment built by cTECs supports the initial (i.e. most immature) stages of intrathymic T cell development and enforces the probing of the TCR affinity required for positive selection. In contrast, mTECs together with DCs enriched at the cortical–medullary junction but also dispersed throughout the medulla are responsible for negative thymic selection.

By virtue of specialized TEC subpopulations, the thymus is able to generate immunological tolerance not only to ubiquitous self-antigens but also to antigens that are typically expressed in a tissue-restricted fashion. Whereas the need for negative selection of TCR specificities recognizing the most common if not all self-antigens was appreciated as a necessity to effect meaningful central T cell tolerance, the molecular control of this vital process remained for a long time largely enigmatic. However, elegant studies have now demonstrated that mTECs have the unique capacity to express in a promiscuous manner a vast array of different organ-specific antigens.[64,65] Medullary epithelial cells thus express and present a "molecular mirror of peripheral self" and hence permit the negative selection of TCRs that recognize with a high affinity these tissue-restricted antigens (TRAs) when complexed to self-MHC molecules.[64,66] Some of these TRAs are in their expression under the control of the transcription factor Aire (autoimmune regulator).[67] Lack of functional Aire expression is the genetic cause of the autoimmune polyendocrinopathy–candidiasis–ectodermal dystrophy (APS-1) syndrome, an autosomal recessive disorder marked by the persistence of autoreactive T cells in the periphery.[68] Direct evidence for a decisive role of Aire in negative thymic selection has been provided by experiments with TCR transgenic mice where expression of the cognate antigen is under the control of Aire.[69,70] Under these experimental conditions, a correlation was established between the level of Aire expression, the number of TRA-specific transcripts controlled by Aire and the extent of negative selection affecting T cells with TCRs specific for a given TRA. The precise regulation of Aire expression is thus indispensable for shaping correctly a TCR repertoire that is devoid of high affinity specificities directed at self-antigens. Since the process of clonal deletion of self-reactive T cells is not entirely efficient, additional mechanisms are fortunately in place that secure the induction of self-tolerance. For example, the thymus generates a population of regulatory T cells (T_{reg}) that are characterized by their signature $CD4^+CD25^+$ phenotype and the expression of the transcription factor Foxp3. The function of T_{reg} cells is to control those self-reactive T cells that have wrongly escaped negative thymic selection and settled in peripheral tissues.[71–73] For their formation, T_{reg} cells require a TCR that binds with a high enough affinity to its cognate p-MHC ligand on TECs and thymic DCs. It remains, however, unknown how this level of TCR affinity shuns the typical fate of such interactions, namely negative selection. The relative contribution of TECs and DCs in fostering this generation of T_{reg} cells is still not settled and awaits to be resolved.[74,75]

Pathways of Posttransplant T Cell Regeneration

Preclinical and clinical studies have examined the role of the thymus in the regeneration of the T cell compartment following conditioning-dependent lymphodepletion and HSCT. As discussed in more detail elsewhere,[1,2,5–9,11,15,35,43,56,76,77] these studies have first and foremost demonstrated that the kinetics of T cell reconstitution is variable owing to differences in the selection of donors and recipients, the regimens employed for the conditioning of recipients and the graft preparation used. Specifically, the following parameters have been identified to play a significant role in clinical practice: the degree of relevant genetic differences between donor and recipient, the age of the recipient, the use of T cell-depleted (TCD) versus unmanipulated grafts, the infusion of bone marrow versus mobilized peripheral blood stem cells (PBSCs), myeloablative versus nonmyeloablative pretreatment, and the presence of transplant-related complications such as GvHD. Despite these factors influencing the kinetics of T cell repletion following HSCT, some general conclusions can be drawn from the studies discussed below.

Thymic-Independent T Cell Regeneration

The early response to severe lymphodepletion is driven by donor and residual host T cells (the former having been transferred as part of the HSC graft or as a delayed lymphocyte infusion[7,56,78–80]). These T cells respond by homeostatic proliferation to low avidity ligand signals.[81] However, high avidity antigenic signals trigger robust cell division.[7] Whereas rapid recovery of CD8[+] T cells can be attained by peripheral homeostatic expansion, this mechanism does not suffice alone to swiftly replenish the CD4[+] T cell pool. Rather, the reconstitution of CD4[+] T cells is primarily dependent on thymic output (see below). Detected in the peripheral blood during the first few months following conditioning or their transfer, T cells are responsive *in vitro* to unspecific mitogenic stimuli such as phytohemagglutinin (PHA) and proliferate *in vivo* upon exposure to previously experienced nominal antigens.[82] Hence, it is the recipient's antigenic milieu that as a consequence of antigen recognition skews the TCR repertoire toward particular specificities.[83,84] The observed T cell expansion is, however, transient and characterized both by clonal exhaustion of cells that have undergone extensive replication, and by a heightened susceptibility to apoptosis.[7,53,56,85,86] Moreover, activation-induced cell death (AICD) of alloreactive donor T cells may be coupled in T-cell-replete HSCT with bystander apoptosis of concomitantly grafted but nonhost-reactive T cells, an aspect that further increases the risk of poor immune reconstitution.[87] Another important issue related to the presence of T cells early after HSCT concerns the observation that the infusion of a TCD bone marrow inoculum is strongly associated with an increased incidence of CMV infections and EBV-associated lymphoproliferative disorders.[88,89] Therefore, memory T cells generated in the donor in response to specific pathogens and transferred with the HSC graft may transiently aid in protecting conditioned recipients from relevant posttransplant infections including CMV and EBV. CD8[+] memory T cells respond more readily to previously encountered pathogens and display an enhanced capacity to enter tissues when compared to naïve T cells. These functional features and their obvious significance for the T lymphopenic phase early after HSCT can be therapeutically exploited. For example, genetically engineered cytotoxic T lymphocytes (CTLs) have been successfully employed that are specific for certain viral and fungal infections.[90,91]

Thymic-dependent T Cell Regeneration: The Phenotype...

Independent of an inadvertent or intentionally therapeutic transfer of mature T cells, sustained immunity with a high TCR diversity can only be achieved over time in HSCT recipients by a sizeable pool of naïve T cells. Reconstitution with naïve T cells is lacking in both experimental animal models and transplant recipients in the absence of a thymus or is severely impaired under conditions where thymus function is compromised.[38,44,56,78,92–95] Although there is some evidence for extrathymic differentiation at various anatomical sites,[96] the intrathymic maturation of new (and hence naïve) T cells constitutes the only relevant pathway by which the T cell compartment is regenerated in a robust and functional fashion. The relative contributions of the thymus-dependent pathway launched by bone-marrow-derived precursors and the thymus-independent pathway of peripheral T cell expansion are variable and influenced by different factors such as age, the development of transplant-related complications and their treatment (see below). The potential for thymic renewal is unquestionably present in younger individuals but restricted or absent in older patients (> 50 years of age).[11] Following HSCT, an enlargement of the thymus can be observed in the first few months after engraftment, a phenomenon occasionally referred to as "thymic rebound".[97,98] The kinetics and extent of thymopoietic reconstitution following lymphodepletion and HSCT are predictive for the number of naïve T cells that will be exported to and detected in the periphery.

The number of peripheral T cells is, under physiological conditions, primarily regulated by the mechanisms of homeostatic expansion.[56,81] Hence, *de novo* T cell export from the thymus plays only a minor role in maintaining peripheral T cell numbers in a healthy individual, even in the face of the several million naïve T cells that are exported daily from a normal thymus at young age.[99] However, under conditions of severe lymphopenia, the thymus plays a critical role in T cell homeostasis, and the extent of thymic insufficiency as caused by aging, cytoreductive treatment or transplant-related toxicities (TRTs) will determine the efficiency with which the peripheral T cell compartment is reconstituted. Because several weeks are required before mature thymic T cells arise from bone-marrow-resident precursors even under optimal conditions,[99,100] it is not surprising that a substantial restoration of the T cell compartment with naïve cells is a very time-consuming process. The immunophenotypic analysis of peripheral blood mononuclear cells (PBMCs) does not disclose meaningful numbers of circulating naïve CD3$^+$ T cells until 2–3 months after transplantation of allogeneic, TCD bone marrow.[82] Intriguingly, this length of time is comparable to the 8–12 weeks required during human fetal development for the most immature thymocytes to progress to mature T cells that can now be detected in the peripheral blood. Independent of specific transplantation protocols employed, peripheral T cell recovery is typically represented by the emergence of CD45RA$^+$, CD62L$^+$ T cells that harbor TRECs.[2,3,6,9,13,15,16,19,38,43,44,46,56,76–78,80,94,101–108] The number of these phenotypically naïve T cells continues to rise for at least 2 years following autologous HSCT. Focusing on total peripheral T cell numbers, normal numbers of CD8$^+$ T cells can be observed as early as 3–6 months following HSCT, depending on the transplant setting, whereas at least 6–12 months are required for CD4$^+$ T cells to reach normal cellularity in the peripheral blood.[1,109] In general, the *de novo* generation of a normally sized T cell pool will require — even under favorable conditions — at least 1–2 years.[77] Although a normal T cell-immune status can be observed in long-term survivors (> 20 years) of allogeneic and syngeneic HSCT,[110] thymopoiesis is frequently limited following transplantation. This obvious constraint on thymopoietic capacity (see below) is consequently responsible for the variable degree of T cell immunodeficiency noted in conditioned transplant recipients.[16,111,112]

... and the Quality

Over and above restoring T cellularity, rebuilding a diverse TCR repertoire constitutes a key element in the functional recovery of the immune system following HSCT. As already delineated above, TCR selection depends on the exposure of developing lymphoid precursors to self-p-MHC. Under nontransplant conditions, the MHC haplotype expressed by hematopoietic and epithelial stromal cells is identical and this constellation ensures that the MHC molecules on which positive and negative selection occur are the same as those used for foreign antigen presentation by bloodborne, professional antigen-presenting cells (APCs) in peripheral tissues. This physiological situation is contrasted by conditions that arise in HSCT recipients. Because cTECs are radioresistant, these positively selecting stromal cells are in transplanted recipients of host origin, whereas the mTECs and bone-marrow-derived DCs involved in negative thymic selection are host- and donor-derived, respectively. Because DCs are radiosensitive, they are relatively quickly replaced by donor type cells following intensive myeloablative therapy and HSCT. In autologous HSCT or under conditions of a complete MHC match between donor and host, the HLA molecules will remain identical for positive and negative thymic selection. In haploidentical HSCT, radioresistant TECs will express the recipients' haplotype but the bone-marrow-derived cells will be of donor origin and hence of a different haplotype. This variance in MHC restriction is thought to influence thymic T cell repertoire selection and, in consequence, that of the peripheral T cell pool.

The posttransplant quality of the T cell compartment is at present most precisely measured by functional T cell assays such as the measurement of pathogen-specific T cell proliferation[106,113] and by the assessment of TCR diversity using either flow cytometric quantification of TCRVβ usage or PCR-based spectratyping of the complementarity determining region 3 (CDR3) of the TCR-β chain.[9,77,114,115] It is, however, of note that measurements of CDR3 diversity alone are insufficient to assess the TCR repertoire and its probable skewing toward certain specificities.[113] Using these and additional methods (e.g. TREC analysis), the complexity of the TCR was investigated by several studies and related to the particular conditions used for HSCT.[9,38,104,105,109,116–118] Results of these investigations suggest that TCR repertoire diversity is only mildly perturbed in recipients of unmanipulated bone marrow from HLA-identical related donors. In contrast, a skewed TCR repertoire (at least for the first four years after transplantation) is noted in recipients of unrelated or HLA-mismatched, related donors, particularly under conditions where the bone marrow inoculum was depleted of T cells.[105,119,120] Importantly, the degree of TCR repertoire contraction is correlated to the extent of immune incompetence, demonstrating that gaps in the TCR diversity contribute to the clinical outcome.[115]

Several specific aspects related to the difficulty of predicting TCR repertoire selection and T cell function in HLA-mismatched transplant recipients need to be discussed in more detail. Although naïve T cells emerge after intense conditioning and haploidentical HSCT,[121–123] little is known with reference to the TCR complexity generated, the MHC restriction and the functional competence of the emerging T cells. Given the disparity in HLA expression between the epithelial cells required for positive selection and the hematopoietic cells involved in negative thymic selection, a distortion of the regenerating TCR repertoire is to be expected; indeed, autoreactive T cells can be recovered at a relatively high frequency in mice that express a particular MHC class II molecule only on cTECs, but not on DCs or mTECs.[124,125] Related to this situation are observations that an unopposed positive selection due to the absence of MHC class II expression on mouse thymic DCs generates a T cell repertoire which causes either autoimmune colitis,[126] autologous GvHD in normal syngeneic mice[127] or chronic GvHD in MHC-disparate recipient mice.[128] These experimental findings underscore the necessity for correct negative thymic selection and suggest (at least in the syngeneic transplant model) that an only positively selected TCR repertoire includes autoreactive TCR specificities with the evident potential to cause autoimmune pathology. Hence, a difference in the set of MHC-restricting elements between positively selecting cTECs and negatively selecting DCs may indeed allow the survival and thymic export of autoreactive T cells. In this context it is, however, interesting to note that an effective reconstitution of TCR diversity and function appears to be possible in some patients following the engraftment of TCD haploidentical bone marrow cells.[17,129–136] Disease-free survivors from such transplants produce within 2–3 years a repertoire of TREC-positive T cells that displays a normal complexity of $V\beta$ usage. While further studies with larger patient cohorts will be needed to confirm independently these results, the data so far suggest that thymic positive and negative selection can nonetheless remain undisturbed after engraftment of HLA-mismatched HSCs. Specifically, these results imply that the emerging T cell compartment exhibits a TCR repertoire comparable to that of recipients of TCD and HLA-matched grafts.[137] Although encouraging, these results are difficult to interpret and the role of thymic selection will need to be investigated in more detail. Nonetheless, the principle still stands that MHC-restricted T cell selection is most efficient and robust under conditions where stromal cells and bone-marrow-derived cells share an identical set of MHC molecules.[138,139]

The notion that cTECs are responsible for positive selection whereas mTECs and hematopoietic APCs (and here, mainly DCs) effect negative selection is, however, challenged by the formation of a functional T cell repertoire in patients grafted with haploidentical HSCs. Indeed, evidence exists both from experimental animal models and from transplanted immunodeficient patients that cells other than TECs can execute positive thymic selection. The intrathymic injection of fibroblasts or medullary epithelium-like cells selects T cells that are restricted to the MHC present on the transferred cells.[140–142] Reconstitution of athymic mice with allogeneic thymic stromal cells results in the formation of mature, functionally competent T effector cells that are restricted to donor but not thymic recipient MHC molecules.[139] Alternatively, developing thymocytes can be positively selected by hematopoietic cells, and the transgenic expression of MHC class II molecules on immature thymocytes of the mouse is sufficient to select functionally competent CD4$^+$ T cells with a mature phenotype and a polyclonal TCR repertoire.[143] While the first experimental evidence described above argues that thymus stromal defects can be efficiently corrected by allogeneic (and possibly xenogeneic) thymic grafts, it is the second set of data that claims thymocyte–thymocyte interactions to suffice for positive selection of CD4-positive T cells (at least in the mouse, where MHC class II molecules are not normally expressed by thymocytes and T cells). Generally speaking, these experimental models may have uncovered a previously unappreciated, independent pathway of positive thymocyte selection that may play a physiological role in species such as man where thymocytes physiologically express MHC class II molecules. Importantly, the selection, MHC-dependent amplification and survival of mature T cells educated either on thymic or nonthymic epithelial MHC appear to be equivalent, at least under the experimental conditions tested.[144] The notion that the thymus holds the capacity to generate a TCR repertoire which is not restricted to the MHC haplotype expressed by TECs comes also from patients with a complete DiGeorge anomaly that have been transplanted with a postnatal, HLA-nonmatched thymus graft to achieve reconstitution of their T cell compartment.[145,146] In these patients, mature host-type T cells are detected as early as six months after transplantation. These cells respond to nominal, T cell-dependent antigens, which indicates that they are (if not exclusively, then at least sufficiently) restricted to host-type MHC molecules.[145,147] Although not yet formally demonstrated in transplanted patients with the complete DiGeorge anomaly, indirect evidence would indicate that positive thymic selection is mediated in these patients by bone-marrow-derived cells. However, it needs to be stressed that the vigor and efficiency of this "noncanonical" selection process is far from clear. It will therefore be important to address in more detail the MHC restriction bestowed on T cells of athymic individuals grafted with non-HLA-matched thymic stroma and to test the functionality of their peripheral T cells.

While it is tempting to speculate on the main function of the thymic epithelial cells as a microenvironment to promote TCR expression in an MHC-unspecific fashion whereas the organ's hematopoietic components control the TCR repertoire through an MHC-dependent mechanism, several important issues related to selection and hence central tolerance induction remain unresolved. For example, the role of tissue-restricted antigens expressed by mTECs is not considered in this alternative model although such antigens and accordingly the mechanism by which they are expressed are critical to prevent autoimmunity (Shikama, Nusspaumer and Holländer, in press). The epithelial thymic microenvironment is, indeed, unique and cannot be replaced by hematopoietic cells.[64,67] Hence, any concept concerning the role of the thymic microenvironment in fostering thymopoiesis and selecting a nonautoreactive TCR repertoire will have to take these particular details into account.

Limitations on Thymus-dependent T Cell Regeneration

Restriction of thymus-dependent T cell development has been directly linked to ineffective generation of the peripheral T cell compartment. This obvious deficiency has been emphasized as the major cause of defects in the adaptive immunity system. Among the parameters that influence thymus-dependent T cell regeneration, the age of the transplant recipient and the treatment-related toxicities confound thymic function the most. Here we discuss the impact of the transplant-related toxicity stemming from GvHD.

Human Thymic Function in the Context of Acute GvHD

The presence of acute GvHD in allogeneic HSCT recipients constitutes a major predictor for an increased probability to be diagnosed with an opportunistic infection.[3,10,45,105,137,148–151] Indeed GvHD severity is inversely correlated with the capacity to recover immune competence.[152] This situation is worsened by pharmacological immunosuppression to treat GHVD. As the pool of potential HSC donors increasingly includes individuals that are largely disparate in their HLA haplotype with the prospective recipient, both the frequency and the severity of GvHD are rising. Consequently, clinically relevant immunodeficiency is likely to be on the upsurge in HSCT recipients as a whole. Understanding the GvHD-related pathomechanisms leading to a compromised immune competence will thus be decisive for improving the clinical outcome in transplant recipients. To this end, both new preclinical models of acute GvHD and the close molecular monitoring of transplant recipients have provided novel and important data for a better understanding of GvHD pathophys-iology[10,153–158]: in brief, mature alloresponsive T cells present in the donor inoculum are known to initiate the events leading in due course to full-scale acute GvHD. Host DCs in their function as professional APCs play a critical role in stimulating donor T cells.[157] Activated donor T cells consequently instigate an inflammatory response that engages multiple effector cells and proinflammatory cytokines that when combined cause cell injury in a limited number of target tissues. Cytokines are important for all phases of GvHD, with donor-derived interferon(IFN)-γ specifically promoting this pathology.[154,159–162] While clinical practice focuses on the involvement of the skin, liver and gastrointestinal tract, it is now broadly accepted that the host lymphohematopoietic system serves as a primary target of acute GvHD.[163]

In the presence of acute GvHD, the reconstitution of the human adaptive immune system is characterized for an extended time by a reduced number of phenotypically naïve T cells.[3,45,118] The two main reasons for this deficiency are (1) the immunosuppressive measures taken for GvHD prophylaxis/treatment[6] and (2) the detrimental immune-mediated effects of acute GvHD itself.[45] The etiology of the latter defect is undoubtedly multifactorial, as GvHD impairs both peripheral and thymic T cell compartments by disparate mechanisms.[87,160,164] As early as 30 years ago, clinical observations had identified the thymus as a target of GvHD, which was evidenced by morphological aberrations in both lymphoid and epithelial components of the patients's thymi following allogeneic bone marrow transplantation.[165–169] The typical histological features of GvHD-induced thymic dysplasia include the depletion of cortical and medullary thymocytes, changes in the number and composition of the different thymic epithelial cell subpopulations, disappearance of the corticomedullary demarcation, phagocytosis of cellular debris, and the elimination of Hassall's bodies.[165,170,171] Loss of the regular tissue architecture is paralleled by deficits in thymopoiesis as confirmed by a distorted TCR repertoire and lower TREC levels when compared with healthy controls.[3,42,44,45,172] Low TREC levels in recipients of HSCT have been interpreted as decreased thymic output secondary to acute or chronic GvHD. Although chronic GvCD and a history of resolved GvCD were, for example, associated with low TREC values in two studies,[3,44] this observation could not be confirmed by Storek *et al.*[42] Difficulties in interpretation of TREC data probably account for this fact as these studies assessed only sjTREC. Indeed, a study by Hazenberg and coworkers demonstrated that sjTREC contents in circulating T cells after transplantation are also determined by peripheral cell divisions.[49] To circumvent this problem, a recent study now assessed both $D\beta$-$J\beta$ TREC and sjTREC in the presence of acute GvCD and demonstrated that lower thymic output is a consequence of both early (at the pre-TN cell stage) and late (apoptosis of postrearrangement thymocytes) defects of thymocyte maturation.[52,172] This data is consistent with the defects seen in a murine haploidentical transplantation model.[173]

Pathomechanisms of Thymic Insufficiency: Insights from Preclinical GvHD Models

Experimentally induced thymic dysplasia in preclinical models mimics the corresponding thymic features observed in human GvHD (i.e. a loss of cortical cellularity, a lack of the cortex/medulla demarcation, an absence of the regular composition and organization of the different TEC subpopulations, the loss of a regular TCR repertoire selection, and diminished numbers of TREC$^+$ cells in both the thymus and the periphery).[3,4,45,62,80,161,162,164,166–169,173–182] Pretransplant conditioning and the antihost immune response by donor T cells are both considered to play a role in thymic injury. Whereas the impact of chemo/radiotherapy on thymic function has been well studied,[183–185] the immunological mechanisms underlying thymic injury have only recently begun to be investigated in detail. Specially adapted preclinical transplantation models that do not necessitate radiation have been successfully employed to decipher the impact of GvHD on thymic architecture and function. For example, the transfer of parental T cells (C57BL/6) into haploidentical F_1 progeny (BDF$_1$) results in cellular injury of typical GvHD target organs secondary to an acute graft-vs-host response (GvHR) which is mediated by antihost CTL and by inflammatory cytokines.[153,162,186–189] Under the given conditions, thymocyte hypocellularity is primarily the consequence of depletion of the largest DP thymocyte population, which appears to be effected by two independent mechanisms. Firstly, pro- and pre-T cells enter the cell cycle in the presence of acute GvHD only intermittently[161] and the nondividing cells at this maturational stage fail to rearrange and express the locus encoding the TCR β chain — a prerequisite for their survival and developmental transition to the next maturational stage (i.e. DP thymocytes). Secondly, DP thymocytes themselves are subject to increased programmed cell death in the presence of acute thymic GvHD, which contributes further to thymic lymphopenia. Interestingly, antigen-nonspecific factors such as high systemic concentrations of proinflammatory cytokines or corticosteroids (both of which when given exogenously are toxic to DP cells) have been determined not to play a significant role in increasing the rate of apoptosis among DP thymocytes.[182]

The alloantigen-specific immune response of donor T cells against host thymic cells is now considered to be the principal reason why T cell maturation and intrathymic survival are severely impaired in recipients of experimental haploidentical HSCT.[151,161,162] In fact, mature donor T cells infiltrating the thymus have long been recognized to constitute a typical feature of acute GvHD.[167] In more recent experiments, we have found that donor MHC-disparate T cells can infiltrate the thymi of recipients even when they are unconditioned, and their number *in situ* correlates directly with the extent to which thymopoiesis is disturbed.[161,162] Although histological studies revealed early on that both lymphoid and stromal cells in the thymus are affected by acute GvHD, the precise sequence of how this pathology occurs was not established. The developing thymocytes can, however, not be the direct targets of the alloimmune response, since these cells are also of donor origin and are hence not recognized for their MHC disparity by the GvHD-inducing T cells transferred with the HSC inoculum.

A more precise understanding of the molecular and cellular events that result in the loss of thymic function has recently been gained from different experimental mouse models. In-depth analyses of the architecture and composition of the TEC compartment in unconditioned mice with acute GvHD reveal an increased frequency of epithelial cell apoptosis.[162] Whereas these descriptive results do not establish whether TECs are the direct or indirect target of the alloimmune response, directing the GVHR exclusively to TECs (i.e. by use of bone marrow chimeras and the transfer of mature T cells from the same donor strain) is sufficient to impair thymopoiesis.[162] This result indicates that TECs are the direct thymic target of allorecognition and suggests that TECs are secondary to their unique biology competent to directly prime naïve allogeneic T cells, even in the absence of hematopoietic, professional APCs.[162] The potent role of TECs as intrathymic APCs to activate donor T cells is also reflected in the fact that experimental thymic GvHD can occur in the absence of other organ pathologies. Following their activation, donor

T cells secrete in the thymus IFN-γ, which in turn initiates via signal transducer and activator of transcription (STAT)-1 the apoptosis of both cortical and medullary TECs. These local but relevant changes to the thymic structure and consequently function are not easily assessed by readily available diagnostic tools, so that monitoring thymic GvHD is not straightforward. The detailed understanding of the primary cellular target of thymic GvHD offers also practical implications for the design of novel strategies to prevent allorecognition by mature donor T cells. In fact, because TECs act as competent APCs it is unlikely that vigorous depletion of host-derived hematopoietic APCs as part of pretransplant conditioning will be sufficient to prevent the activation of alloresponsive donor T cells and the ensuing cell injury to TECs. With TECs efficiently recognized by donor T cells, future diagnostic efforts may therefore want to focus on strategies that prevent and/or repair epithelial damage (see below). If successful, such endeavors are likely to shed light on the current uncertainty as to whether the increased susceptibility to infections and the incomplete reconstitution of the adapted immune system in recipients of unrelated donor HSCT are caused by subclinical GvHD that is exclusively restricted to the thymus.

Thymic Dysfunction as a Link to Autoimmunity/Chronic GvHD?

The number of allogeneic HSCT recipients who have now survived for two to three decades is increasing. However, only a few of these individuals have fully regained their premorbid state of immunological health. Although the pathogenesis for late complications of HSCT is multifactorial, some of these disorders are clearly autoimmune in origin.[190] Whilst infectious complications can be easily related to defective and/or delayed reconstitution of the adaptive immune system, the mechanisms responsible for the long-term defects in adaptive immunity remain at present largely unknown. Autoimmunity after HSCT has many hallmarks of chronic GvHD, the latter being a pleiomorphic syndrome with the onset originally occurring between 3 and 24 months after allogeneic HSCT.[191]

Indeed, while not all HSCT recipients with autoimmune syndromes experience also symptoms of chronic GvHD, there is a strong association between the development of chronic GvHD and autoimmune disease in HSCT recipients.[192] Experimental studies have thus far proposed at least four distinct pathomechanisms to explain chronic GvHD,[193] implicating (1) regulatory cytokines such as transforming growth factor β (TGF-β),[194] (2) autoreactive B cells,[195] (3) T_{reg} deficiency,[196] or (4) a failure in negative thymocyte selection to play critical roles (see below).

Reliable evidence for a role of the thymus in the pathogenic events leading to chronic GvHD has been gained from different mouse transplantation models. In one model, thymic injury in recipients (C57BL/6) is caused by the infusion of MHC-mismatched donor $CD8^+$ T cells (C3H.SW). As a result, TCR repertoire selection among recipient-type $CD4^+$ T cells is severely altered by the damaged thymic microenvironment and now includes reactivity to self-antigens.[197] In addition, these donor T cells induce all the hallmarks of chronic GvHD when adoptively transferred into secondary B6 recipients but elicit an acute form of GvHD when injected into C3H.SW mice. Hence, thymic damage in the course of acute GvHD will select a repertoire of T cells that is in due course able to cause autoimmune manifestations reminiscent of chronic GvHD. In keeping with these observations are results from bone marrow chimeric mice in which negative thymic selection of $CD4^+$ T cells by hematopoietic APCs is impaired due to the absence of MHC class II expression on DCs but not TECs.[127,128] As a consequence, the T cells are autoreactive and will induce in a thymus-dependent manner chronic GvHD in MHC-mismatched recipients (C57BL/6-MHC II$^{-/-}$ → C3H) and an "autoimmune GvHD"-like syndrome in matched (C57BL/6-MHC II$^{-/-}$ → C57BL/6) chimeras. Importantly, acute GvHD not only affects negative T cell selection in the thymus but also impairs development of T_{reg},[198] which have been successfully used in mice to prevent chronic GvHD.[195] Taken together, this experimental data strongly support a model in which acute GvHD causes thymic injury and consequently harms TCR repertoire selection. As a result, T cells exported to the periphery can mediate the evolution from acute to chronic GvHD through either direct targeting of specific organs or, indirectly, the lack of T_{reg} control. Although not all cases of human acute GvHD evolve into chronic GvHD, the former has nonetheless been recognized as a risk for the latter. It is therefore intriguing to speculate that the early posttransplant impairment of TEC function and hence TCR selection provide an etiological link between the alloreactivity of acute GvHD and aspects of autoimmunity typically seen in the course of chronic GvHD.[151] Here, the loss of Aire+ TECs may constitute a crucial mechanism by which central tolerance induction is disturbed, since this particular subpopulation of TECs is instrumental both in negative selection of autoreactive TCRs and in generation of natural T_{reg}. Preliminary data from our laboratory certainly indicate a dysregulation of Aire expression in experimental acute GvHD. Detailed work is, however, still required to confirm under experimental and clinical conditions that such a mechanism is indeed operational in the induction and/or the maintenance of chronic GvHD. Although caveats remain regarding the clinical relevance of improving thymus function, preclinical models would indicate that measures to enhance thymic function in the context of allogeneic HSCT may ameliorate GvHD not only in its acute but also in its chronic form.[193]

Interventions to Improve Immune Regeneration via Protection of Thymic Epithelium by Fibroblast Growth Factor 7

Strategies aimed at enhancing thymic function hold the promise of ameliorating posttransplant T cell immunodeficiency. Specifically, prophylactic and therapeutic approaches could either be directed at enhancing the (residual) thymic function or employed to (re)generate new thymic stromal elements. Several strategies to improve immune reconstitution have so far been developed in preclinical models but only a few have for now been successfully translated to clinical practice (reviewed in Refs. 4, 12 and 199). As TEC damage by radiation,[183,200–202] chemotherapy,[185,203] GvHD,[62,162] or infection[4,204] precludes normal T cell development, interventions will be discussed that seek to intervene with

TEC dysfunction and attempt to enhance TEC recovery after allogeneic HSCT.

Fibroblast growth factor Fgf 7 (aka keratinocyte growth factor, KGF) is a potent epithelial cell mitogen that belongs to the large family of the structurally related Fgf's,[205] Fgf 7 is currently an approved drug for the prophylaxis of oral mucositis in conditioned transplant recipients.[206,207] Its action as a trophic factor and its potential to protect against radio- and chemotherapeutic damage[205] serve as the rationale for testing the impact of Fgf 7 on recovery of TECs following conditioning and HSCT. This concept has received further support by the contention that the postnatal thymic epithelial compartment may continue to require growth-regulating signals, including possibly endogenous Fgf 7. Since postmitotic TECs are continuously replaced by the progeny of immature TEC precursors,[58] thymic expression of Fgf 7 is sustained throughout life.[208] To exert its biological activity, Fgf 7 binds to and activates the IIIb variant of the FgfR2 receptor (FgfR2IIIb), which in the thymus is exclusively expressed on TECs.[62,63,209,210] In response to systemic treatment of normal mice with exogenous Fgf 7, the postnatal thymic microenvironment undergoes specific changes. These *in vivo* alterations are characterized by a robust expansion of both mature and immature TECs within days of Fgf 7 exposure even as the architectural organization of all TEC populations remains unchanged.[63] Due to an increased proliferation rate following Fgf 7 stimulation, the resultant enlargement of the TEC scaffold accommodates a higher lymphoid cellularity while keeping a normal thymocyte:TEC ratio. In addition, it is also likely that the exposure of TECs to a pharmacological dose of Fgf 7 results in a qualitative change of the TEC compartment. In support of such potential are results from experimental models where a single course of Fgf 7 suffices to reverse the age-related decrease in thymocyte numbers and to restore the architecture and cellular composition of the thymic stromal microenvironment.[211] Moreover, exposure of mice of any age to exogenous Fgf 7 also causes an increase in thymopoietic activity and reconstitution of the peripheral T cell compartment in syngeneic or allogeneic transplant recipients preconditioned with chemo- or radiotherapy.[208,212] Similarly, rhesus macaques engrafted with autologous

HSCs and treated with Fgf7 display an enhanced T cell recovery as assessed by an increase in TREC$^+$ cells.[213] When used in preclinical models of acute GvHD, the systemic administration of Fgf7 preserves TEC architectural organization, cellularity and function.[62] As a result, normal T cell development is maintained regardless of alloreactive donor T cells in the thymus and ongoing GvHD in other typical target organs. In consequence, the administration of Fgf7 prevents the emergence of a repertoire of autoreactive T cells that promotes the development of experimental chronic GvHD.[197] Exploiting these effects for clinical use in lymphopenic HSCT recipients, studies are now underway to assess whether Fgf7 as a growth and differentiation factor can enhance T cell recovery in either the presence or absence of a chemical androgen blockade used to further protect TECs.[199,202,214,215] This latter intervention has previously been proposed as an independent measure to correct the transplant-related immune deficiency, because the senescence-driven thymic involution has been linked to physiological changes in sex steroid hormone production.[59,216,217] Indeed, androgen receptors are expressed on TECs and their binding to sex steroid ligands inhibits thymopoiesis although the molecular mechanisms by which this occurs are not yet precisely known.[218] These data raise a reasonable hope that Fgf7 alone or in combination with other agents (such as an androgen blockade) can be used to enhance T cell reconstitution in lymphopenic recipients of allogeneic HSCT.

The molecular mechanisms by which Fgf7 influences TEC function are currently under investigation. Given physiological conditions, Fgf7 is expressed within the thymus both by stromal cells and by T cells at specific developmental stages.[209,219] Experiments using mice deficient in FgfR2IIIb expression or *in vitro* conditions where mesenchymal cells are physically removed from embryonic thymus lobes have revealed the importance of Fgf signaling during early thymus organogenesis.[209,220,221] The postnatal thymic epithelial compartment may, however, continue to require growth-regulating signals, including endogenous Fgf7, whose thymic expression is sustained throughout life. A recent study designed to examine the molecular and cellular mechanisms by which Fgf7 stimulates thymic T lymphopoiesis in normal adult TECs has concluded that FgfR2IIIb is expressed by both mature cortical and medullary as well as immature thymic epithelia.[63] Upon exposure to exogenous Fgf7, these stromal cell subsets proliferate and express several growth and differentiation factors, including different members of the family of Wnt molecules and bone-morphogenetic proteins.[63] In consequence, a robust and sustained increase in thymopoiesis occurs which is initiated as a single wave affecting first the number of the most immature T cell precursors and subsequently that of more mature thymocytes. This effect of enhanced thymopoiesis is uniquely dependent on the exposure of the stromal microenvironment to Fgf7, as the transfer of the earliest intrathymic T cell precursor from Fgf7-treated donor mice to naïve (i.e. untreated) recipients fails to impart enhanced thymopoiesis and export of mature T cells to the periphery.

An increase in thymopoiesis and thymic T cell export appears to be highly beneficial for lymphopenic individuals, not least because the thymus neither senses peripheral T lymphopenia nor gauges its T cell export accordingly. Hence, any changes in thymic output should positively affect the process of replenishing the peripheral T cell pool. Enhanced thymic function should also secure a diverse T cell repertoire, as it will concurrently offset an otherwise homeostatic expansion of a limited number of mature T cells. Thus, the clinical use of Fgf7 in transplantation medicine may efficiently restore the T cell compartment and its competence for an effective adaptive immune response. Based on the understanding that interactions between developing thymocytes and TECs determine thymic function, enhanced endogenous production of the cytoprotective Fgf7 may thus constitute an adjunct strategy for the treatment of thymic GvHD. However, expression of Fgf7 is subject to negative regulation by glucocorticoids, a standard component of GvHD therapy as steroids decrease Fgf7 mRNA in a time- and concentration-dependent manner.[222] The administration of pharmacological doses of Fgf7 prior to conditioning may therefore be needed to compensate at least for the loss of the physiological production of Fgf7 secondary to GvHD prophylaxis with corticosteroids.

Conclusion

A wealth of data from preclinical models and clinical allogeneic HSCT studies has identified the thymus as a typical target of transplant-related toxicities. An enhanced understanding of the immune regenerative pathways operational in the thymus is essential for the development of new approaches that correct posttransplant immune deficiency. This knowledge is expected to form a rational basis for devising novel strategies that maintain regular thymopoietic function via the protection of thymic stromal cells, a condition pivotal for the reconstitution of a functionally competent adaptive immune system.

References

1. Mackall CL. (2000) T-cell immunodeficiency following cytotoxic antineoplastic therapy: A review. *Stem Cells* **18**: 10–18.
2. Haynes BF, Markert ML, Sempowski GD *et al.* (2000) The role of the thymus in immune reconstitution in aging, bone marrow transplantation, and HIV-1 infection. *Annu Rev Immunol* **18**: 529–560.
3. Weinberg K, Blazar BR, Wagner JE *et al.* (2001) Factors affecting thymic function after allogeneic hematopoietic stem cell transplantation. *Blood* **97**: 1458–1466.
4. Van den Brink MR, Alpdogan O, Boyd RL. (2004) Strategies to enhance T-cell reconstitution in immunocompromised patients. *Nat Rev Immunol* **4**: 856–867.
5. Auletta JJ, Lazarus HM. (2005) Immune restoration following hematopoietic stem cell transplantation: An evolving target. *Bone Marrow Transplant* **35**: 835–857.
6. Antin JH. (2005) Immune reconstitution: The major barrier to successful stem cell transplantation. *Biol Blood Marrow Transplant* **11**: 43–45.
7. Muraro PA, Douek DC. (2006) Renewing the T cell repertoire to arrest autoimmune aggression. *Trends Immunol* **27**: 61–67.

8. Crooks GM, Weinberg K, Mackall C. (2006) Immune reconstitution: from stem cells to lymphocytes. *Biol Blood Marrow Transplant* **12**: 42–46.

9. Peggs KS. (2006) Reconstitution of adaptive and innate immunity following allogeneic hematopoietic stem cell transplantation in humans. *Cytotherapy* **8**: 427–436.

10. Welniak LA, Blazar BR, Murphy WJ. (2007) Immunobiology of allogeneic hematopoietic stem cell transplantation. *Annu Rev Immunol* **25**: 139–170.

11. Chidgey A, Dudakov J, Seach N, Boyd R. (2007) Impact of niche aging on thymic regeneration and immune reconstitution. *Semin Immunol* **19**: 331–340.

12. Zakrzewski JL, Goldberg GL, Smith OM, Van den Brink MRM. (2008) Enhancing T cell reconstitution after hematopoietic stem cell transplantation: A brief update of the latest trends. *Blood Cells Mol Dis* **40**: 44–47.

13. Toubert A. (2008) Immune reconstitution after allogeneic HSCT. In *Hematopoietic Stem Cell Transplantation* European School of Haematology, Paris.

14. Krenger W, Holländer GA. (2008) The thymus in GVHD pathophysiology. *Best Pract Res Clin Haematol* **21**: 119–128.

15. Storek J. (2008) Immunological reconstitution after hematopoietic cell transplantation — its relation to the contents of the graft. *Expert Opin Biol Ther* **8**: 583–597.

16. Small TN, Papadopoulos EB, Boulad F *et al.* (1999) Comparison of immune reconstitution after unrelated and related T-cell-depleted bone marrow transplantation: Effect of patient age and donor leukocyte infusions. *Blood* **93**: 467–480.

17. Haddad E, Landais P, Friedrich W *et al.* (1998) Long-term immune reconstitution and outcome after HLA-nonidentical T-cell-depleted bone marrow transplantation for severe combined immunodeficiency: A European retrospective study of 116 patients. *Blood* **91**: 3646–3653.

18. Porrata LF, Litzow MR, Tefferi A *et al.* (2002) Early lymphocyte recovery is a predictive factor for prolonged survival after autologous hematopoietic stem cell transplantation for acute myelogenous leukemia. *Leukemia* **16**: 1311–1318.

19. Clave E, Rocha V, Talvensaari K *et al.* (2005) Prognostic value of pretransplantation host thymic function in HLA-identical sibling hematopoietic stem cell transplantation. *Blood* **105**: 2608–2613.

20. Parkman R, Cohen G, Carter SL *et al.* (2006) Successful immune reconstitution decreases leukemic relapse and improves survival in recipients of unrelated cord blood transplantation. *Biol Blood Marrow Transplant* **12**: 919–927.

21. Ege H, Gertz MA, Markovic SN *et al.* (2008) Prediction of survival using absolute lymphocyte count for newly diagnosed patients with multiple myeloma: A retrospective study. *Br J Haematol* **141**: 792–798.

22. Gill J, Malin M, Sutherland J *et al.* (2003) Thymic generation and regeneration. *Immunol Rev* **195**: 28–50.

23. Guidos C. (2006) Thymus and T-lymphocyte development: What is new in the 21st century? *Immunol Rev* **209**: 5–9.

24. Holländer G, Gill J, Zuklys S *et al.* (2006) Cellular and molecular events during early thymus development. *Immunol Rev* **209**: 28–46.

25. Boehm T. (2008) Thymus development and function. *Curr Opin Immunol* **20**: 178–184.

26. Rothenberg EV, Moore JE, Yui MA (2008) Launching the T-cell-lineage developmental programme. *Nat Rev Immunol* **8**: 9–21.

27. Anderson G, Lane PJ, Jenkinson EJ (2007) Generating intrathymic microenvironments to establish T-cell tolerance. *Nat Rev Immunol* **7**: 954–963.

28. Rodewald HR. (2008) Thymus organogenesis. *Annu Rev Immunol* **26**: 355–388.

29. Palmer E. (2003) Negative selection-clearing out the bad apples from the T-cell repertoire. *Nat Rev Immunol* **3**: 383–391.

30. Petrie HT, Zúñiga-Pflücker JC. (2007) Zoned out: Functional mapping of stromal signaling microenvironments in the thymus. *Annu Rev Immunol* **25**: 649–679.

31. Gabor MJ, Scollay R, Godfrey DI. (1997) Thymic T cell export is not influenced by the peripheral T cell pool. *Eur J Immunol* **27**: 2986–2993.

32. Michie CA, McLean A, Alcock C, Beverley PC. (1992) Lifespan of human lymphocyte subsets defined by CD45 isoforms. *Nature* **360**: 264–265.

33. Picker LJ, Treer JR, Ferguson-Darnell B *et al.* (1993) Control of lymphocyte recirculation in man. I. Differential regulation of the peripheral lymph node homing receptor L-selectin on T cells during the virgin to memory cell transition. *J Immunol* **150**: 1105–1121.

34. McFarland RD, Douek DC, Koup RA, Picker LJ. (2000) Identification of a human recent thymic emigrant phenotype. *Proc Natl Acad Sci USA* **97**: 4215–4220.

35. Peggs KS, Mackinnon S. (2004) Immune reconstitution following hematopoietic stem cell transplantation. *Br J Haematol* **124**: 407–420.

36. Douek DC, McFarland RD, Keiser PH *et al.* (1998) Changes in thymic function with age and during the treatment of HIV infection. *Nature* **396**: 690–695.

37. Douek DC, Koup RA, McFarland RD *et al.* (2000) Effect of HIV on thymic function before and after antiretroviral therapy in children. *J Infect Dis* **181**: 1479–1482.

38. Douek DC, Vescio RA, Betts MR *et al.* (2000) Assessment of thymic output in adults after haematopoietic stem-cell transplantation and prediction of T-cell reconstitution. *Lancet* **355**: 1875–1881.

39. Patel DD, Gooding ME, Parrott RE *et al.* (2000) Thymic function after hematopoietic stem-cell transplantation for the treatment of severe combined immunodeficiency. *N Engl J Med* **342**: 1325–1332.

40. Markert ML, Hicks CB, Bartlett JA *et al.* (2000) Effect of highly active antiretroviral therapy and thymic transplantation on

immunoreconstitution in HIV infection. *AIDS Res Hum Retroviruses* **16**: 403–413.

41. Steffens CM, Al-Harthi L, Shott S *et al.* (2000) Evaluation of thymopoiesis using T cell receptor excision circles (TRECs): differential correlation between adult and pediatric TRECs and naive phenotypes. *Clin Immunol* **97**: 95–101.

42. Storek J, Joseph A, Dawson MA *et al.* (2002) Factors influencing T-lymphopoiesis after allogeneic hematopoietic cell transplantation. *Transplantation* **73**: 1154–1158.

43. Hochberg EP, Chillemi AC, Wu CJ. (2001) Quantitation of T-cell neogenesis *in vivo* after allogeneic bone marrow transplantation. *Blood* **98**: 1116–1121.

44. Lewin SR, Heller G, Zhang L *et al.* (2002) Direct evidence for new T-cell generation by patients after either T-cell-depleted or unmodified allogeneic hematopoietic stem cell transplantation. *Blood* **100**: 2235–2242.

45. Hakim FT, Gress RE. (2002) Reconstitution of thymic function after stem cell transplantation in humans. *Curr Opin Hematol* **9**: 490–496.

46. Hazenberg MD, Otto SA, de Pauw ES *et al.* (2002) T-cell receptor excision circle and T-cell dynamics after allogeneic stem cell transplantation are related to clinical events. *Blood* **99**: 3449–3353.

47. Ye P, Kirschner DE. (2002) Reevaluation of T cell receptor excision circles as a measure of human recent thymic emigrants. *J Immunol* **169**: 4968–4979.

48. Svaldi M, Lanthaler AJ, Dugas M *et al.* (2003) T-cell receptor excision circles: A novel prognostic parameter for the outcome of transplantation in multiple myeloma patients. *Br J Haematol* **122**: 795–801.

49. Hazenberg MD, Borghans JA, de Boer RJ, Miedema F. (2003) Thymic output: A bad TREC record. *Nat Immunol* **4**: 97–99.

50. Ribeiro RM, Perelson AS. (2007) Determining thymic output quantitatively: Using models to interpret experimental T-cell receptor excision circle (TREC) data. *Immunol Rev* **216**: 21–34.

51. Dion ML, Poulin JF, Bordi R *et al.* (2004) HIV infection rapidly induces and maintains a substantial suppression of thymocyte proliferation. *Immunity* **21**: 757–768.

52. Fry TJ. (2009) Is a little GVHD a good thing? *Blood* **113**: 6274–6275.

53. Almeida AR, Borghans JA, Freitas AA. (2001) T cell homeostasis: Thymus regeneration and peripheral T cell restoration in mice with a reduced fraction of competent precursors. *J Exp Med* **194**: 591–599.

54. Jamieson BD, Douek DC, Killian S *et al.* (1999) Generation of functional thymocytes in the human adult. *Immunity* **10**: 569–575.

55. Douek DC, Koup RA. (2000) Evidence for thymic function in the elderly. *Vaccine* **18**: 1638–1641.

56. Hakim FT, Memon SA, Cepeda R *et al.* (2005) Age-dependent incidence, time course, and consequences of thymic renewal in adults. *J Clin Invest* **115**: 930–939.

57. Ortman CL, Dittmar KA, Witte PL, Le PT. (2002) Molecular characterization of the mouse involuted thymus: Aberrations in expression of transcription regulators in thymocyte and epithelial compartments. *Int Immunol* **14**: 813–822.

58. Gray D, Seach N, Ueno T *et al.* (2006) Developmental kinetics, turnover, and stimulatory capacity of thymic epithelial cells. *Blood* **108**: 3777–3785.

59. Taub DD, Longo DL. (2005) Insights into thymic aging and regeneration. *Immunol Rev* **205**: 72–93.

60. Hakim FT, Gress RE. (2007) Immunosenescence: Deficits in adaptive immunity in the elderly. *Tissue Antigens* **70**: 179–189.

61. Hakim FT, Gress RE. (2007) Thymic involution: Implications for self-tolerance. *Methods Mol Biol* **380**: 377–390.

62. Rossi S, Blazar BR, Farrell CL *et al.* (2002) Keratinocyte growth factor preserves normal thymopoiesis and thymic microenvironment during experimental graft-versus-host disease. *Blood* **100**: 682–691.

63. Rossi SW, Jeker LT, Ueno T *et al.* (2007) Keratinocyte growth factor (KGF) enhances postnatal T-cell development via enhancements in

proliferation and function of thymic epithelial cells. *Blood* **109**: 3803–3811.

64. Anderson MS, Venanzi ES, Klein L *et al.* (2002) Projection of an immunological self shadow within the thymus by the Aire protein. *Science* **298**: 1395–1401.

65. Derbinski J, Gabler J, Brors B *et al.* (2005) Promiscuous gene expression in thymic epithelial cells is regulated at multiple levels. *J Exp Med* **202**: 33–45.

66. Kyewski B, Klein L. (2006) A central role for central tolerance. *Annu Rev Immunol* **24**: 571–606.

67. Anderson MS, Venanzi ES, Chen Z *et al.* (2005) The cellular mechanism of Aire control of T cell tolerance. *Immunity* **23**: 227–239.

68. Pereira LE, Bostik P, Ansari AA. (2005) The development of mouse APECED models provides new insight into the role of AIRE in immune regulation. *Clin Dev Immunol* **12**: 211–216.

69. Park Y, Moon Y, Chung HY. (2003) AIRE-1 (autoimmune regulator type 1) as a regulator of the thymic induction of negative selection. *Ann NY Acad Sci* **1005**: 431–435.

70. Liston A, Gray DH, Lesage S *et al.* (2004) Gene dosage — limiting role of Aire in thymic expression, clonal deletion, and organ-specific autoimmunity. *J Exp Med* **200**: 1015–1026.

71. Fontenot JD, Rudensky AY. (2005) A well-adapted regulatory contrivance: Regulatory T cell development and the forkhead family transcription factor Foxp3. *Nat Immunol* **6**: 331–337.

72. Von Boehmer H. (2005) Mechanisms of suppression by suppressor T cells. *Nat Immunol* **6**: 338–344.

73. Miyara M, Sakaguchi S. (2007) Natural regulatory T cells: Mechanisms of suppression. *Trends Mol Med* **13**: 108–116.

74. Aschenbrenner K, D'Cruz LM, Vollmann EH *et al.* (2007) Selection of Foxp3$^+$ regulatory T cells specific for self antigen expressed and presented by Aire$^+$ medullary thymic epithelial cells. *Nat Immunol* **8**: 351–358.

75. Nomura T, Sakaguchi S. (2007) Foxp3 and Aire in thymus-generated Treg cells: A link in self-tolerance. *Nat Immunol* **8**(4): 333–334.

76. Hakim FT, Gress RE. (2005) Reconstitution of the lymphocyte compartment after lymphocyte depletion: A key issue in clinical immunology. *Eur J Immunol* **35**: 3099–3102.

77. Williams KM, Hakim FT, Gress RE. (2007) T cell immune reconstitution following lymphodepletion. *Semin Immunol* **19**: 318–330.

78. Mackall CL, Granger L, Sheard MA *et al.* (1993) T-cell regeneration after bone marrow transplantation: Differential CD45 isoform expression on thymic-derived versus thymic-independent progeny. *Blood* **82**: 2585–2594.

79. Bahceci E, Epperson D, Douek DC *et al.* (2003) Early reconstitution of the T-cell repertoire after non-myeloablative peripheral blood stem cell transplantation is from post-thymic T-cell expansion and is unaffected by graft-versus-host disease or mixed chimerism. *Br J Haematol* **122**: 934–943.

80. Fallen PR, McGreavey L, Madrigal JA *et al.* (2003) Factors affecting reconstitution of the T-cell compartment in allogeneic hematopoietic cell transplant recipients. *Bone Marrow Transplant* **32**: 1001–1014.

81. Jameson SC. (2005) T cell homeostasis: Keeping useful T cells alive and live T cells useful. *Semin Immunol* **17**: 231–237.

82. Parkman R, Weinberg KI. (1997) Immunological reconstitution following bone marrow transplantation. *Immunol Rev* **157**: 73–78.

83. De Gast GC, Verdonck LF, Middeldorp JM *et al.* (1985) Recovery of T cell subsets after autologous bone marrow transplantation is mainly due to proliferation of mature T cells in the graft. *Blood* **66**: 428–431.

84. Gaschet J, Denis C, Milpied N *et al.* (1995) Alterations of T cell repertoire after bone marrow transplantation: Characterization of over-represented subsets. *Bone Marrow Transplant* **16**: 427–435.

85. Brugnoni D, Airò P, Pennacchio M *et al.* (1999) Immune reconstitution after bone marrow transplantation for combined immunodeficiencies: Down-modulation of Bcl-2 and high expression of CD95/Fas account for increased susceptibility to spontaneous and activation-induced lymphocyte cell death. *Bone Marrow Transplant* **23**: 451–457.

86. Lin MT, Tseng LH, Frangoul H *et al.* (2000) Increased apoptosis of peripheral blood T cells following allogeneic hematopoietic cell transplantation. *Blood* **95**: 3832–3839.

87. Brochu S, Rioux-Mass B, Roy J *et al.* (1999) Massive activation-induced cell death of alloreactive T cells with apoptosis of bystander postthymic T cells prevents immune reconstitution in mice with graft-versus-host disease. *Blood* **94**: 390–400.

88. Curtis RE, Travis LB, Rowlings PA *et al.* (1999) Risk of lympho-proliferative disorders after bone marrow transplantation: A multi-institutional study. *Blood* **94**: 2208–2216.

89. Wagner JE, Thompson JS, Carter SL, Kernan NA. (2005) Effect of graft-versus-host disease prophylaxis on 3-year disease-free survival in recipients of unrelated donor bone marrow (T-cell depletion trial): A multi-centre, randomised phase II–III trial. *Lancet* **366**: 733–741.

90. Einsele. (2005) T-cell therapy for viral and fungal infections. *Blood* **106**: 4023.

91. Gress RE, Komanduri KV, Einsele H, Cooper LJ. (2007) Lymphoid reconstruction and vaccines. *Biol Blood Marrow Transplant* **13**: 17–22.

92. Heitger A, Neu N, Kern H *et al.* (1997) Essential role of the thymus to reconstitute naive (CD45RA$^+$) T-helper cells after human allo-geneic bone marrow transplantation. *Blood* **90**: 850–857.

93. Heitger A, Greinix H, Mannhalter C *et al.* (2000) Requirement of residual thymus to restore normal T-cell subsets after human allo-geneic bone marrow transplantation. *Transplantation* **69**: 2366–2373.

94. Klein AK, Patel DD, Gooding ME *et al.* (2001) T-cell recovery in adults and children following umbilical cord blood transplantation. *Biol Blood Marrow Transplant* **7**: 454–466.

95. Chen X, Barfield R, Benaim E *et al.* (2005) Prediction of T-cell reconstitution by assessment of T-cell receptor excision circle before allogeneic hematopoietic stem cell transplantation in pediatric patients. *Blood* **105**: 886–893.

96. Sato K, Ohtsuka K, Hasegawa K *et al.* (1995) Evidence for extrathymic generation of intermediate T cell receptor cells in the

liver revealed in thymectomized, irradiated mice subjected to bone marrow transplantation. *J Exp Med* **182**: 759–767.

97. Mackall CL, Fleisher TA, Brown MR *et al.* (1995) Age, thymopoiesis, and CD4⁺ T-lymphocyte regeneration after intensive chemotherapy. *N Engl J Med* **332**: 143–149.

98. Hara M, McAdams HP, Vredenburgh JJ *et al.* (1999) Thymic hyperplasia after high-dose chemotherapy and autologous stem cell transplantation: Incidence and significance in patients with breast cancer. *AJR Am J Roentgenol* **173**: 1341–1344.

99. Scollay R, Godfrey DI. (1995) Thymic emigration: Conveyor belts or lucky dips? *Immunol Today* **16**: 268–273.

100. Benz C, Martins VC, Radtke F, Bleul CC. (2008) The stream of precursors that colonizes the thymus proceeds selectively through the early T lineage precursor stage of T cell development. *J Exp Med* **205**: 1187–1199.

101. Weinberg K, Annett G, Kashyap A *et al.* (1995) The effect of thymic function on immunocompetence following bone marrow transplantation. *Biol Blood Marrow Transplant* **1**: 18–23.

102. Kook H, Goldman F, Padley D *et al.* (1996) Reconstruction of the immune system after unrelated or partially matched T-cell-depleted bone marrow transplantation in children: immunophenotypic analysis and factors affecting the speed of recovery. *Blood* **88**: 1089–1097.

103. Dumont-Girard F, Roux E, van Lier RA *et al.* (1998) Reconstitution of the T-cell compartment after bone marrow transplantation: Restoration of the repertoire by thymic emigrants. *Blood* **92**: 4464–4471.

104. Douek DC. (2002) The contribution of the thymus to immune reconstitution after hematopoietic stem-cell transplantation. *Cytotherapy* **4**: 425–426.

105. Roux E, Dumont-Girard F, Starobinski M *et al.* (2000) Recovery of immune reactivity after T-cell-depleted bone marrow transplantation depends on thymic activity. *Blood* **96**: 2299–2303.

106. Storek J, Dawson MA, Storer B *et al.* (2001) Immune reconstitution after allogeneic marrow transplantation compared with blood stem cell transplantation. *Blood* **97**: 3380–3389.

107. Muraro PA, Douek DC, Packer A *et al.* (2005) Thymic output generates a new and diverse TCR repertoire after autologous stem cell transplantation in multiple sclerosis patients. *J Exp Med* **201**: 805–816.

108. Fry TJ, Mackall CL. (2005) Immune reconstitution following hematopoietic progenitor cell transplantation: Challenges for the future. *Bone Marrow Transplant* **35**(Suppl. 1): S53-S57.

109. Mackall CL, Gress RE. (1997) Pathways of T-cell regeneration in mice and humans: Implications for bone marrow transplantation and immunotherapy. *Immunol Rev* **157**: 61–72.

110. Storek J, Joseph A, Espino G *et al.* (2001) Immunity of patients surviving 20 to 30 years after allogeneic or syngeneic bone marrow transplantation. *Blood* **98**: 3505–3512.

111. Mackall CL, Stein D, Fleisher TA *et al.* (2000) Prolonged CD4 depletion after sequential autologous peripheral blood progenitor cell infusions in children and young adults. *Blood* **96**: 754–762.

112. Komanduri KV, St John LS, De Lima M *et al.* (2007) Delayed immune reconstitution after cord blood transplantation is characterized by impaired thymopoiesis and late memory T-cell skewing. *Blood* **110**: 4543–4551.

113. Hentschke P, Omazic B, Mattsson J *et al.* (2005) T-cell receptor Vβ repertoire after myeloablative and reduced intensity conditioning allogeneic haematopoietic stem cell transplantation. *Scand J Immunol* **61**: 285–294.

114. Pannetier C, Cochet M, Darche S *et al.* (1993) The sizes of the CDR3 hypervariable regions of the murine T-cell receptor beta chains vary as a function of the recombined germ-line segments. *Proc Natl Acad Sci USA* **90**: 4319–4323.

115. Gorski J, Yassai M, Zhu X *et al.* (1994) Circulating T cell repertoire complexity in normal individuals and bone marrow recipients analyzed by CDR3 size spectratyping: Correlation with immune status. *J Immunol* **152**: 5109–5119.

116. Mackall CL, Hakim FT, Gress RE. (1997) T-cell regeneration: all repertoires are not created equal. *Immunol Today* **18**: 245–251.

117. Roux E, Helg C, Dumont-Girard F *et al.* (1996) Analysis of T-cell repopulation after allogeneic bone marrow transplantation: Significant differences between recipients of T-cell depleted and unmanipulated grafts. *Blood* **87**: 3984–3992.

118. Talvensaari K, Clave E, Douay C *et al.* (2002) A broad T-cell repertoire diversity and an efficient thymic function indicate a favorable long-term immune reconstitution after cord blood stem cell transplantation. *Blood* **99**: 1458–1464.

119. Godthelp BC, van Tol MJ, Vossen JM, van Den Elsen PJ. (1999) T-cell immune reconstitution in pediatric leukemia patients after allogeneic bone marrow transplantation with T-cell-depleted or unmanipulated grafts: Evaluation of overall and antigen-specific T-cell repertoires. *Blood* **94**: 4358–4369.

120. Eyrich M, Croner T, Leiler C *et al.* (2002) Distinct contributions of CD4$^+$ and CD8$^+$ naive and memory T-cell subsets to overall T-cell-receptor repertoire complexity following transplantation of T-cell-depleted CD34-selected hematopoietic progenitor cells from unrelated donors. *Blood* **100**: 1915–1918.

121. Dey BR, Spitzer TR. (2006) Current status of haploidentical stem cell transplantation. *Br J Haematol* **135**: 423–437.

122. Koh LP, Chao NJ. (2008) Nonmyeloablative allogeneic hematopoietic stem cell transplant using mismatched/haploidentical donors: A review. *Blood Cells Mol Dis* **40**: 20–24.

123. Aversa F. (2008) Haploidentical haematopoietic stem cell transplantation for acute leukaemia in adults: Experience in Europe and the United States. *Bone Marrow Transplant* **41**: 473–481.

124. Laufer TM, DeKoning J, Markowitz JS *et al.* (1996) Unopposed positive selection and autoreactivity in mice expressing class II MHC only on thymic cortex. *Nature* **383**: 81–85.

125. Laufer TM, Fan L, Glimcher LH. (1999) Self-reactive T cells selected on thymic cortical epithelium are polyclonal and are pathogenic *in vivo*. *J Immunol* **162**: 5078–5084.

126. Tivol E, Komorowski R, Drobyski WR. (2005) Emergent autoimmunity in graft-versus-host disease. *Blood* **105**: 4885–4891.

127. Teshima T, Reddy P, Liu C *et al.* (2003) Impaired thymic negative selection causes autoimmune graft-versus-host disease. *Blood* **102**: 429–435.

128. Sakoda Y, Hashimoto D, Asakura S *et al.* (2007) Donor-derived thymic-dependent T cells cause chronic graft-versus-host disease. *Blood* **109**: 1756–1764.

129. Knobloch C, Friedrich W. (1991) T cell receptor diversity in severe combined immunodeficiency following HLA-haploidentical bone marrow transplantation. *Bone Marrow Transplant* **8**: 383–387.

130. Sarzotti M, Patel DD, Li X *et al.* (2003) T cell repertoire development in humans with SCID after nonablative allogeneic marrow transplantation. *J Immunol* **170**: 2711–2718.

131. Woodard P, Cunningham JM, Benaim E *et al.* (2004) Effective donor lymphohematopoietic reconstitution after haploidentical CD34$^+$-selected hematopoietic stem cell transplantation in children with refractory severe aplastic anemia. *Bone Marrow Transplant* **33**: 411–418.

132. Caillat-Zucman S, Le Deist F, Haddad E *et al.* (2004) Impact of HLA matching on outcome of hematopoietic stem cell transplantation in children with inherited diseases: A single-center comparative analysis of genoidentical, haploidentical or unrelated donors. *Bone Marrow Transplant* **33**(11): 1089–1095.

133. Chen X, Hale GA, Barfield R *et al.* (2006) Rapid immune reconstitution after a reduced-intensity conditioning regimen and a CD3-depleted haploidentical stem cell graft for paediatric refractory haematological malignancies. *Br J Haematol* **135**: 524–532.

134. Friedrich W, Hönig M, Müller SM. (2007) Long-term follow-up in patients with severe combined immunodeficiency treated by bone marrow transplantation. *Immunol Res* **38**: 165–173.

135. Fu YW, Wu de P, Cen JN *et al.* (2007) Patterns of T-cell reconstitution by assessment of T-cell receptor excision circle and T-cell receptor clonal repertoire after allogeneic hematopoietic stem cell

transplantation in leukemia patients — a study in Chinese patients. *Eur J Haematol* **79**: 138–145.

136. Touraine JL, Plotnicky H, Roncarolo MG *et al.* (2007) Immunological lessons learnt from patients transplanted with fully mismatched stem cells. *Immunol Res* **38**: 201–209.

137. Verfuerth S, Peggs K, Vyas P *et al.* (2000) Longitudinal monitoring of immune reconstitution by CDR3 size spectratyping after T-cell-depleted allogeneic bone marrow transplant and the effect of donor lymphocyte infusions on T-cell repertoire. *Blood* **95**: 3990–3995.

138. Hashimoto F, Sugiura K, Inoue K, Ikehara S. (1997) Major histo-compatibility complex restriction between hematopoietic stem cells and stromal cells *in vivo*. *Blood* **89**: 49–54.

139. Zinkernagel RM, Althage A. (1999) On the role of thymic epithelium vs. bone marrow-derived cells in repertoire selection of T cells. *Proc Natl Acad Sci USA* **96**: 8092–8097.

140. Vukmanovic S. (1992) Positive selection of T lymphocytes induced by intrathymic injection of a thymic epithelial cell line. *Nature* **359**: 729–732.

141. Hugo P, Kappler JW, McCormack JE, Marrack P. (1993) Fibroblasts can induce thymocyte positive selection *in vivo*. *Proc Natl Acad Sci USA* **90**: 10335–10339.

142. Pawlowski T, Elliott JD, Loh DY, Staerz UD. (1993) Positive selection of T lymphocytes on fibroblasts. *Nature* **364**: 642–645.

143. Choi EY, Jung KC, Park HJ *et al.* (2005) Thymocyte–thymocyte interaction for efficient positive selection and maturation of CD4 T cells. *Immunity* **23**: 387–396.

144. Martinic MM, Rülicke T, Althage A *et al.* (2003) Efficient T cell repertoire selection in tetraparental chimeric mice independent of thymic epithelial MHC. *Proc Natl Acad Sci USA* **100**: 1861–1866.

145. Markert ML, Boeck A, Hale LP *et al.* (1999) Transplantation of thymus tissue in complete DiGeorge syndrome. *N Engl J Med* **341**: 1180–1189.

146. Markert ML, Devlin BH, Alexieff MJ *et al.* (2007) Review of 54 patients with complete DiGeorge anomaly enrolled in protocols

for thymus transplantation: Outcome of 44 consecutive transplants. *Blood* **109**: 4539–4547.

147. Markert ML, Kostyu DD, Ward FE *et al.* (1997) Successful formation of a chimeric human thymus allograft following transplantation of cultured postnatal human thymus. *J Immunol* **158**: 998–1005.

148. Ochs L, Shu XO, Miller J *et al.* (1995) Late infections after allogeneic bone marrow transplantations: Comparison of incidence in related and unrelated donor transplant recipients. *Blood* **86**: 3979–3986.

149. Wu CJ, Chillemi A, Alyea EP *et al.* (2000) Reconstitution of T-cell receptor repertoire diversity following T-cell depleted allogeneic bone marrow transplantation is related to hematopoietic chimerism. *Blood* **95**: 352–359.

150. Bacigalupo A. (2007) Management of acute graft-versus-host disease. *Br J Haematol* **137**: 87–98.

151. Weinberg KI. (2007) Protection from posttransplantation immune deficiency? *Blood* **109**: 3617–3618.

152. Sale GE, Alavaikko M, Schaefers KM, Mahan CT. (1992) Abnormal CD4:CD8 ratios and delayed germinal center reconstitution in lymph nodes of human graft recipients with graft-versus-host disease (GVHD): An immunohistological study. *Exp Hematol* **20**: 1017–1021.

153. Krenger W, Ferrara JL. (1996) Graft-versus-host disease and the Th1/Th2 paradigm. *Immunol Res* **15**: 50–73.

154. Krenger W, Hill GR, Ferrara JL. (1997) Cytokine cascades in acute graft-versus-host disease. *Transplantation* **64**: 553–558.

155. Blazar BR, Murphy WJ. (2005) Bone marrow transplantation and approaches to avoid graft-versus-host disease (GVHD). *Philos Trans R Soc Lond B Biol Sci* **360**: 1747–1767.

156. Ferrara JL, Reddy P. (2006) Pathophysiology of graft-versus-host disease. *Semin Hematol* **43**: 3–10.

157. Shlomchik WD. (2007) Graft-versus-host disease. *Nat Rev Immunol* **7**: 340–352.

158. Riddell SR, Appelbaum FR. (2007) Graft-versus-host disease: a surge of developments. *PLoS Med* **4**: 1174–1177.

159. Krenger W, Snyder KM, Byon JC *et al.* (1995) Polarized type 2 alloreactive CD4$^+$ and CD8$^+$ donor T cells fail to induce experimental acute graft-versus-host disease. *J Immunol* 1995; **155**: 585–593.

160. Krenger W, Falzarano G, Delmonte J *et al.* (1996) Interferon-gamma suppresses T-cell proliferation to mitogen via the nitric oxide pathway during experimental acute graft-versus-host disease. *Blood* **88**: 1113–1121.

161. Krenger W, Rossi S, Piali L, Holländer GA. (2000) Thymic atrophy in murine acute graft-versus-host disease is effected by impaired cell cycle progression of host pro-T and pre-T cells. *Blood* **96**: 347–354.

162. Hauri-Hohl MM, Keller MP, Gill J *et al.* (2007) Donor T-cell alloreactivity against host thymic epithelium limits T-cell development after bone marrow transplantation. *Blood* **109**: 4080–4088.

163. Ferrara JLM. (2006) GVHD: *In vivo veritas. Blood* **106**: 772–773.

164. Dulude G, Roy DC, Perreault C. (1999) The effect of graft-versus-host disease on T cell production and homeostasis. *J Exp Med* **189**: 1329–1342.

165. Beschorner WE, Hutchins GM, Elfenbein GJ, Santos GW. (1978) The thymus in patients with allogeneic bone marrow transplants. *Am J Pathol* **92**: 173–181.

166. Seddik M, Seemayer TA, Lapp WS. (1980) T cell functional defect associated with thymic epithelial cell injury induced by a graft-versus-host reaction. *Transplantation* **29**: 61–66.

167. Seemayer TA, Lapp WS, Bolande RP. (1978) Thymic epithelial injury in graft-versus-host reactions following adrenalectomy. *Am J Pathol* **93**: 325–338.

168. Lapp WS, Ghayur T, Mendez M *et al.* (1985) The functional and histological basis for graft-versus-host-induced immunosuppression. *Immunol Rev* **88**: 107.

169. Ghayur T, Seemayer T, Lapp WS *et al.* (1990) Histologic correlates of immune functional deficits in graft-vs.-host disease. In: Burakoff SJ, Deeg HJ, Ferrara J, Atkinson K (eds.) *Graft-vs.-Host*

Disease: Immunology, Pathophysiology, and Treatment, pp. 109–132. Marcel Dekker, New York.

170. Seemayer TA, Bolande RP. (1980) Thymic involution mimicking thymic dysplasia: A consequence of transfusion-induced graft versus host disease in a premature infant. *Arch Pathol Lab Med* **104**: 141–144.

171. Gartner JG. (1991) Thymic involution with loss of Hassall's corpuscles mimicking thymic dysplasia in a child with transfusion-associated graft-versus-host disease. *Pediatr Pathol* **11**: 449–456.

172. Clave E, Busson M, Douay C *et al.* (2009) Acute graft versus host disease transiently impairs thymic output in young patients after allogeneic hematopoietic stem cell transplantation. *Blood* **113**: 6477–6484.

173. Krenger W, Schmidlin H, Cavadini G, Holländer GA. (2004) On the relevance of TCR rearrangement circles as molecular markers for thymic output during experimental graft-versus-host disease. *J Immunol* **172**: 7359–7367.

174. Seemayer TA, Lapp WS, Bolande RP. (1977) Thymic involution in murine graft-versus-host reaction: Epithelial injury mimicking human thymic dysplasia. *Am J Pathol* **88**: 119–133.

175. Fukuzawa M, Via CS, Shearer GM. (1988) Defective thymic education of L3T4$^+$ T helper cell function in graft-vs-host mice. *J Immunol* **141**: 430–439.

176. Ghayur T, Seemayer TA, Xenocostas A, Lapp WS. (1988) Complete sequential regeneration of graft-vs.-host-induced severely dysplastic thymuses: Implications for the pathogenesis of chronic graft-vs.-host disease. *Am J Pathol* **133**: 39–46.

177. Fukushi N, Arase H, Wang B *et al.* (1990) Thymus: A direct target tissue in graft-versus-host reaction after allogeneic bone marrow transplantation that results in abrogation of induction of self-tolerance. *Proc Natl Acad Sci USA* **87**: 6301–6305.

178. Desbarats J, Lapp WS. (1993) Thymic selection and thymic major histocompatibility complex class II expression are abnormal in

mice undergoing graft-versus-host reactions. *J Exp Med* **178**: 805–814.

179. Holländer GA, Widmer B, Burakoff SJ. (1994) Loss of normal thymic repertoire selection and persistence of autoreactive T cells in graft vs. host disease. *J Immunol* **152**: 1609–1617.

180. Van den Brink MR, Moore E, Ferrara JL, Burakoff SJ. (2000) Graft-versus-host-disease-associated thymic damage results in the appearance of T cell clones with anti-host reactivity. *Transplantation* **69**: 446–449.

181. Morohashi T, Ogasawara K, Kitaichi N *et al.* (2000) Abrogation of negative selection by GVHR induced by minor histocompatibility antigens or H-2D antigen alone. *Immunobiology* **202**: 268–279.

182. Krenger W, Rossi S, Holländer GA. (2000) Apoptosis of thymocytes during acute graft-versus-host disease is independent of glucocorticoids. *Transplantation* **69**: 2190–2193.

183. Huiskamp R, van Ewijk W. (1985) Repopulation of the mouse thymus after sublethal fission neutron irradiation. I. Sequential appearance of thymocyte subpopulations. *J Immunol* **134**: 2161–2219.

184. Huiskamp R, Davids JA, van Ewijk W. (1988) The effect of graded doses of fission neutrons or X rays on the stromal compartment of the thymus in mice. *Radiat Res* **113**: 25–39.

185. Kumamoto T, Inaba M, Toki J *et al.* (1995) Cytotoxic effects of irradiation and deoxyguanosine on fetal thymus. *Immunobiology* **192**: 365–381.

186. Via CS, Sharrow SO, Shearer GM. (1987) Role of cytotoxic T lymphocytes in the prevention of lupus-like disease occurring in a murine model of graft-versus-host disease. *J Immunol* **139**: 1840–1849.

187. Via CS, Finkelman FD. (1993) Critical role of interleukin-2 in the development of acute graft-versus-host disease. *Int Immunol* **5**: 565–572.

188. Via CS, Rus V, Gately MK, Finkelman FD. (1994) IL-12 stimulates the development of acute graft-versus-host disease in mice that

would normally develop chronic, autoimmune graft-versus-host disease. *J Immunol* **153**: 4040–4047.

189. Garside P, Reid S, Steel M, Mowat AM. (1994) Differential cytokine production associated with distinct phases of murine graft-versus-host reaction. *Immunology* **82**: 211–214.

190. Daikeler T, Tyndall A. (2007) Autoimmunity following haematopoietic stem-cell transplantation. *Best Pract Res Clin Haematol* **20**: 349–360.

191. Filipovich AH, Weisdorf D, Pavletic S *et al.* (2005) National Institutes of Health consensus development project on criteria for clinical trials in chronic graft-versus-host disease: I. Diagnosis and staging working group report. *Biol Blood Marrow Transplant* **11**: 945–956.

192. Mackey JR, Desai S, Larratt L *et al.* (1997) Myasthenia gravis in association with allogeneic bone marrow transplantation: Clinical observations, therapeutic implications and review of literature. *Bone Marrow Transplant* **19**: 939–942.

193. Chu YW, Gress RE. (2008) Murine models of chronic graft-versus-host disease: Insights and unresolved issues. *Biol Blood Marrow Transplant* **14**: 365–378.

194. McCormick LL, Zhang Y, Tootell E, Gilliam AC. (1999) Anti-TGF-beta treatment prevents skin and lung fibrosis in murine sclerodermatous graft-versus-host disease: A model for human scleroderma. *J Immunol* **163**: 5693–5699.

195. Zhang C, Todorov I, Zhang Z *et al.* (2006) Donor CD4$^+$ T and B cells in transplants induce chronic graft-versus-host disease with autoimmune manifestations. *Blood* **107**: 2993–3001.

196. Anderson BE, McNiff JM, Matte C *et al.* (2004) Recipient CD4$^+$ T cells that survive irradiation regulate chronic graft-versus-host disease. *Blood* **104**: 1565–1573.

197. Zhang Y, Hexner E, Frank D, Emerson SG. (2007) CD4$^+$ T cells generated *de novo* from donor hemopoietic stem cells mediate the evolution from acute to chronic graft-versus-host disease. *J Immunol* **179**: 3305–3314.

198. Chen X, Vodanovic-Jankovic S, Johnson B *et al.* (2007) Absence of regulatory T-cell control of TH1 and TH17 cells is responsible for the autoimmune-mediated pathology in chronic graft-versus-host disease. *Blood* **110**: 3804–3813.

199. Goldberg G. (2007) Clinical strategies to enhance T cell reconstitution. *Semin Immunol* **19**: 289–296.

200. Adkins B, Gandour D, Strober S, Weissman I. (1988) Total lymphoid irradiation leads to transient depletion of the mouse thymic medulla and persistent abnormalities among medullary stromal cells. *J Immunol* **140**: 3373–3379.

201. Chung B, Barbara-Burnham L, Barsky L, Weinberg K. (2001) Radiosensitivity of thymic interleukin-7 production and thymopoiesis after bone marrow transplantation. *Blood* **98**: 1601–1606.

202. Kelly RM, Highfill SL, Panoskaltsis-Mortari A *et al.* (2008) Keratinocyte growth factor and androgen blockade work in concert to protect against conditioning regimen-induced thymic epithelial damage and enhance T-cell reconstitution after murine bone marrow transplantation. *Blood* **111**: 5734–5744.

203. Van Vliet E, Melis M, Van Ewijk W. (1986) The influence of dexamethasone treatment on the lymphoid and stromal composition of the mouse thymus: A flow cytometric and immunohistological analysis. *Cell Immunol* **103**: 229–240.

204. Savino W. (2006) The thymus is a common target organ in infectious diseases. *PLoS Pathog* **2**: e62.

205. Finch PW, Rubin JS. (2004) Keratinocyte growth factor/fibroblast growth factor 7, a homeostatic factor with therapeutic potential for epithelial protection and repair. *Adv Cancer Res* 69–115.

206. Radtke ML, Kolesar JM. (2005) Palifermin (Kepivance) for the treatment of oral mucositis in patients with hematologic malignancies requiring hematopoietic stem cell support. *J Oncol Pharm Pract* **11**: 121–125.

207. Siddiqui MA, Wellington K. (2005) Palifermin: In myelotoxic therapy-induced oral mucositis. *Drugs* **65**: 2139–2146.

208. Alpdogan O, Hubbard VM, Smith OM *et al.* (2006) Keratinocyte growth factor (KGF) is required for post-natal thymic regeneration. *Blood* **107**: 2453–2460.

209. Revest JM, Suniara RK, Kerr K *et al.* (2001) Development of the thymus requires signaling through the fibroblast growth factor receptor r2-iiib. *J Immunol* **167**: 1954–1961.

210. Guo L, Degenstein L, Fuchs E. (1996) Keratinocyte growth factor is required for hair development but not for wound healing. *Genes Dev* **10**: 165–175.

211. Min D, Panoskaltsis-Mortari A, Kuro OM *et al.* (2007) Sustained thymopoiesis and improvement in functional immunity induced by exogenous KGF administration in murine models of aging. *Blood* **109**: 2529–2537.

212. Min D, Taylor PA, Panoskaltsis-Mortari A *et al.* (2002) Protection from thymic epithelial cell injury by keratinocyte growth factor: A new approach to improve thymic and peripheral T-cell reconstitution after bone marrow transplantation. *Blood* **99**: 4592–4600.

213. Seggewiss R, Loré K, Guenaga FJ *et al.* (2007) Keratinocyte growth factor augments immune reconstitution after autologous hematopoietic progenitor cell transplantation in rhesus macaques. *Blood* **110**: 441–449.

214. Blazar BR, Weisdorf DJ, DeFor TE *et al.* (2006) Phase 1/2 randomized, placebo-control trial of palifermin to prevent graft-versus-host disease (GVHD) after allogeneic hematopoietic stem cell transplantation (HSCT). *Blood* **108**: 3216–3222.

215. Seggewiss R, Einsele H. (2007) Hematopoietic growth factors including keratinocyte growth factor in allogeneic and autologous stem cell transplantation. *Semin Hematol* **44**: 203–211.

216. Heng TS, Goldberg GL, Gray DH *et al.* (2005) Effects of castration on thymocyte development in two different models of thymic involution. *J Immunol* **175**: 2982–2993.

217. Sutherland JS, Goldberg GL, Hammett MV *et al.* (2005) Activation of thymic regeneration in mice and humans following androgen blockade. *J Immunol* **175**: 2741–2753.

218. Olsen NJ, Olson G, Viselli SM *et al.* (2001) Androgen receptors in thymic epithelium modulate thymus size and thymocyte development. *Endocrinology* **142**: 1278–1283.

219. Erickson M, Morkowski S, Lehar S *et al.* (2002) Regulation of thymic epithelium by keratinocyte growth factor. *Blood* **100**: 3269–3278.

220. Suniara RK, Jenkinson EJ, Owen JJ. (2000) An essential role for thymic mesenchyme in early T cell development. *J Exp Med* **191**: 1051–1056.

221. Revest JM, Spencer-Dene B, Kerr K *et al.* (2001) Fibroblast growth factor receptor 2-IIIb acts upstream of Shh and Fgf4 and is required for limb bud maintenance but not for the induction of Fgf8, Fgf10, Msx1, or Bmp4. *Dev Biol* **231**: 47–62.

222. Brauchle M, Fässler R, Werner S. (1995) Suppression of keratinocyte growth factor expression by glucocorticoids *in vitro* and during wound healing. *J Invest Dermatol* **105**: 579–584.

Chapter 15

Human T Cell Differentiation: New Techniques, Old Challenges

Jean Plum, Magda De Smedt, Georges Leclercq, Bart Vandekerckhove and Tom Taghon*

Basic studies of human T lymphocyte differentiation are subject to a number of constraints. Therefore, insufficient knowledge is available on the differentiation of human stem cells into T cells in order to be able to efficiently generate immune-competent cells. As a result, animal models, particularly the mouse model, are the driving force in immunology. Recent technical advances, however, have made it possible to pursue the goal of generating functional human T cells *in vitro* as a novel culture system has been developed that supports the early stages of their development. Here, we review the *in vivo* and *in vitro* models that have been used in our laboratory to study various aspects of human T cell differentiation. Despite their critical contributions, these models still have several limitations. Therefore, we are currently developing novel approaches that will illuminate critical aspects of human T cell biology and should enhance the *in vitro* generation of functional human T cells.

Introduction

T cells are critical mediators of the immune system and are essential for protecting our body against pathogens and tumor cells. In a number of clinical cases, for example, after myeloablative therapy prior to stem cell transplantation or in the case of HIV infection, patients have reduced

*Corresponding author. Department of Clinical Chemistry, Microbiology and Immunology, University of Ghent, 4BlokA, De Pintelaan 185, B-9000 Gent, Belgium. Tel: 32 9 3323658, Fax: 32 9 3323659. E-mail: jean.plum@ugent.be.

T cell numbers, making them highly susceptible to opportunistic infections. Providing such patients with functional T cells could help to strengthen their immune system, generating a new therapeutic breakthrough. Furthermore, if one was able to manipulate these T cells in such a manner that they specifically recognize tumor cells, new avenues of specific immune therapy with multiple applications would open up. T cell development is initiated when precursor cells from the bone marrow (BM) migrate toward the thymus. However, the precursor cells that are responsible for human T cell development are poorly characterized, despite being of considerable therapeutic interest. When they are provided in sufficient numbers, their presence during stem cell transplantations should significantly enhance T cell generation in these patients.[1–3] Furthermore, progenitor cells from adults seem to lose T cell potential compared to progenitors at a younger age. Thus, characterizing T cell precursors, enabling their *in vitro* expansion and generating functional T cells *in vitro* are critical aspects of T cell biology that have important clinical implications.

Our understanding of human developmental processes is limited, in comparison with some animal models, for several obvious reasons, such as ethical constraints, the complexity of genetic background, or lack of *in vivo* models. It is heartwarming to observe that editors of leading journals stimulate consciousness that "mice are not man" and encourage human immunological research.[4] With respect to T cell development, several differences between mouse and man have been observed.[4,5]

To fill the gap in our knowledge of human T cell differentiation, we have tools that are nearly as powerful as the one available for murine studies. First, with the availability of monoclonal antibodies, it is possible to delineate different populations in bone marrow, thymus, peripheral lymphoid organs and blood. The key monoclonal antibodies for addressing T lymphocyte differentiation are CD34, present on early multipotent progenitors; CD1a, which defines cells that are T-cell-committed; and CD4 and CD8, for delineating successive steps in T cell differentiation. Secondly, molecular techniques gave the opportunity to match these phenotypes with the genotypes for rearrangement of the TCR genes important for the developmental characterization of these populations.[6] The use of a

352

quantitative estimation was instrumental in estimating the degree of rearrangements that was achieved in the different subpopulations. Thirdly, *in vitro* and *in vivo* studies allow the analysis of successive steps in differentiation and the testing of the T lymphocyte potential of precursor cells. The models used are (a) the infusion of cells in NOD-SCID mice, (b) the injection of cells in reconstituted SCID/hu mice, (c) the growth and differentiation of cells in fetal thymus organ culture (FTOC), (d) culture on thymic stromal layers, and (e) differentiation on BM-derived engineered stromal cell layers expressing the Notch ligand delta-like 1 (DLL1). Finally, molecular techniques allow the examination of the role of proteins in human T cell differentiation. A powerful approach similar to that for transgenic mice or knockout mice can be achieved for human progenitor cells by the use of virus-based knockin or RNAi and shRNA knockout technology, although the level of knockdown is never as efficient and long-lasting as in gene-deficient mice.

Here, we will present data from our lab that illustrate how different aspects of human T cell biology can be addressed experimentally and how existing models could improve our knowledge in this field. Using mixed human–murine FTOC we showed (a) that TCR$\alpha\beta$, TCR$\gamma\delta$ lymphocytes, NK cells and dendritic cells complete their differentiation, (b) that IL-7Rα signaling and IL-7 are essential, (c) a detailed phenotypic and functional analysis of discrete successive steps of positively selected thymocytes, (d) that an efficient transduction of genes in HSCs with persistent gene expression throughout the T lymphocyte differentiation can be realized, (e) that enforced expression of the active form of Notch causes an increased ratio of $\gamma\delta$ to $\alpha\beta$ T cells, and (f) that cord blood and BM-derived CD34$^+$ Lin$^-$ hematopoietic precursor cells are able to generate human T cells on OP9-DLL1 cells. Another approach is the *in vivo* SCID-hu reconstitution model. With this method small fragments of the human fetal liver and thymus are implanted under the kidney capsule of an adult SCID mouse, which results in an impressive human thymus organ six months after transplantation. We use this model to study thymus T cell developmental kinetics, development of gene-marked precursor cells and thymic homing of precursor cells. Finally, we have developed systems that allow us to address positive and negative selection of human thymo-cytes *in vitro*.

The Multipotent Hematopoietic Stem Cell and T Cell Potency

Culture techniques have been instrumental in testing the T cell potential of human hematopoietic stem cells (HSCs). It is now accepted that a single type of cell, the multipotent stem cell, is the precursor of all major hematopoietic lineages.[7–9] Stem cells divide to replicate themselves (self-renewal), as well as to produce progeny that will further differentiate into mature blood cells (multipotency). The search for HSCs began with the use of *in vivo* assays in mice in which lethally irradiated animals were reconstituted with candidate precursor cells and tested for radioprotection and long term reconstitution.[9] These assays cannot be performed in man, but some have been performed in baboons. In this way, it was demonstrated that CD34-bearing cells contain the HSCs. However, the CD34$^+$ population is very heterogenous and only a minor fraction is considered to contain actual stem cells.[10]

The nature of T cell precursors is a long-standing debate, questioning whether T cell development is dependent on a clonogenic lymphoid-restricted stem cell [common lymphoid progenitor (CLP)] or whether they derive from multipotent progenitors. Very stimulating but confusing has been the discovery that IL-7Rα is present on a subset of murine BM cells and that this Lin$^-$IL7Rα^+Thy-1$^-$Sca-1^{lo}c-kit^{lo} subpopulation possesses a rapid lymphoid-restricted (T, B, NK) reconstitution capacity and lacks myeloid differentiation potential.[11] Based on these findings the model was proposed wherein B, NK and T cells are derived from CLPs that have lost myeloid potential. A human counterpart of this population with CLP-like properties has been described as a minor subset with a CD34$^+$CD38$^-$CD7$^+$ phenotype in human cord blood.[12] However, the T cell potential of this population was not addressed at that time. Recently, we have shown that this population has indeed T cell potential,[13] but molecular analysis showed that this population expressed genes that are expressed in one or more consecutive stages of early human T and B cell development. This suggests that CLPs are not bipotent at the clonal level but are composed of a mixed population of T and B early precursor cells. This "classical" model of hematopoiesis, in which T cells are derived from CLPs, has recently been challenged by murine studies that support a myeloid-based model instead, for both adult and fetal hematopoiesis.[14–16] These experiments showed that the earliest thymic progenitors (ETPs) retain their myeloid potential and suggested that either multipotent BM progenitors can lose their myeloid potential when they develop into early B cells in the bone marrow, thereby generating CLPs, or, after seeding the thymus, these lymphomyeloid precursors differentiate into ETPs. This implies that selection of CLPs in extrathymic populations enriches for B-cell-engaged cells and should be contraproductive to enrich for progenitors that will differentiate into T cells. However, it still offers the opportunity to generate precursor cells from multipotent progenitor cells that would differentiate more rapidly into a larger number of T cells. This could be of interest in alleviating the T cell deficiency that is seen after myeloablative therapy and stem cell transplantation.

In this respect, Galy *et al.*[17,18] have shown that the $CD10^+CD34^+Lin^-$ c-kit$^-$Thy-1$^-$ population in human BM gives rise to T, B, NK and lymphoid dendritic cells, but very few myeloerythroid cells. As this work was not performed at the clonal level, the clonogenic nature of this population is still unknown. Recently, the subdivision of the $Lin^-CD34^+CD10^+$ progenitor population according to CD24 expression has identified a $CD24^+$ subset that appeared to be exclusively restricted to the B lineage whereas the $CD24^-$ subset has CLP activity and low myeloid potential. These populations were present in cord blood (CB) and adolescent and adult BM, although the staining intensity of CD10 was highest in adolescent BM.[19] It is also important to note that a $CD34^+CD45RA^{hi}CD7^+$ subset has been described in FL, fetal BM and CB that is T/NK-polarized.[20,21] As this population is present in fetal BM but declines around birth, it is possible that this population is no longer present in adults.

A very exciting new development has been the demonstration that Notch signaling is critical for T/B lineage specification, which has been reviewed elsewhere.[22–24] Mammalian Notch proteins constitute a family of transmembrane receptors (Notch 1–4) and ligands [jagged 1–2, delta-like (DLL) 1, 3, 4], conserved throughout evolution and involved in cell fate decisions in many tissues. Upon ligand binding, the Notch protein undergoes a series of proteolytical cleavages, one of them mediated by presenilin, a member of the γ-secretase complex. This cleavage releases the Notch intracellular domain (ICN), which represents the activated form of Notch. ICN translocates to the nucleus and binds to the transcriptional repressor protein CSL, a DNA-binding protein that normally represses transcription through binding with several corepressor complexes. Binding of ICN converts CSL into a transcriptional activator through recruitment of several proteins, such as the proteins of the mastermind-like (MAML) family.

Notch triggering induces mouse hematopoietic progenitors[25] and even mouse embryonic stem (ES) cells[26] to adopt a T cell fate *in vitro* when cocultured on stromal cell lines that express the Notch ligand DLL1. This is astonishing if one considers that complete T cell differentiation, until the end stage of single positive CD8 T cells, has been realized under these *in vitro* conditions. This is also possible for human hematopoietic progenitors. Whereas initially only a progression to the first stages of T cell development was achieved on coculture of CB progenitors with a stromal S17 cell line engineered to express DLL1,[27] further steps of T cell differentiation were obtained in coculture with OP9-DLL1 stromal cells.[28] We have shown that this is also possible with human HSCs from adolescent BM[29] or from granulocyte macrophage–colony stimulating factor–mobilized blood (unpublished data from La Motte-Mohs[30] and De Smedt) and human ES cells.[31]

Human T Cell Differentiation and Development in the Thymus

The development of human T cells in FTOC or on OP9-DLL1 stromal cells has been important for studying the kinetics of the different steps of T cell differentiation. The most immature intrathymic T cell precursors are phenotypically similar to the extrathymically derived progenitor cells. These cells express CD34, are negative for lineage markers (CD3, CD4, CD8), and a subset of those cells is CD38 dim.

We have addressed the phenotypic and lineage potential changes during early T cell development by introducing CD34$^+$CD38$^-$ FL cells in FTOC.[32] We showed that the CD34$^+$CD38$^-$ precursor cells, which are CD4$^-$CD7$^-$cytoplasmatic(cy)CD3$^-$HLA-DR$^{-/++}$, differentiate into a CD4$^+$ population which remains CD7$^-$cyCD3$^-$HLA-DR^{++} and a CD4$^-$ population which expresses CD7 and cyCD3. The CD4$^+$CD7$^-$cyCD3$^-$ cells differentiate into phenotypically and functionally mature dendritic cells, but do not differentiate into T or NK cells. The CD4$^-$CD7$^+$cyCD3$^+$ population later differentiates into a CD4$^+$CD7$^+$cyCD3$^+$HLA-DR$^-$ population, which has no potential to differentiate into dendritic cells, but is able to differentiate into NK cells and $\gamma\delta$ and $\alpha\beta$ T lymphocytes. These findings support the notion that the T/NK split occurs downstream of the NK/dendritic split and were recently confirmed by Crooks and colleagues.[33]

Upregulation of CD1a expression in CD34$^+$ thymocytes marks T lineage commitment, providing the cells with the option to become TCR-$\alpha\beta$ cells and/or TCR-$\gamma\delta$ T cells. Upon further differentiation, human thymocytes start to express CD4, in the absence of CD3, and these cells are called CD4 immature single positive (CD4ISP) cells. These cells express high levels of RAG proteins, necessary for TCR rearrangements, as well as pTα, which will combine with TCRβ to allow pre-TCR signaling. This process is called β selection and allows the immature thymocytes to further differentiate along the TCR-$\alpha\beta$ lineage into CD4$^+$CD8α^+CD8β^+ double positive (DP) thymocytes. If TCR-γ and TCR-δ rearrangements occur prior to β selection, the cells will most likely develop into TCR-$\gamma\delta$ T cells.

The confrontation of these phenotypic changes with gene rearrangements has been done recently by the group of F. Staal.[6] They have selected the following phenotypes as successive steps of T cell differentiation: CB CD34$^+$Lin$^-$ as the most immature progenitors and within the thymus CD34$^+$CD38$^-$CD1a$^-$; CD34$^+$CD38$^+$CD1a$^-$; CD34$^+$CD38$^+$CD1a$^+$; ISPCD4$^+$CD3$^-$; DPCD3$^-$; DPCD3$^+$ and the mature single positive (SP) CD4$^+$CD3$^+$

and the SP CD8α^+CD8β^+CD3$^+$ subsets. It was shown that TCR loci rearrange in a highly ordered way (TCRD-TCRG-TCRB-TCRA). The initiating Dδ2–Dδ3 rearrangements occur at the most immature CD34$^+$CD38$^-$CD1a$^-$ intrathymic stage. TCRB rearrangements start at the next CD34$^+$CD38$^+$CD1a$^-$ stage and complete in-frame TCRB is first detected in ISPCD4$^+$CD3$^-$. Together with the expression of the pTα chain, these data show that human TCRβ selection can initiate at the CD34$^+$CD38$^+$CD1a$^+$ stage, but mainly occurs at the ISP4 stage. This is the first round of selection that allows the survival, expansion and further differentiation of the thymocytes with productive TCRβ rearrangements. It is clear that phenotypic changes during T lymphopoiesis are correlated with important stages of T cell development.

We have done a careful analysis of the phenotypic changes that occur in CD4/CD8 lineage commitment.[34,35] At the DP stage, thymocytes rearrange the TCRα locus and from these DP TCR-$\alpha\beta^+$CD3$^+$ precursors mature functional CD4 or CD8 SP thymocytes differentiate through a process of positive selection and terminal differentiation. Based on the differential expression of CD27, CD1 and CD45RA/RO, human postselection CD69$^+$ thymocytes could be separated into distinct subpopulations, which represent transitional stages of a common differentiation pathway. Phenotypically, CD69$^+$ thymocytes, which are initially CD27$^-$CD1$^+$CD45RA$^-$, sequentially upregulate CD27, downregulate CD1, and eventually acquire CD45RA upon maturation.

Examination of CD4 and CD8 expression on these CD69$^+$ subsets identified an early postselection CD69$^+$CD27$^-$CD4SP population that gives rise to both CD4SP and CD8SP mature T cells when cultured in mouse thymus organs. This indicates that postselection both CD4- and CD8-committed cells downregulate CD8, soon after CD69 is upregulated and before the cells become CD27$^+$. The CD4-committed cells stop the production of CD8 permanently and will acquire CD27. Likewise, the CD8-committed cells will acquire CD27 but stop CD4 production permanently. However, at that stage CD4 molecules already present on the cell surface are retained for a certain period of time, so that the cells appear to be CD4$^+$CD8$^+$. This explains why we can identify a CD4$^+$CD8$^+$ DP cell population that is CD69[+] and CD27[+], which only gives rise to CD8SP progeny upon culture.[36]

In contrast to thymic differentiation of human TCR $\alpha\beta$ cells, differentiation stages of human TCR $\gamma\delta$ cells are only partially known. We have shown that CD1, a known marker of immature TCR $\alpha\beta$ thymocytes, is expressed on a subpopulation of postnatal TCR $\gamma\delta$ thymocytes. Only CD1[+]TCR $\gamma\delta$ thymocytes express recombination-activating gene-1 mRNA, and differentiate into CD1[−] TCR $\gamma\delta$ thymocytes. Interestingly, in contrast to CD1[−] TCR $\alpha\beta$ cells, CD1[−] TCR $\gamma\delta$ thymocytes proliferate extensively when cultured with exogenous rIL-2 or rIL-15 alone. Flow-cytometric analysis as well as reverse transcription-PCR analysis showed that only CD1[−] TCR $\gamma\delta$ thymocytes express IL-2Rβ protein and mRNA. The differential expression of maturation markers, such as CD27, CD45RO and CD45RA, as a function of the expression of CD1, is similar in TCR $\gamma\delta$ and TCR $\alpha\beta$ thymocytes. An important exception is the expression of CD4 and CD8. TCR $\alpha\beta$ thymocytes are mainly CD4[+]CD8[+] DP at the immature CD1[+] stage and CD4 or CD8 SP at the mature CD1[−] stage. On the contrary, CD1[bright] TCR $\gamma\delta$ thymocytes all expressed CD4, but only some of them expressed CD8. Some CD1[−] TCR $\gamma\delta$ thymocytes also expressed CD8, but were negative for CD4. Collectively, our data clearly show that CD1 is a useful marker for distinguishing immature human TCR $\gamma\delta$ thymocytes from functional mature $\gamma\delta$ cells based on recombination-activating gene-1 expression, *in vitro* differentiation, and phenotypic and functional characteristics.[37]

Models for Selection of Human Developing T Cells

The composition of self-peptide ligands present in the thymus plays a critical role in shaping the preimmune T cell repertoire.[38] Immature thymocytes expressing TCRs with low affinity for self-peptide/MHC survive and undergo further maturation (positive selection). Overtly, autoreactive T cells are deleted by induction of programmed cell death (negative selection). Thereby, mature thymocytes with low affinity for self-peptide/MHC migrate to the periphery, founding a highly diverse T cell repertoire.[39]

Additionally, self-peptide/MHC ligands deliver survival signals to naive T cells for their persistence in the periphery[40,41] The recognition of self-peptides by T cells through the TCR has exquisite specificity, as demonstrated by the drastic effects of single amino acid substitutions.[42] However, the high degree of peptide cross-reactivity built in the T cell repertoire ensures recognition of virtually any presentable peptide. Synthetic peptide libraries contributed to the identification of multiple ligands that stimulate the same T cell clone without necessarily displaying sequence homology.[41] It has been estimated that the frequency of individual epitope-specific naive T cells ranges around $1–5 \times 10^{-5}$,[43] which is below the limit of direct detection with currently available assays. TCR-transgenic approaches provide model systems for monitoring the selection process and *in vivo* fate of naive antigen-specific T cells.[44] In humans, however, the low frequency of self-peptide–specific T cells in the preimmune repertoire has so far precluded their precise investigation.

Naturally Occurring Selection Processes Allow the Addressing Positive and Negative Selection of Human Thymocytes

Positive Selection

The melanocyte differentiation antigen Melan-A/MART-1 (Melan-A)* is a self-protein of unknown function that is expressed by melanocytes and the majority of malignant melanoma cells, but not by other tissues.[45,46] HLA-A2–restricted Melan-A–specific CD8 T cells have been shown to primarily recognize the Melan-A 26–35 and 27–35 peptides.[46,47] The use of HLA-A2 multimers synthesized around the Melan-A 26–35 A27L peptide analog enabled identification of Melan-A–specific T cells *ex vivo* in both tumor-infiltrated lymph nodes and circulating lymphocytes of melanoma patients, as well as healthy individuals.[48] In the latter, Melan-A–specific T cells are phenotypically naive ($CCR7^+$ $CD45RA^{high}$ $CD45RO^-CD28^+$), and surprisingly comprise $\sim10^{-3}$ of circulating CD8 T cells. This frequency is at least 10^2 times higher than the one currently estimated for naive antigen-specific lymphocyte precursors, and is comparable to that of epitope-specific memory CD8 T cells. In collaboration with the group of P. Romero (Lausanne, Switzerland) we have recently discovered how this unexpected large T cell pool is established and maintained. Using MHC/peptide multimers, Melan-A–specific T cells in the thymus and periphery of newborns and adults were enumerated. The contribution of thymic production to this large self-specific T cell pool was estimated by combined A2/Melan-A multimer labeling with measurement of the postthymic replicative history by quantification of T cell receptor excision circles (TRECs) and telomere length in antigen-specific CD8 T cells. Both parameters provided direct evidence that a high frequency of thymic precursors is the predominant mechanism shaping the Melan-A–specific T cell preimmune repertoire.[49]

Identification of antigen-specific cells in both the DP and SP stages of T cell development by staining with A2/peptide multimers showed that neither A2/Melan-A$^+$ nor A2/Flu-MA$^+$ cells were detected in the pool of DP thymocytes. However, staining of CD4-depleted thymocytes from nine HLA-A2$^-$ individuals with A2/Melan-A multimers did not detect CD8 SP cells, whereas similar analysis with HLA-A2$^+$ thymocytes revealed significant numbers of A2/Melan-A$^+$ CD8 SP cells in two-thirds of the individuals. As expected, A2/Melan-A$^+$ cells were not detectable in CD4 SP cells. Furthermore, A2/Flu$^-$MA$^+$ cells were not detected in the thymus. Altogether, our results indicated that a high frequency of Melan-A, but not influenza-specific CD8 SP precursors, is generated in the human thymus, so that all the conditions are fulfilled to trace positively selected human thymocytes.

Negative Selection

In collaboration with the group of B. Conrad (Geneve, Switzerland) we have shown that the human endogenous retrovirus K-18 (HERV-K18) region on chromosome 1 provides an excellent model for exploring central tolerance in human.[50] HERV-K18 encodes a superantigen (SAg) stimulating Vβ7CD4 T cells. We showed that this HERV-K18 SAg is constitutively expressed in immature DPCD3⁻ thymocytes. HERV-K18 exists as three alleles, encoding secreted or cell surface membrane proteins. The surface protein complexes are unstable and are shed from cells.[51] As a result, in all cases, SAg can become available for presentation by MHC class 2 in *trans*. We developed an *in vitro* model wherein A20 murine B lymphoma cells, to function as APCs, were added to human thymocytes and cultured overnight. Either A20 cells transduced with HERVK18 or exogenously added soluble SAg SEB resulted in a SAg dose-dependent decrease of either $V\beta7$ or $V\beta17$ CD4 T cells, whereas the nonreactive $V\beta2$ CD4 population remained unchanged as compared to the thymocytes that were cultured with A20 cells alone. In our hands the induced negative selection affected the targeted $V\beta7$ or $V\beta17$ CD4 cells which were semimature CD4SP in transition between CD4CD8DP and CD4SP. This model offers the opportunity to address negative selection in human T cell differentiation.

More or Less Notch Matters

The OP9-DLL1 coculture system was developed with the knowledge that Notch signaling is a major driving force for T cell development. We were able to show that this is also the case for human T cell development as CD4⁺CD8⁺CD1⁺TCR$\alpha\beta$⁺ T cells differentiate in the BM of SCID mice that have been injected with human CB HSCs, after transduction with the gene encoding for the constitutive active form of Notch1 (ICN1).[51] This indicates that extrathymic differentiation of human T cells is possible, if the Notch pathway is sufficiently triggered. Therefore, we concluded that a strong Notch signal is essential for adopting the T cell fate. Unexpectedly, we also observed that in FTOC, ICN1-transduced CD34⁺ progenitors from CB or the thymus consistently generated more TCR-$\gamma\delta$ T cells at the expense of TCR-$\alpha\beta$ T cells. This observation suggested that Notch signaling intensities are critical for the developmental outcome of human T cell precursors.[52] Therefore, we modulated the intensity of the Notch signaling pathway during human T cell development by various methods. Strong Notch signals were provided in OP9-DLL1 coculture, and in FTOC through the mouse thymic microenvironment or through transduction of the human progenitor cells with ICN1. Notch signaling was reduced or inhibited with the γ-secretase inhibitor 7 (N-[N-(3,5-difluorophenyl)-L-alanyl]-S-phenyl-glycine t-butyl ester) (DAPT) or by transducing human T cell precursors with a dominant negative form of MAML protein.[53] With these approaches we could show: (1) that cell fate decisions in human CD34[+] progenitor cells toward T, NK and B cells are influenced by the intensity or absence of the Notch signal, (2) that Notch signaling intensities are important in TCR-$\alpha\beta$ versus TCR-$\gamma\delta$ lineage decisions in a manner that is the opposite compared to murine T cell development, (3) and that lowering Notch signaling in CD34[+] or CD4 ISP thymocytes with the γ-secretase inhibitor DAPT induces the development of aberrant CD4[+]CD8[+] DP T lymphocytes that do not succeed in the rearrangement of the TCR-β chain.[54] Thus, Notch signaling critically influences human hematopoietic cell fate decisions.

The intensity of the Notch signal is the result of the interaction between the Notch receptor and its ligand, in combination with a complex molecular network. Subsequently, it will vary throughout development within the cell, and the Notch signaling pathway must therefore be viewed as a rheostat, rather than as an "on–off" switch. Thus, during T cell differentiation, it is simply not sufficient for the Notch signal to be present — it must also be present at the appropriate level at the appropriate stage of differentiation. Although a detailed expression topography of the Notch ligands in the thymus is lacking, it is clear that the developing T cell will encounter different Notch signal intensities during its passage through different zones of the thymus.[55] Altering these signaling intensities will influence the cell fate as well as important developmental checkpoints such as TCR $\alpha\beta$ versus TCR $\gamma\delta$ diversification or positive and negative selection of TCR $\alpha\beta$ cells. It is important to realize that culturing T cell precursors on OP9-DLL1 cells could affect normal T cell development because the normal *in vivo* regulation in the intensity of Notch signaling by the different ligand interactions is absent. Therefore, the OP9-DLL1 model needs further in-depth studies that address these fine-tunings.

Notch and Human NK Cell Development

T cells and NK cells are closely related, not only functionally but also developmentally as T/NK cell precursors have been described in the thymus of both mouse and man. It has been proposed that this thymic pathway of NK cell differentiation generates NK cells that are distinct, in both phenotype and function, compared to the mainstream BM-derived NK cells.[56] Since Notch signaling is abundantly present in the thymus, we investigated the impact of this pathway on human NK cell development and provided a link between Notch signaling and the generation of intracellular CD3ε (cyCD3)–expressing NK cells in humans.[57] We obtained a high percentage of cyCD3$^+$ NK cells from human CD34$^+$ CB progenitors that differentiated in IL-15–supplemented FTOC or OP9-DLL1 coculture. In contrast, blocking Notch signaling in these conditions with the γ-secretase inhibitor DAPT mainly yields cyCD3$^-$ NK cells. The requirement for Notch signaling to generate cyCD3$^+$ NK cells was further substantiated by transduction of CD34$^+$CB cells with ICN1 (to stimulate Notch signaling) or the dominant-negative mutant of MAML1 (to inhibit Notch signaling), which results in the generation of NK cells with respectively high and low frequencies of cyCD3. Human thymic CD34$^+$ progenitor cells have the potential to generate cyCD3$^+$ NK cells in the absence of Notch/DLL1 signaling, indicating that those cells had already received a sufficient strong Notch signal prior to initiation of the cultures. Since peripheral blood NK cells are unable to induce cyCD3 expression after DLL1 exposure, this shows that Notch-dependent cyCD3 expression can only be achieved during the early phase of NK cell differentiation. *In vivo*, the cyCD3$^+$ NK cells are found at high frequency in the NK cell populations of the human postnatal thymus (~30%) and CB (~25%), and at lower frequency in peripheral blood (~3%).

Although it was tempting to relate the cyCD3$^+$ NK cell subset to the described thymus-dependent CD56^{bright}CD16$^-$ cytokine–producing NK cell subset and the cyCD3$^-$NK cell subset to the BM-derived CD56^{low}CD16$^+$ cytolytic NK cell subset, we were not able to show these distinct functions in the NK cells we generated on OP9-DLL1. CyCD3$^+$ NK cells display both a higher cytolytic and cytokine-producing capacity than the cyCD3$^-$NK cells that are generated on OP9 control cells. This potential discrepancy could be explained by a difference in the stem cell source. Since cyCD3 expression is clearly dependent on signals during early stages of NK cell development, the difference in the environment between the fetal liver and adult BM can certainly influence the NK cell potential of the residing stem cells. Alternatively, additional components of the thymic microenvironment are lacking in the OP9-DLL1 coculture system that might influence the development and functional capacities of the resulting NK cells.

When we generate NK cells from precursors in the postnatal thymus, we also obtain a population that is highly enriched for cyCD3[+] NK cells, even in the absence of Notch signaling. Therefore, we consider that cyCD3[+] NK cells represent the offspring of precursor cells that received a Notch signal during the very early stages of differentiation. This indicates that, during early fetal life, NK cells are generated in the fetal liver, and later in the thymus, that differ from the postnatal NK cells that are generated in the BM. The significance of this early wave with distinct characteristics remains to be established, but is in line with the properties of the CD34[+]CD45RA[hi]CD7[+] subset which has been described by the group of Canque.[21] However, it is important to note that in adult peripheral blood a small population of cyCD3[+]NK cells is present. Those NK cells are of interest because they could be derived from precursors that resemble early T cell precursors, thereby helping us to discover a precursor cell population that is possibly endowed with the capacity of rapid thymus restoration. However, a major drawback is the fact that cyCD3 is an intracellular marker which necessitates permeabilization of the cells. Therefore, because the cells are no longer viable after their identification, it is impossible to test if cyCD3 characterizes precursor cells that efficiently differentiate into T cells. We are currently looking for membrane antigens that allow the characterization of these cyCD3[+] precursor cells.

Conclusion and Future Directions

There are many techniques available for generating and studing human T cell differentiation *in vitro* and *in vivo*. The availability of the

OP9-DLL1 stromal cell line, which allows human T cell differentiation *in vitro*, is instrumental because it allows the study of T cell potential at the clonal level. In addition, the possibility of transducing TCR genes from well-characterized human T cell clones into precursor cells allows the generation of T cells with a clonal TCR and the investigation of the cell fate on OP9-DLL1 stromal cells that have been engineered to express human HLA class I or class II molecules. Addition of the selecting peptide will give a powerful approach to investigating positive and negative selection. However, we must keep in mind that T cell differentiation in a thymus microenvironment is a far more complex and subtle process wherein multiple variables, including an important variability of Notch ligand interaction, result in the fine-tuning of Notch signaling in the developing cell. All these variables will ultimately shape T cell differentiation and T cell and TCR selection in a coordinated manner. Therefore, we will have to interpret with caution the data that we obtain in our models, especially when we want to use these *in-vitro*-generated T cells in clinical applications.

Acknowledgments

This study was supported by grants from the Fund for Scientific Research–Flanders (FWO), the Flemish Institute for the Advancement of Scientific–Technological Research in the Industry (IWT), the Concerted Research Action of Ghent University (GOA), the Interuniversity Attraction Pole of the Belgian Federal Science Policy, and the Foundation Against Cancer (a foundation of public interest).

References

1. Zakrzewski JL, Goldberg GL, Smith OM, van den Brink MR. (2008) Enhancing T cell reconstitution after hematopoietic stem cell transplantation: A brief update of the latest trends. *Blood Cells Mol Dis* **40**: 44.
2. Zakrzewski JL, Kochman AA, Lu SX *et al.* (2006) Adoptive transfer of T-cell precursors enhances T-cell reconstitution after allogeneic hematopoietic stem cell transplantation. *Nat Med* **12**: 1039.

3. Zakrzewski JL, Suh D, Markley JC *et al.* (2008) Tumor immunotherapy across MHC barriers using allogeneic T-cell precursors. *Nat Biotechnol* **26**: 453.

4. Editorial. (2008) Assessing the status of human immunology. *Nat Immunol* **9**: 569.

5. Payne KJ, Crooks GM. (2007) Immune-cell lineage commitment: Translation from mice to humans. *Immunity* **26**: 674.

6. Dik WA, Pike-Overzet K, Weerkamp F *et al.* (2005) New insights on human T cell development by quantitative T cell receptor gene rearrangement studies and gene expression profiling. *J Exp Med* **201**: 1715.

7. Dexter M, Allen T. (1992) Haematopoiesis: Multi-talented stem cells? *Nature* **360**: 709.

8. Huang S, Terstappen LW. (1994) Lymphoid and myeloid differentiation of single human CD34$^+$, HLA-DR$^+$, CD38$^-$ hematopoietic stem cells. *Blood* **83**: 1515.

9. Keller G. (1992) Hematopoietic stem cells. *Curr Opin Immunol* **4**: 133.

10. Bender JG, Unverzagt KL, Walker DE *et al.* (1991) Identification and comparison of CD34-positive cells and their subpopulations from normal peripheral blood and bone marrow using multicolor flow cytometry. *Blood* **77**: 2591.

11. Kondo M, Weissman IL, Akashi K. (1997) Identification of clonogenic common lymphoid progenitors in mouse bone marrow. *Cell* **91**: 661.

12. Hao Q-L, Zhu J, Price MA *et al.* (2001) Identification of a novel, human multilymphoid progenitor in cord blood. *Blood* **97**: 3683.

13. Hoebeke I, De Smedt M, Stolz F *et al.* (2007) T-, B- and NK-lymphoid, but not myeloid cells arise from human CD34(+)CD38(−)CD7(+) common lymphoid progenitors expressing lymphoid-specific genes. *Leukemia* **21**: 311.

14. Bell JJ, Bhandoola A. (2008) The earliest thymic progenitors for T cells possess myeloid lineage potential. *Nature* **452**: 764.

15. Wada H, Masuda K, Satoh R *et al.* (2008) Adult T-cell progenitors retain myeloid potential. *Nature* **452**: 768.

16. Schwarz BA, Bhandoola A. (2004) Circulating hematopoietic progenitors with T lineage potential. *Nat Immunol* **5**: 953.

17. Galy A, Travis M, Cen D, Chen B. (1995) Human T, B, natural killer, and dendritic cells arise from a common bone marrow progenitor cell subset. *Immunity* **3**: 459.

18. Galy AH, Cen D, Travis M *et al.* (1995) Delineation of T-progenitor cell activity within the CD34$^+$ compartment of adult bone marrow. *Blood* **85**: 2770.

19. Six EM, Bonhomme D, Monteiro M *et al.* (2007) A human postnatal lymphoid progenitor capable of circulating and seeding the thymus. *J Exp Med* **204**: 3085.

20. Haddad R, Guardiola P, Izac B *et al.* (2004) Molecular characterization of early human T/NK and B-lymphoid progenitor cells in umbilical cord blood. *Blood* **104**: 3918.

21. Haddad R, Guimiot F, Six E *et al.* (2006) Dynamics of thymus-colonizing cells during human development. *Immunity* **24**: 217.

22. Radtke F, Wilson A, MacDonald HR. (2004) Notch signaling in T- and B-cell development. *Curr Opin Immunol* **16**: 174.

23. Radtke F, Wilson A, Mancini SJ, MacDonald HR. (2004) Notch regulation of lymphocyte development and function. *Nat Immunol* **5**: 247.

24. Maillard I, Fang T, Pear WS. (2005) Regulation of lymphoid development, differentiation, and function by the Notch pathway. *Annu Rev Immunol* **23**: 945.

25. Schmitt TM, Zuniga-Pflucker JC. (2002) Induction of T cell development from hematopoietic progenitor cells by delta-like-1 *in vitro*. *Immunity* **17**: 749.

26. de Pooter RF, Cho SK, Carlyle JR, Zuniga-Pflucker JC. (2003) *In vitro* generation of T lymphocytes from embryonic stem cell-derived prehematopoietic progenitors. *Blood* **102**: 1649.

27. Jaleco AC, Neves H, Hooijberg E *et al.* (2001) Differential effects of Notch ligands delta-1 and jagged-1 in human lymphoid differentiation. *J Exp Med* **194**: 991.

28. La Motte-Mohs RN, Herer E, Zuniga-Pflucker JC. (2005) Induction of T-cell development from human cord blood hematopoietic stem cells by delta-like 1 *in vitro*. *Blood* **105**: 1431.

29. De Smedt M, Hoebeke I, Plum J. (2004) Human bone marrow CD34$^+$ progenitor cells mature to T cells on OP9-DL1 stromal cell line without thymus microenvironment. *Blood Cells Mol Dis* **33**: 227.

30. Awong G, La Motte-Mohs RN, Zuniga-Pflucker JC. (2007) Generation of pro-T cells *in vitro*: Potential for immune reconstitution. *Semin Immunol* **19**: 341.

31. Frank Timmermans, Imke Velghe, Lieve Vanwallegham, *et al.* (2009) Generation of T cells from embryonic stem cell-derived hematopoietic zones. *J Immuno* **182**: 6879–6888.

32. Plum J, De Smedt M, Verhasselt B *et al.* (1999) *In vitro* intrathymic differentiation kinetics of human fetal liver CD34$^+$CD38$^-$ progenitors reveals a phenotypically defined dendritic/T-NK precursor split. *J Immunol* **162**: 60.

33. Hao QL, George AA, Zhu J *et al.* (2008) Human intrathymic lineage commitment is marked by differential CD7 expression: Identification of CD7$^-$ lympho-myeloid thymic progenitors. *Blood* **111**: 1318.

34. Vanhecke D, Leclercq G, Plum J, Vandekerckhove B. (1995) Characterization of distinct stages during the differentiation of human CD69$^+$CD3$^+$ thymocytes and identification of thymic emigrants. *J Immunol* **155**: 1862.

35. Vanhecke D, Verhasselt B, De Smedt M *et al.* (1997) MHC class II molecules are required for initiation of positive selection but not during terminal differentiation of human CD4 single positive thymocytes. *J Immunol* **158**: 3730.

36. Vanhecke D, Verhasselt B, De Smedt M *et al.* (1997) Human thymocytes become lineage committed at an early postselection CD69$^+$ stage, before the onset of functional maturation. *J Immunol* **159**: 5973.

37. Offner F, Van Beneden K, Debacker V *et al.* (1997) Phenotypic and functional maturation of TCR gamma-delta cells in the human thymus. *J Immunol* **158**: 4634.

38. Goldrath AW, Bogatzki LY, Bevan MJ. (2000) Naive T cells transiently acquire a memory-like phenotype during homeostasis-driven proliferation. *J Exp Med* **192**: 557.

39. Sandberg JK, Franksson L, Sundback J *et al.* (2000) T cell tolerance based on avidity thresholds rather than complete deletion allows maintenance of maximal repertoire diversity. *J Immunol* **165**: 25.

40. Viret C, Wong FS, Janeway CA, Jr. (1999) Designing and maintaining the mature TCR repertoire: The continuum of self-peptide:self-MHC complex recognition. *Immunity* **10**: 559.

41. Ernst B, Lee DS, Chang JM *et al.* (1999) The peptide ligands mediating positive selection in the thymus control T cell survival and homeostatic proliferation in the periphery. *Immunity* **11**: 173.

42. Hemmer B, Pinilla C, Gran B *et al.* (2000) Contribution of individual amino acids within MHC molecule or antigenic peptide to TCR ligand potency. *J Immunol* **164**: 861.

43. Mason D. (1998) A very high level of crossreactivity is an essential feature of the T-cell receptor. *Immunol Today* **19**: 395.

44. Bouneaud C, Kourilsky P, Bousso P. (2000) Impact of negative selection on the T cell repertoire reactive to a self-peptide: A large fraction of T cell clones escapes clonal deletion. *Immunity* **13**: 829.

45. Coulie PG, Brichard V, Van Pel A *et al.* (1994) A new gene coding for a differentiation antigen recognized by autologous cytolytic T lymphocytes on HLA-A2 melanomas. *J Exp Med* **180**: 35.

46. Kawakami Y, Eliyahu S, Delgado CH *et al.* (1994) Identification of a human melanoma antigen recognized by tumor-infiltrating lymphocytes associated with *in vivo* tumor rejection. *Proc Natl Acad Sci USA* **91**: 6458.

47. Romero P, Gervois N, Schneider J *et al.* (1997) Cytolytic T lymphocyte recognition of the immunodominant HLA-A*0201-restricted Melan-A/MART-1 antigenic peptide in melanoma. *J Immunol* **159**: 2366.

48. Romero P, Dunbar PR, Valmori D *et al.* (1998) *Ex vivo* staining of metastatic lymph nodes by class I major histocompatibility complex tetramers reveals high numbers of antigen-experienced tumor-specific cytolytic T lymphocytes. *J Exp Med* **188**: 1641.

49. Zippelius A, Bioley G, Le Gal FA *et al.* (2004) Human thymus exports naive CD8 T cells that can home to nonlymphoid tissues. *J Immunol* **172**: 2773.

50. Meylan F, De Smedt M, Leclercq G *et al.* (2005) Negative thymocyte selection to HERV-K18 superantigens in humans. *Blood* **105**: 4377.

51. Fass D, Kim PS. (1995) Dissection of a retrovirus envelope protein reveals structural similarity to influenza hemagglutinin. *Curr Biol* **5**: 1377.

52. De Smedt M, Reynvoet K, Kerre T *et al.* (2002) Active form of Notch imposes T cell fate in human progenitor cells. *J Immunol* **169**: 3021.

53. Tom Taghon, Inge Van de Walle, Greet De Smet, *et al.* (2009) Notch signaling is required for proliferation but not for differentiation at a well-defined β-selection checkpoint during human T-cell development. *Blood* **113**: 3254–3263.

54. De Smedt M, Hoebeke I, Reynvoet K *et al.* (2005) Different thresholds of Notch signaling bias human precursor cells toward B-, NK-, monocytic/dendritic-, or T-cell lineage in thymus microenvironment. *Blood* **106**: 3498.

55. Ciofani M, Zuniga-Pflucker JC. (2007) The thymus as an inductive site for T lymphopoiesis. *Annu Rev Cell Dev Biol* **23**: 463.

56. Vosshenrich CA, Garcia-Ojeda ME, Samson-Villeger SI *et al.* (2006) A thymic pathway of mouse natural killer cell development characterized by expression of GATA-3 and CD127. *Nat Immunol* **7**: 1217.

57. De Smedt M, Taghon T, Van de Walle I *et al.* (2007) Notch signaling induces cytoplasmic CD3 epsilon expression in human differentiating NK cells. *Blood* **110**: 2696.

Chapter 16

Optimising Adoptive T Cell Therapy Following Allogeneic Hematopoietic Stem Cell Transplantation

*Sara Ghorashian, Graham Wright, Sharyn Thomas,
Daniel P. Hart, Judy King, Cecile Voisine,
Constandina Pospori, Mario Perro, Michela Cesco-Gaspere,
Angelika Holler, Liquan Gao, Shao-An Xue, Emma C. Morris,
Ronjon Chakraverty and Hans J. Stauss**

Introduction

Allogeneic hematopoietic stem cell transplantation (HSCT) is carried out to correct genetic disorders of the hematopoietic system, as well as to treat hematopoietic malignancies. Adoptive T cell therapy has great potential as an adjunct to this treatment modality, and clinical trials have already demonstrated the feasibility and efficacy of this approach. It offers two therapeutic effects in this setting:

(1) Augmentation of anti-tumor responses, such as in the setting of relapsed disease;
(2) Prevention and treatment of transplant-related infections.

Underlying the therapeutic efficacy of adoptive T cell therapy is the demonstration of a graft-vs-leukemia/lymphoma (GvL) effect

*Corresponding author. Department of Immunology and Molecular Pathology, Royal Free Hospital, University College London, Hampstead Campus, Rowland Hill Street, London NW3 2PF, England. E-mail: hstauss@medsch.ucl.ac.uk.

post-allogeneic-HSCT. In other words, patients treated by allogeneic HSCT for certain hematological malignancies have a lower rate of relapse than those receiving their own HSCs or HSCs from a syngeneic twin. Within the transferred allogeneic hematopoietic system, the T lymphocyte population plays an important role in mediating the GvL effect. This principle has been further advanced by the beneficial use of infusions of donor lymphocytes to control relapse post-allogeneic-HSC transplantation in malignancies such as chronic myeloid leukemia and non-Hodgkin lymphoma, where the GvL effect is most prominent.

Adoptive T cell therapy is also an important strategy to treat and prevent peri-transplant viral infections, e.g. cytomegalovirus (CMV). Patients are vulnerable to these infections because of the immunosuppressive nature of the conditioning they receive.

However, until recently, traditional adoptive T cell therapies have been limited in scope. Administration of donor T cells carries with it the risk of graft-vs-host disease (GvHD). The ability to tailor adoptive therapy to an individual's disease, immune status and HLA background could unlock the full potential of this therapeutic modality whilst reducing the risk of GvHD, and hence is the research interest of many groups around the world.

Tailoring could be achieved in two ways:

(1) Transfer of antigen-selected T cells, i.e. a population which expresses a T cell receptor (TCR) with specificity for a certain antigen or tumor cell. This strategy may reduce the risk of GvHD; however, the donor's lymphocyte pool may lack the necessary TCR repertoire — for example, when using a donor that has not previously been exposed to CMV, or does not harbor T cells capable of responding to the tumor in question.
(2) Genetic engineering (transduction) of T cells such that they express a new TCR which confers upon them the ability to target disease.

The first strategy has been extensively examined by groups studying antigen-specific T cell therapy to treat viral infections following allogeneic

HSC transplantation. Viral infections contribute significantly to transplant-related mortality. Drug treatments are effective but limited and are associated with significant toxicity. The incidence of post-transplant viral infection is related to the delay in reconstitution of cell-mediated adaptive immunity, the degree of immunosuppression consequent to donor–recipient HLA mismatch, the viral immune status of the donor, whether the disease is transmitted in the graft and the presence of latent disease in the recipient.

Small clinical studies have demonstrated the safety and efficacy of transfer of virus-specific cytotoxic lymphocytes (CTLs) following allogeneic HSC transplantation for therapy of adenoviral, cytomegalovirus (CMV) and Epstein–Barr virus (EBV) infections (reviewed in Refs. 1 and 2). In addition, trials of prophylaxis for EBV and CMV show promising results. Further work is now focused on:

- Optimization of the CTL population to minimize the risk of GvHD, e.g. via depletion of CTLs with reactivity to the recipient;
- Improvement of selection protocols to avoid the necessity of prolonged stimulation and culture, e.g. use of interferon γ capture technology;
- Generation of multi-virus-specific CTLs with reactivity against a combination of viral epitopes, e.g. for both CMV and EBV;
- Reduction of the risk of GvHD by transduction of virus-specific CTLs with susceptibility genes, such as viral thymidine-kinase or inducible apoptosis pathway mediators, e.g. caspase 9;
- Use of third-party CTLs to overcome a lack of virus-specific CTLs in the HSC donor.

A similar approach to cancer immunotherapy has been to isolate autologous tumor-responsive CTLs from the circulation of patients suffering from cancer, or from the tumor itself, in the case of solid malignancies. This approach, in combination with administration of IL-2, was first used to treat patients with metastatic melanoma in 1988.[3] More recent studies suggest response rates of 50–75%, depending on the concomitant conditioning, such as total body irradiation.[4]

However, use of antigen-selected CTLs is often limited by an absence of high-avidity CTLs to cancer antigens in the natural T cell repertoire. This is because most tumor-associated antigens (TAAs) are also self-antigens, but are up-regulated in tumor cells. The adaptive immune system has evolved this as a necessary "safety feature" whereby high-avidity T cells to self-antigens are deleted or rendered unresponsive by central and peripheral tolerance mechanisms.

Studies published in 1999 by Clay *et al.*[5] demonstrated the proof of principle of TCR gene transfer. This was followed by the work of other groups proving that TCRs of many specificities can be transferred. Thus, there is potential for lymphocytes of any HLA background to be redirected with the specificity of choice, overcoming the lack of a tumor-specific T cell repertoire in the patient and providing an instantly available "off the shelf" therapeutic product. This latter strategy will be the main subject of this chapter.

Having demonstrated the feasibility of tailored adoptive T cell therapy, we are now faced with challenges that include raising the efficiency of these cells to the threshold required for a therapeutic clinical effect, optimizing their mass production so that they are available on a clinically relevant time scale, and achieving all the regulatory requirements for a clinical grade therapeutic product.

This chapter presents the processes involved in generating antigen-redirected T cells by the process of transduction, a review of studies in which this therapy has been used, a discussion on the limitations and potential dangers of this approach and, finally, consideration of ways in which adoptive therapy with TCR-transduced T cells can be optimised.

Identification of an Appropriate Target Antigen

To be presented to a CD8[+] T cell, a target antigen from a tumor cell must be processed into peptides and bind to MHC class 1 in the endoplasmic reticulum. In doing so, it must compete for the various parts of this cellular machinery with peptides derived from normal proteins. This influences the density and range of tumor antigens expressed on any tumor cell. In addition, tumors may evolve ways of bypassing antigen presentation in order to evade recognition by the immune system.

Tumor-specific antigens (TSAs) are those only seen on tumor cells, and never on normal cells. They often arise from mutations due to oncogenesis, such as the BCR–ABL fusion protein generated as a result of the chromosomal rearrangement underlying chronic myeloid leukemia, or as a result of expression of antigens from oncogenic viruses. Theoretically, they represent excellent targets for immune therapy, as they are specific for tumor cells and unlikely to trigger autoimmune damage to normal tissues. However, these antigens are often weakly expressed because of competition with peptides derived from the larger number of normal cellular proteins. In addition, they may only be expressed in a limited number of patients with HLA alleles that are capable of presenting the mutated peptide in their peptide-binding groove.

The majority of tumor antigens recognized by T cells are therefore tumor-associated antigens (TAAs), e.g. Wilms tumor antigen 1 (WT1). These are normal proteins which are over-expressed in tumor cells. The disadvantage of generating T cells redirected against TAAs is the risk of damaging normal tissues expressing the same proteins. In addition, there is a risk of these therapeutic cells becoming "tolerised," either by deletion or peripheral mechanisms which render them non-responsive to their cognate antigen.

TCR Gene Transfer via Transduction Protocols

The antigen specificity of a T cell is dependent on its TCR. The TCR is a heterodimeric protein, consisting of an α and a β chain in 90–95% of T lymphocytes (a rarer T cell population bears a receptor consisting of a γ and a δ chain). The α and β chains each consist of a variable and a constant region domain and are linked by a disulphide bond between cysteine residues in a short hinge region. The variable regions of the TCR are responsible for the diversity of antigen recognition and are encoded by gene segments (V and J for the α chain and V, D and J segments for the β chain). Rearrangement of these gene segments during T cell development leads to the generation of a repertoire of 10^{15} different specificities. Within the variable regions, three complementarity-determining regions (CDRs) contain residues which bind the peptide and the major histocompatibility molecule in which it is presented.

To obtain the rearranged gene sequence from a T cell of a defined specificity, T cells are cultured with the antigen of choice, and processed such that T cell clones are generated from responding cells. Following this, complementary DNA encoding the α and β TCR chains is isolated and amplified by polymerase chain reaction (PCR). The DNA sequences can then be compiled into complete TCR chain genes.

These genes are then incorporated into the DNA sequence of a vector derived from a modified retrovirus. Such retroviruses have been stripped of the genes they need to self-replicate (gag-pol and env) and therefore need to interact with vectors containing these genes within "packaging" cells.[6] This occurs via a process known as transfection, and after 48–72 h complete retroviral particles can be isolated from the supernatant of the packaging cells (see Fig. 1).

These retroviral particles can then infect T cells in culture. Provided that they have been activated and are undergoing cell division (for example using anti-CD3/CD28 monoclonal antibodies and Il-2), the TCR genes encoded by the retroviral vector are incorporated into the replicating DNA of the T cell. This is known as transduction. The exogenous TCR genes are then transcribed under the control of a retroviral promoter, translated and complexed with CD3 sub-units within the endoplasmic reticulum, allowing expression of the exogenous TCR on the surface of the T cell.

Use of monoclonal antibodies allows labelling of the exogenous TCR α or β chain to identify cells which have been transduced. However, to

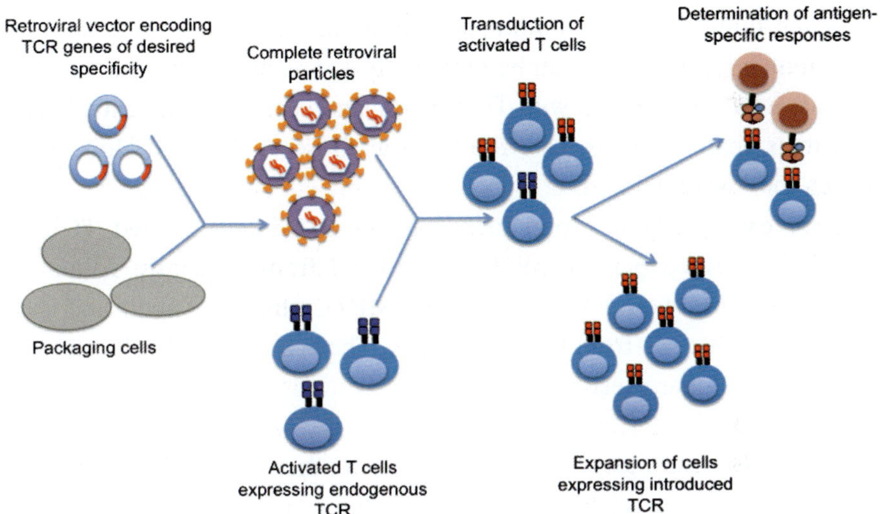

Fig. 1. A TCR of desired specificity is identified and its genes are cloned into a retroviral vector. This vector is capable of transfecting packaging cells which produce viral particles that are capable of infecting or transducing activated T cells. Twenty-four hours after transduction, TCR cell surface expression can be determined by flow cytometry. T cells expressing the introduced TCR expand preferentially when they are stimulated with the cognate antigen. The antigen-specific effector functions of these transduced cells can then be characterized via a number of biological assays.

detect expression of the exogenous α and β TCR together as a heterodimer requires the use of specific peptide-MHC multimers. As we shall discuss later, transduction may lead to the heterodimerization of introduced α or β TCR chains with endogenous partners, a less desirable result of the transduction process.

Use of Transduced T Cells for Adoptive T Cell Therapy

Prior to the first clinical trial of transduced T cells, *in vivo* experiments with murine tumor models demonstrated that TCR-transduced T cells can mediate rejection of tumors expressing their cognate antigen, and persist after the tumor has been eliminated.[7] In addition, many groups showed that human lymphocytes can be effectively redirected towards an antigen of choice by transduction with TCR genes, and *in vitro* studies established that their characteristics were the same as those of the CTL clone from which they were derived.

For example, our group identified an HLA-A2-restricted TCR to the WT-1-derived peptide pWT126, isolated from a healthy volunteer. The TCR genes were inserted into the pMP71 retroviral vector and used to transduce T cells from healthy donors. These transduced cells showed the following characteristics:

(1) HLA-A2-restricted killing of pWT126-loaded target cells;
(2) Specific killing of human tumor cell lines endogenously expressing WT1;
(3) Ability to kill WT-1-expressing leukemic cells from patients with AML and CML.

We also demonstrated that autologous cells transduced with the WT126 TCR are capable of eliminating human leukemia cells engrafted into NOD/SCID mice.[8] On the basis of these exciting discoveries, a clinical trial of the use of WT126-TCR-transduced autologous cells is planned for patients with leukemia.

The first clinical trial of TCR-transduced lymphocytes for the treatment of cancer was published in 2006 by Morgan *et al.*[9] They used a TCR specific for the MART1 antigen to treat patients with metastatic melanoma, and to date 4/31 (13%) patients have shown overall responses, some of which have been durable.[10] This landmark study has established the safety of adoptive therapy with TCR-transduced lymphocytes, as autoimmune toxicity was rare and limited in nature. However, the response rates have been modest. Further progress is therefore aimed at improving clinical efficacy. The same group are hoping to improve the response rate by identifying TCRs of higher affinity, and have already initiated clinical trials employing these.

Limitations and Potential Dangers of Adoptive Therapy Using Transduced T Cells

The functional efficacy of a T cell depends not only on the affinity of the TCR for its cognate antigen, but also on the level of TCR expression, as well as its ability to interact with co-receptors and co-stimulatory molecules. The concept of the immunological synapse explains the supramolecular organization of these interactions when a T cell encounters an antigen-presenting cell (APC) bearing its cognate antigen.[11] Within the synapse, optimal densities of co-receptors such as CD8, co-stimulatory molecules and adhesion molecules are arranged, probably just after TCR signaling occurs, to activate intracellular signaling pathways.

The level of expression of an introduced TCR at the T cell surface is in turn dependent on many factors, such as:

- Strength of the retroviral promoter;
- Efficiency of transcription and translation;
- Stability of tertiary and quaternary structures of the α and β chains, as well as their affinity for each other;
- Competition with endogenous TCR chains for CD3 sub-units within the endoplasmic reticulum.

Work carried out by our group and others[12–14] has established the concept of a "weak" TCR, i.e. one which, when transduced into a T cell, is expressed poorly, despite equivalent transcription and translation. This is in contrast to a "strong" TCR, which is expressed in preference to the endogenous TCR, and when introduced into a T cell converts its specificity to that of the exogenous TCR. The latter is demonstrated by specific killing of cells bearing the antigen, or antigen-dependent cytokine production *in vitro*.

The mechanisms by which the strength of a TCR is determined are not yet understood. It appears to be a post-translational phenomenon, occurring even when intracellular quantities of mRNA and TCR protein are identical for the endogenous and the introduced TCR. Recent work

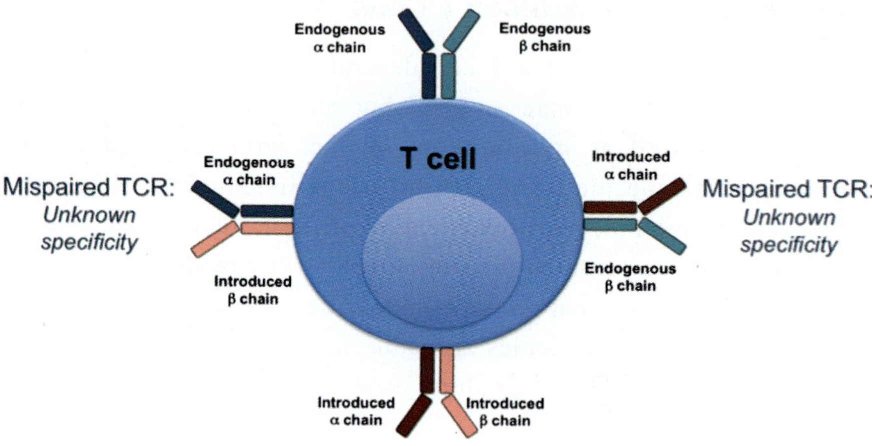

Fig. 2. Mispairing of endogenous and introduced TCR chains after retroviral transduction may lead to expression of TCRs with unknown specificity.

suggests that inter-chain affinity of the TCR affects CD3 binding and, in turn, stability of surface expression.[13]

Another factor limiting the level of expression of the α and β TCR chain of choice is the potential for mispairing of the endogenous and introduced TCR chains (Fig. 2). If the affinity of an introduced chain is greater for an endogenous TCR chain than for its introduced partner, then hybrid TCRs of unknown specificity may be expressed. The introduction of transduced cells with unknown specificity into the host may have more serious consequences: autoimmune damage to normal tissues — so-called "off-target" effects.

Autoimmune disease may also arise from adoptive transfer of transduced cells via a process known as cross-activation. This in theory could occur if tolerised, self-reactive T cells are transduced with a TCR against another antigen with equivalent TCR "strength," such that both TCRs are expressed. Though most self-reactive cells are deleted from the T cell repertoire, some escape this process and circulate in the periphery. Such self-reactive T cells are rendered tolerant to self-antigens by a number of peripheral mechanisms to prevent auto-immune responses. However, if transduced, these lymphocytes may be activated via an introduced TCR and become capable of targeting self-antigens again. Studies confirm that dual-specific T cells are capable of responding to both cognate antigens.[15] More recently, Teague *et al.*[16] clearly demonstrated that activation of such dual-specific T cells via one TCR can overcome tolerance of the cell to the cognate antigen of the second TCR.

A final risk with the use of TCR-transduced cells for adoptive transfer is the risk of insertional mutagenesis. Insertion of a viral promoter into host DNA as a result of transduction may lead to the activation of oncogenes within the genome, triggering malignant transformation. This serious consequence of adoptive transfer of transduced cells was demonstrated by the development of acute T cell lymphoblastic leukemia in five of 20 children treated within two studies for severe combined immunodeficiency disease (SCID-X1).[17,18] The study protocols involved administration of HSCs transduced with the common cytokine receptor gamma chain. Use of molecular techniques suggested that retroviral integration had occurred close to a T cell proto-oncogene, LMO2, in a proportion of the cases, suggesting its activation as the cause of oncogenesis.[19,20] Up to now there has been no evidence of a risk of oncogenesis with the transduction of mature cells, in either animal studies or clinical trials undertaken to date.

Strategies to Improve TCR-Transduced T Cells as Adoptive Therapy for Malignancy

Selection of High-Affinity TCRs

We have seen that the affinity of a TCR may be important for determining the anti-tumor efficacy of adoptive therapy in a clinical context. A significant body of murine studies supports this assumption (e.g. Refs. 21 and 22). High-affinity TCRs to TAAs may be deleted from the T cell repertoire, and this mechanism must therefore be bypassed in order to provide TCRs of high affinity for relevant antigens, rather than relying on the natural repertoire within a host to provide them.

There are a number of immune contexts in which TAAs are rendered truly "foreign":

- Crossing species barriers to tolerance. For example, immunization of transgenic mice expressing human MHC class 1 to human TAA peptides raises murine CTLs expressing TCRs recognizing human peptides in the context of human MHC.
- Allo-immunization: use of CTLs of a different MHC background to that of APCs loaded with the peptide in question. Responding CTLs need to be depleted of those that are purely responding to allo-MHC, leaving those that recognize the antigen in the context of the host MHC.

Both of these strategies were employed by Stanislawski *et al.* (2001) in an attempt to raise high-affinity TCRs against an epitope of murine double minute 2 (MDM2) oncoprotein. This work used transgenic mice which express human class I MHC and successfully generated murine cytotoxic lymphocytes (CTLs) specific to the human homolog of MDM2. Cloning of the raised murine TCR genes was followed by transduction of human lymphocytes, which efficiently express the murine TCR. Further groups confirmed this observation with TCRs of other specificities, e.g. against an epitope of human p53.[23]

However, concerns about the unknown immunogenicity of fully murine TCRs within human hosts have led to further adaptations, such as hybrid human–murine TCRs (see below).

Other strategies include *in vitro* mutagenesis to alter the affinity of TCRs present in the natural repertoire.

Optimising Vectors and TCR Constructs

Codon optimization has been shown to improve the expression of transduced TCRs[24] and influence antigen-specific responses in transduced T cells. In this strategy, the codon sequence of a TCR is altered to make maximal use of codons which have been demonstrated to be preferentially translated in that host species, but without changing the overall amino acid sequence. This, along with removal of cryptic splice sites and mRNA instability motifs, can greatly increase the expression of a protein.

Initially, TCR gene transfer was mediated by dual vector transduction protocols, where the α and β chains were present on separate vectors. This relies on a T cell being infected by both retroviral vectors in order that the desired TCR may be expressed. Because each chain is under the control of a separate promoter region, the requirement for dual transduction, in theory, also carries an increased risk of insertional mutagenesis.[25] The development of bicistronic vectors, with the coding sequence for both the α and β chains present in a single vector and with both genes under the control of a common promoter, potentially limits this risk. In addition, these vectors introduce the two TCR chain genes in equal proportions. The IRES motif (internal ribosomal entry site) mimicks the 5′ ribosomal cap, allowing ribosomal binding midway along the mRNA, such that the two genes can be simultaneously translated. In practice, the gene positioned after the IRES site tends to be expressed at a lower level. Introduction of a picornavirus-derived 2A sequence instead of the IRES motif allows stoichiometric expression of both peptides.[26] In this case, the 2A sequence causes failure of the peptide bond between the two chains, so that they are effectively cleaved as translation progresses.

A further refinement towards the goal of generating therapeutic transduced lymphocytes involved the construction of hybrid TCRs. Here, murine TCR constant regions are linked to the human variable regions conferring the TCR specificity of choice (Fig. 3). Such hybrid constructs have been demonstrated to be expressed in preference to human TCR chains,[12] and confer superior anti-tumor responses compared to fully human TCRs.[27] This latter observation, seen in lymphocytes transduced with a p53-specific TCR, as well as a TCR recognizing the melanoma TAA MART-1, was supported by evidence for improved pairing of the hybrid TCR chains and increased stability of the TCRs with CD3 sub-units.

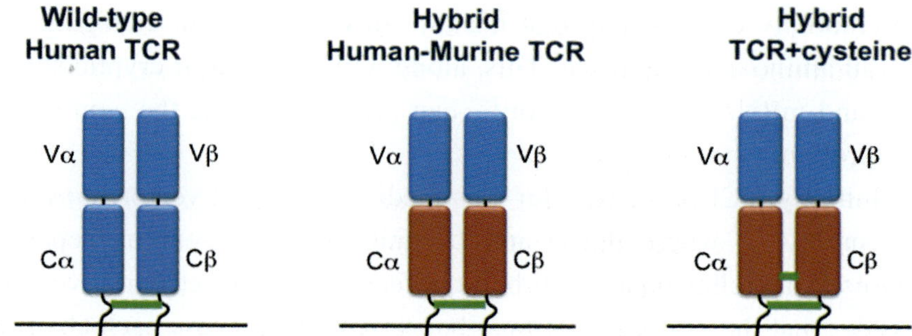

Fig. 3. Strategies to reduce mispairing of endogenous and introduced TCR chains include incorporating murine constant regions (middle) and extra cysteine-cysteine disulphide bonds (right). These alterations may also favor expression of the introduced TCR over that of the endogenous TCR.

A concern with the use of hybrid TCRs is their unknown immunogenicity in humans. Other modifications of the introduced TCR chains to reduce mispairing include the use of additional cysteine residues within the extracellular constant domains of the α and β chains (Fig. 3). These residues induce additional disulphide bonds but only when the introduced chains pair with each other, rather than the endogenous TCR α or β. Kuball *et al.*[28] demonstrated preferential pairing of exogenous TCR chains, improved expression of exogenous TCR and improved antigen-specific responses with a cysteine-modified WT-1-specific TCR. Work by our group and others has confirmed some of these findings with cysteine-modified TCRs to this and other antigens.[29,30]

Optimising T Cell Populations Used for Adoptive Transfer

An ideal lymphocyte population for adoptive transfer would have the following characteristics:

- High functional avidity for the antigen in question;
- Long-term survival and self-renewal capability, rather like the endogenous memory lymphocyte population;

- Rapid activation and proliferation to provide an effector population on antigen re-encounter.

Use of clonal, tumor-specific CD8$^+$ lymphocytes expanded under prolonged culture conditions for the adoptive therapy of melanoma was initially clinically unsuccessful and failed to provide long-lasting persistence of adoptively transferred cells in the host.[31] Better response rates and persistence were obtained from the same investigators when they utilized tumor-infiltrating lymphocytes generated under more rapid culture conditions and when they transferred a mixture of CD4$^+$ and CD8$^+$ populations.[32]

These observations indicated that the lymphocyte culture conditions and the populations transferred are hugely important for the efficacy of adoptive therapy. More recently, research efforts have been directed to identifying a lymphocyte subtype which fulfils the above criteria, and to determining in turn the conditions required to selectively produce cells of this phenotype.

Murine studies involving adoptive transfer of transgenic lymphocytes to mice bearing B16, a form of melanoma, demonstrated that lymphocytes of a naïve or early effector phenotype show improved anti-tumor responses compared to effector populations.[33] This was an unexpected finding given that effector populations generally show increased antigen-specific IFNγ release and cytolysis *in vitro*. The lymphocyte populations most effective on adoptive transfer showed increased expression of markers such as CD62L, CCR7 and IL-7Rα, consistent with a central memory phenotype and ability to home to secondary lymphoid organs. Studies by the same group confirmed the superiority of central memory versus effector memory lymphocytes in adoptive transfer experiments to B16 melanoma-bearing mice.[34] Retrospectively, it is clear that the conditions under which lymphocytes are commonly expanded *in vitro* (such as by repeated rounds of stimulations and in the presence of Il-2) favor terminal effector differentiation, which is now known to confer poor survival and proliferative capacity on adoptive transfer.

It is clear then that optimisation of lymphocyte populations for adoptive transfer also requires optimization of culture and transduction protocols. Excessive activation or cytokine-driven proliferation may cause terminal differentiation of lymphocytes with an effector phenotype and compromise their *in vivo* activity. Animal studies have suggested that IL-7, IL-15 and IL-21, rather than IL-2, are capable of supporting lymphocyte populations that are superior for adoptive therapy in terms of the phenotype, and in terms of improved anti-tumor responses.[33–35] Much work is now focused on determining which characteristics reliably identify the best population for transfer, e.g. CD27, CD28, telomere length, IL-7Rα.

Activation to induce proliferation is a requirement of T cell transduction using retroviral vectors. Therefore, a further strategy to avoid excessive activation of lymphocytes prior to adoptive transfer is the use of HIV1-based lentiviral vectors. These are able to efficiently transduce T lymphocytes which have progressed from the G0 to the G1 phase of the cell cycle after exposure to IL-2 and IL-7, without loss of a naïve or memory phenotype.[36] Many groups are now assessing the feasibility of using these vectors in animal and clinical studies.

Optimizing the Host Environment

One limitation of adoptive T cell transfer is limited persistence. As discussed above, this may be due to the differentiation state of the lymphocytes. Various observations have also suggested that the lymphopenic environment generated by conditioning regimens administered at the time of adoptive transfer can improve the persistence and expansion of the transferred population. There is evidence that this in turn contributes to improved clinical efficacy. For example, compilation of data from clinical trials involving adoptive transfer of tumor-infiltrating lymphocytes with anti-melanoma activity has shown an increase in response rates with an increased dose of total body irradiation (TBI). NB: This effect is not a directly therapeutic one, as melanoma is considered resistant to these doses of irradiation.[37]

There are various mechanisms which may be involved:

- The lymphopaenia induced by TBI or chemotherapy (e.g. cyclophosphamide, fludarabine) provides an environment in which *lymphopenia-induced proliferation* occurs. This proliferation appears to be dependent on certain cytokines, e.g. Il-7 and Il-15, and appears to cause a shift towards a "memory" phenotype of the lymphocyte population generated (reviewed in Ref. 38).
- Other beneficial effects on the host immune environment may include depletion of host regulatory immune elements and removal of lymphocyte populations that might compete for pro-survival cytokines.[39]

Thus, it appears that the host immune environment in which adoptively transferred T cells are introduced can dramatically alter their persistence and phenotype. These factors are being investigated in the context of clinical trials of adoptive therapy to determine the most effective conditioning strategies.

Conclusions

The paradigm underlying adoptive cell therapy developed from the application of allogeneic HSCs to generate a GvL effect. As for the field of allogeneic HSC transplantation, advances made in the clinical application of adoptive cell therapy have often occurred before a detailed scientific understanding of the immune environment in which these cells are introduced. However, clinical therapies are constantly being refined as our understanding increases.

The two arms of adoptive therapy — use of antigen-selected CTLs and gene-modified lymphocytes — provide different ways of overcoming the lack of an effective immune repertoire against malignancy or infectious agents and, as such, potentially have an important role in extending the efficacy and safety of allogeneic HSCT.

Investigators have been able to show some efficacy of gene-modified lymphocytes in the first clinical trial to date. In addition, many lessons learnt from the use of antigen-selected autologous T cells have been applied and the results of further clinical trials employing these refinements are eagerly awaited.

Future Directions

There are many more areas of T cell biology which may be exploited to improve the efficacy of transduced T cell populations in the future. They include:

- *Provision of antigen-specific CD4+ T cell help.* Many observations have suggested that the responses of CD8+ T cells are augmented by co-presence of antigen-specific CD4+ populations, including use of cloned CD8+ cells for clinical trials of melanoma therapy,[31] as well as in allogeneic HSC recipients receiving CMV-specific lymphocytes.[40] The proposed mechanisms underlying this include production of cytokines such as IL-2, improved persistence of antigen-specific CD8+ cells, reduced anergy in the face of persistent antigens, and augmented CD8+ memory responses. Unfortunately, very few MHC class II–restricted TAAs are known, so isolating T cells with specific TCRs to these antigens is difficult. Strategies to overcome this problem include transducing CD4+ T cells with CD8-independent TCRs, or co-transduction with the CD8 co-receptor.[41] In addition, endogenous T helper populations can be recruited through vaccination regimens (and have been effective in overcoming tolerance to TAAs[42]) as well as by providing an inflammatory immune environment with Toll-like receptor (TLR) agonists.
- *Optimizing co-stimulatory signals at the time of antigen ligation by transferred T cell populations.* Many strategies have been employed, including co-transduction with CD28, co-administration of agonist antibodies to CD40, as well as other co-stimulatory receptors.
- *Improving the functional avidity of transduced lymphocytes for their specific antigen by co-transduction with CD3 sub-units.*

- *TCR transduction of hematopoietic stem cell populations.* The rationale behind this approach is that the introduced TCR is expressed early in T cell differentiation within the thymus, and silences the recombination events required to generate an endogenous TCR, thus indirectly reducing mispairing of endogenous and exogenous TCR chains.
- *Manipulation of the suppressive immune axis.* This can be done, for example, by selectively depleting Treg populations within the host, or rendering transduced lymphocytes resistant to suppressive signals by manipulating intracellular mediators (such as the phosphatase enzymes which interact with the CD3-TCR complex and set a threshold for TCR signaling).

It remains to be seen whether these interventions will improve the efficacy of transduced T lymphocytes as adoptive therapy for cancer. However, the technologies utilised in generating these cells also have a broader application as adjuncts to allogeneic HSCT — for example, as therapy for GvHD by the generation of alloantigen-specific T regulatory cells.

References

1. Fujita Y, Rooney CM, Heslop HE. (2007) Adoptive cellular immunotherapy for viral diseases. *Bone Marrow Transplant* **41**(2): 193–198.
2. Kennedy-Nasser AA, Brenner MK. (2007) T cell therapy after hematopoietic stem cell transplantation. *Curr Opin Hematol* **14**(6): 616–624.
3. Rosenberg SA, Packard BS, Aebersold PM *et al.* (1988) Use of tumor-infiltrating lymphocytes and interleukin-2 in the immunotherapy of patients with metastatic melanoma: A preliminary report. *N Engl J Med* **319**(25): 1676–1680.
4. Rosenberg SA, Restifo NP, Yang JC *et al.* (2008) Adoptive cell transfer: A clinical path to effective cancer immunotherapy. *Nat Rev Cancer* **8**(4): 299–308.

5. Clay TM, Custer MC, Sachs J *et al.* (1999) Efficient transfer of a tumor antigen-reactive TCR to human peripheral blood lymphocytes confers anti-tumor reactivity. *J Immunol* **163**(1): 507–513.

6. Pear WS, Nolan GP, Scott ML, Baltimore D. (1993) Production of high-titer helper-free retroviruses by transient transfection. *Proc Natl Acad Sci USA* **90**(18): 8392–8396.

7. Kessels HW, Wolkers MC, van den Boom MD *et al.* (2001) Immunotherapy through TCR gene transfer. *Nat Immunol* **2**(10): 957–961.

8. Xue S, Bendle GM, Holler A, Stauss HJ. (2008) Generation and characterization of transgenic mice expressing a T cell receptor specific for the tumor-associated antigen MDM2. *Immunology* Jan 24.

9. Morgan RA, Dudley ME, Wunderlich JR *et al.* (2006) Cancer regression in patients after transfer of genetically engineered lymphocytes. *Science* **314**(5796): 126–129.

10. Rosenberg SA, Restifo NP, Yang JC *et al.* (2008) Adoptive cell transfer: A clinical path to effective cancer immunotherapy. *Nat Rev Cancer* **8**(4): 299–308.

11. Monks CR, Freiberg BA, Kupfer H *et al.* (1998) Three-dimensional segregation of supramolecular activation clusters in T cells. *Nature* **395**(6697): 82–86.

12. Hart DP, Xue S, Thomas S *et al.* (2008) Retroviral transfer of a dominant TCR prevents surface expression of a large proportion of the endogenous TCR repertoire in human T cells. *Gene Ther* **15**(8): 625–631.

13. Heemskerk MHM, Hagedoorn RS, van der Hoorn MAWG *et al.* (2007) Efficiency of T cell receptor expression in dual-specific T cells is controlled by the intrinsic qualities of the TCR chains within the TCR-CD3 complex. *Blood* **109**(1): 235–243.

14. Sommermeyer D, Neudorfer J, Weinhold M *et al.* (2006) Designer T cells by T cell receptor replacement. *Eur J Immunol* **36**(11): 3052–3059.

15. Heemskerk MHM, Hoogeboom M, Hagedoorn R *et al.* (2004) Reprogramming of virus-specific T cells into leukemia-reactive T cells using T cell receptor gene transfer. *J Exp Med* **199**(7): 885–894.

16. Teague RM, Greenberg PD, Fowler C *et al.* (2008) Peripheral CD8[+] T cell tolerance to self-proteins is regulated proximally at the T cell receptor. *Immunity* **28**(5): 662–674.

17. Cavazzana-Calvo M, Hacein-Bey S, de Saint Basile G *et al.* (2000) Gene therapy of human severe combined immunodeficiency (SCID)-X1 disease. *Science* **288**(5466): 669–672.

18. Gaspar HB, Parsley KL, Howe S *et al.* Gene therapy of X-linked severe combined immunodeficiency by use of a pseudotyped gammaretroviral vector. *Lancet* **364**(9452): 2181–2187.

19. Hacein-Bey-Abina S, Von Kalle C, Schmidt M *et al.* (2003) LMO2-associated clonal T cell proliferation in two patients after gene therapy for SCID-X1. *Science* **302**(5644): 415–419.

20. Hacein-Bey-Abina S, von Kalle C, Schmidt M *et al.* (2003) A serious adverse event after successful gene therapy for X-linked severe combined immunodeficiency. *N Engl J Med* **348**(3): 255–256.

21. Johnson LA, Heemskerk B, Powell DJ *et al.* (2006) Gene transfer of tumor-reactive TCR confers both high avidity and tumor reactivity to nonreactive peripheral blood mononuclear cells and tumor-infiltrating lymphocytes. *J Immunol* **177**(9): 6548–6559.

22. Zeh HJ, Perry-Lalley D, Dudley ME *et al.* (1999) High avidity CTLs for two self-antigens demonstrate superior *in vitro* and *in vivo* antitumor efficacy. *J Immunol* **162**(2): 989–994.

23. Kuball J, Schmitz FW, Voss R *et al.* (2005) Cooperation of human tumor-reactive CD4[+] and CD8[+] T cells after redirection of their specificity by a high-affinity p53A2.1-specific TCR. *Immunity* **22**(1): 117–129.

24. Scholten KBJ, Kramer D, Kueter EWM *et al.* (2006) Codon modification of T cell receptors allows enhanced functional expression in transgenic human T cells. *Clin Immunol* **119**(2): 135–45.

25. Fehse B, Kustikova OS, Bubenheim M, Baum C. (2004) Pois(s)on — it's a question of dose[hellip]. *Gene Ther* **11**(11): 879–881.

26. Szymczak AL, Workman CJ, Wang Y *et al.* (2004) Correction of multi-gene deficiency *in vivo* using a single "self-cleaving" 2A peptide-based retroviral vector. *Nat Biotech* **22**(5): 589–594.

27. Cohen CJ, Zhao Y, Zheng Z *et al.* (2006) Enhanced antitumor activity of murine–human hybrid T cell receptor (TCR) in human lymphocytes is associated with improved pairing and TCR/CD3 stability. *Cancer Res* **66**(17): 8878–8886.

28. Kuball J, Dossett ML, Wolfl M *et al.* (2007) Facilitating matched pairing and expression of TCR chains introduced into human T cells. *Blood* **109**(6): 2331–2338.

29. Cohen CJ, Li YF, El-Gamil M *et al.* (2007) Enhanced antitumor activity of T Cells engineered to express T cell receptors with a second disulfide bond. *Cancer Res* **67**(8): 3898–3903.

30. Thomas S, Xue S, Cesco-Gaspere M *et al.* (2007) Targeting the Wilms tumor antigen 1 by TCR gene transfer: TCR variants improve tetramer binding but not the function of gene-modified human T cells. *J Immunol* **179**(9): 5803–5810.

31. Dudley ME, Wunderlich JR, Yang JC *et al.* A phase I study of non-myeloablative chemotherapy and adoptive transfer of autologous tumor antigen-specific T lymphocytes in patients with metastatic melanoma. *J Immunother* **25**(3): 243–251.

32. Dudley ME, Wunderlich JR, Robbins PF *et al.* (2002) Cancer regression and autoimmunity in patients after clonal repopulation with antitumor lymphocytes. *Science* **298**(5594): 850–854.

33. Gattinoni L, Klebanoff CA, Palmer DC *et al.* (2005) Acquisition of full effector function *in vitro* paradoxically impairs the *in vivo* antitumor efficacy of adoptively transferred CD8$^+$ T cells. *J Clin Invest* **115**(6): 1616–1626.

34. Klebanoff CA, Gattinoni L, Torabi-Parizi P *et al.* (2005) Central memory self/tumor-reactive CD8$^+$ T cells confer superior antitumor immunity compared with effector memory T cells. *Proc Natl Acad Sci USA* **102**(27): 9571–9576.

35. Hinrichs CS, Spolski R, Paulos CM *et al.* (2008) IL-2 and IL-21 confer opposing differentiation programs to CD8$^+$ T cells for adoptive immunotherapy. *Blood* **111**(11): 5326–5333.

36. Cavalieri S, Cazzaniga S, Geuna M *et al.* (2003) Human T lymphocytes transduced by lentiviral vectors in the absence of TCR

activation maintain an intact immune competence. *Blood* **102**(2): 497–505.

37. Dudley ME, Yang JC, Sherry R *et al.* (2008) Adoptive cell therapy for patients with metastatic melanoma: Evaluation of intensive myelo-ablative chemoradiation preparative regimens. *J Clin Oncol* **26**(32): 5233–5239. Epub 2008 Sep 22.

38. Jameson SC. (2005) T cell homeostasis: Keeping useful T cells alive and live T cells useful. *Semi Immunol* **17**(3): 231–237.

39. Gattinoni L, Jr DJP, Rosenberg SA, Restifo NP. (2006) Adoptive immunotherapy for cancer: Building on success. *Nat Rev Immunol* **6**(5): 383–393.

40. Walter EA, Greenberg PD, Gilbert MJ *et al.* (1995) Reconstitution of cellular immunity against cytomegalovirus in recipients of allogeneic bone marrow by transfer of T cell clones from the donor. *N Engl J Med* **333**(16): 1038–1044.

41. Morris EC, Tsallios A, Bendle GM *et al.* (2005) A critical role of T cell antigen receptor–transduced MHC class I–restricted helper T cells in tumor protection. *Proc Natl Acad Sci USA* **102**(22): 7934–7939.

42. Overwijk WW, Theoret MR, Finkelstein SE *et al.* (2003) Tumor regression and autoimmunity after reversal of a functionally tolerant state of self-reactive CD8$^+$ T cells [Internet]. *J Exp Med* **198**(4) [cited May 13, 2008]. Available from http://www.pubmedcentral.nih.gov/articlerender.fcgi?artid=2194177.

Chapter 17

Alloreactive T Cells for the Treatment of Leukemia

J. H. Frederik Falkenburg

Introduction

Following allogeneic stem cell transplantation (SCT), T cells derived from the healthy stem cell donor can mediate a curative immune response resulting in elimination of (residual) hematopoietic tumor cells in the patient.[1] The observation that autologous SCT and allogeneic SCT using homozygous twins as donors resulted in decreased control of the hematological malignancy after transplantation, compared to allogeneic SCT, indicated that the mere presence of T cells in the graft does not result in a graft versus leukemia (GvL) reactivity.[2–4] Apparently, the genetic differences between donors and patients are not only responsible for the development of graft versus host disease (GvHD) but also capable of eliciting a GvL response. After partially HLA-matched allogeneic SCT, T cell responses of donor origin directed against polymorphic antigens in the patient are likely to be mainly directed against the mismatched HLA allele, since the number of alloreactive T cells in the peripheral blood of normal individuals can exceed 1% of circulating T cells. After HLA-matched allogeneic SCT, minor histocompatibility antigens (mHags) are the target antigens for alloimmune reactivity of T cells.[5] T cell responses against HLA or mHags can result in both GvHD and GvL. However,

Department of Hematology, Leiden University Medical Center, PO Box 9600, 2300 RC Leiden, The Netherlands. Tel.: +31 71 526 2267. E-mail: Falkenburg.hematology@lumc.nl.

laboratory studies and clinical observations have demonstrated that GvHD responses can be separated from GvL, and that characterization of the fine specificity of the T cell reactivities involved in these alloresponses may lead to the development of T cell therapy resulting in eradication of the disease without severe side effects.

Minor Histocompatibility Antigens

Minor histocompatibility antigens (mHags) can be defined as alloantigens that are capable of inducing an allogeneic T cell reponse between HLA-identical individuals.[5–8] More precisely, they are polymorphic peptides presented in the context of self HLA molecules, which can be recognized by fully HLA-matched allogeneic donors. MHags are encoded by polymorphic genes. The human genome contains many single nucleotide polymorphisms (SNPs), part of which is present within the coding region of genes. These polymorphisms may lead to polymorphisms in the protein which may result in the presence in HLA molecules of peptides that show amino acid differences between individuals. In addition, polymorphisms in the protein may lead to impaired presentation of peptides in HLA molecules, resulting in a "null allele", which is defined by the absence of the specific peptide in HLA due to inappropriate processing and/or presentation. If a peptide derived from a polymorphic gene is differentially presented in HLA molecules, the difference may lead to the induction of an immune response from an HLA-matched donor.[5–8]

Not every polymorphism in proteins will lead to development of an mHag. A prerequisite for an mHag to be recognized by alloreactive T cells is obviously the presentation in HLA molecules expressed on the cell membrane. Most knowledge has been obtained on mHags that are presented in the context of HLA class I molecules.[5] First, the protein must be degraded by intracellular proteases (the proteasome) into small peptide fragments, which should then be transported by the "transporter in antigen processing" (TAP) into the endoplasmatic reticulum and bound to HLA class I molecules. The likelihood that a specific peptide is presented by HLA molecules is dependent on a variety of intracellular processes, including the activity of intracellular proteases, trimming of the protein by amino peptidases, binding to TAP, and binding to the HLA molecules. For instance, peptides that potentially may bind to the groove of HLA but are subject to cleavage within the peptide by the proteosome will not be presented. Alternatively, polymorphisms that may lead to reduced binding of the peptide to the groove of HLA molecules will also result in absence of presentation on the cell membrane. In most cases, mHag alleles are defined by single or multiple amino acid substitutions that will lead to a three-dimensional structure that can be differentially recognized by T cell receptors (TCRs) from different individuals. In summary, an mHag may result from the presence or absence of a specific peptide in HLA molecules, or polymorphisms in amino acids present in peptides presented in the context of HLA molecules. Whether or not these polymorphic complexes will be recognized by a specific donor will depend on the T cell repertoire of the individuals. As with the presentation in HLA class I molecules, polymorphic peptides of various lengths can be presented by HLA class II molecules. Although the intracellular mechanism by which these endogenous proteins are processed in HLA class II molecules is less well understood, polymorphisms in endogenous proteins can also act as mHags presented in HLA class II molecules recognized by CD4$^+$ T cells.

Tissue Distribution of mHags

The tissue distribution of the polymorphic antigens plays an essential role in the clinical effect of the T cell responses against these structures.[5–9] The recognition of target tissues by mHag-specific T cells will depend on the presentation of the HLA molecules as well as the expression of the genes encoding the polymorphic peptides. Since most nucleated cells express HLA class I molecules, the presentation of an HLA class I–associated mHag is mainly dependent on the expression of the polymorphic gene encoding the peptide. The expression of HLA class II molecules is more restricted. Many cells of hematopoietic origin constitutively express HLA class II molecules, whereas other cell populations express these molecules only during inflammatory reactions.[10–12] Therefore, only co-ordinated expression of HLA class II molecules and the gene encoding the poly-morphic peptide will lead to presentation of the HLA class II–associated mHags in target tissues of GvL and GvHD. Under steady state conditions, expression of HLA class II–associated mHags may be restricted to the hematopoietic system but during inflammation nonhematopoietic tissues may be recognized by mHag/HLA class II–specific T cells. Furthermore, recognition of mHags on target tissues will depend not only on the expres-sion of these molecules but also on the expression of accessory molecules, including costimulatory and adhesion molecules and/or inhibitory mole-cules which play a role in both the induction phase and the effector phase of the immune response.

Clinical Relevance of mHags

Following allogeneic hematopoietic SCT, hematopoiesis from the recipient is replaced by donor hematopoiesis. Obviously, residual hematopoietic tumor cells are of recipient origin, whereas, depending on the intensity of the conditioning regimen, some residual normal hematopoietic cells may also be derived from the patient. Allogeneic donor-derived T cells recog-nizing polymorphic antigens expressed on hematopoietic cells from the recipient, including hematopoietic tumor cells, will lead to eradication of the tumor with concurrent elimination of residual recipient-derived hematopoietic cells. In contrast, donor-derived T cells recognizing poly-morphic antigens on recipient cells will not impair donor hematopoiesis in the patient. The tissue distribution of the mHag/HLA complex will determine whether this GvL response will be accompanied by GvHD. If the T cell response is directed against mHag/HLA restricted to hematopoietic tissues, the immune response will lead to destruction of the hematopoietic (tumor) cells from the recipient without direct attack of nonhematopoietic tissues. Several mHags have been found to be relatively restricted to hematopoietic tissues, including the HLA class I–restricted mHags, HA-1, HA-2, HB1, BCL2A1, LRH1, PANE and ECGF-1.[13–19] In addition, T cell responses against HLA class II–restricted mHags, includ-ing the recently characterized phosphatidyl inositol 4 kinase 2B (PI4K2B) mHag recognized in the context of HLA-DQ, may recognize only hematopoietic (tumor) cells under noninflammatory conditions.[20] In contrast, T cell responses against broadly expressed mHags may result in the development of severe GvHD.

The *in vivo* induction of an mHag-specific T cell response will probably depend on the presentation of these antigens by professional antigen-presenting cells (APCs).[21–24] Most of the mHags characterized thus far have been demonstrated to be highly expressed in dendritic cells (DCs) or cells of B cell origin, which may also act as APCs. Murine studies have illustrated that the presentation of the alloantigens in professional APCs may be essential for the development of both GvHD and GvL. Thus, not only the expression of the mHags on target tissues during the effector phase of the immune response is relevant for the clinical outcome, but also the expression of these antigens on APCs during *in vivo* development of alloimmune responses. The latter prerequisite can be bypassed by the induction of *in vitro* immune responses against these antigens followed by adoptive transfer.[25]

Beneficial Alloreactive T Cell Responses

The characterization of immune responses in patients successfully treated with donor lymphocyte infusion (DLI) for persistent or relapsed hematological malignancies after allo-SCT has illustrated that the development of T cell responses against hematopoiesis-associated mHags may result in a potent antitumor effect, and conversion to full donor chimerism with no or only temporary GvHD.[9,26–31]

T cells directed against hematopoiesis-associated mHags can also result in an inflammatory response in target tissues of GvHD, since many hematopoietic cells, including DCs, are present within these normal tissues. Therefore, especially target tissues containing high frequencies of hematopoietic cells may be targets for GvHD, although the severity of GvHD in the case of alloimmune responses specifically directed against hematopoiesis-associated mHags is likely to be limited. Analyses of patients successfully treated with DLI have demonstrated development of hematopoiesis-associated mHag specific T cell responses with kinetics resembling immune responses against viral infections.[9] Following an initial rise of antigen-specific T cells to high frequencies that may exceed 10% of all circulating T cells, the immune response declined after eradication of antigen-expressing cells, which may be followed by a memory T cell response.[9,32] Persistence of the T cell response and the development of a memory response may be essential for sustained and prolonged suppression of the tumor. In summary, the development of a T cell response against hematopoiesis-associated mHags *in vivo* with the development of a memory response may result in tumor reduction with limited GvHD, and even sustained suppression of the tumor.

HLA Class II–Restricted T Cell Responses

HLA class II–restricted mHag-specific T cell responses are also likely to play a significant role in the development and sustenance of beneficial T cell responses after transplantation. We recently characterized the first autosomal HLA class II–restricted mHag as a polymorphic peptide derived from the PI4K2B gene, which is relatively broadly expressed in many tissues.[20] Due to the fact that the restriction molecule HLA-DQ is mainly expressed by cells of hematopoietic origin, including professional APCs, such HLA class II–restricted mHags may play a role in the development of a beneficial T cell response as well as the sustenance of the alloreactivity. Recently, it has been demonstrated that CD4 T cells not only play a role in the induction of the immune response but also allow greater persistence of HLA class I–specific T cells.[33,34] Since HLA class II molecules are not only restricted to normal cells of the hematopoietic system under steady state conditions but also can be highly expressed on hematological tumors, especially tumors of B cell origin, we hypothesized that alloreactive T cells recognizing HLA class II molecules may directly eradicate hematopoietic tumors.[12] Therefore, we investigated whether allo–HLA class II responses may result in GvL reactivity in the absence of GvHD. In the case of HLA-identical unrelated SCT, donor and recipient are usually matched for HLA A, B, C, DR and DQ, but not for HLA-DP.

To analyze whether DP-specific T cell responses could result in GvL without GvHD, we investigated whether patients treated with DLI from HLA-ABC, HLA-DR and HLA-DQ matched, but HLA-DP-mismatched donors could develop an HLA-DP-specific T cell response resulting in a beneficial outcome. In a patient with a chronic B cell malignancy we could demonstrate that HLA-DP-specific T cells specifically eradicated the hematological tumor without development of GvHD.[35] In this case, no inflammatory environment was present. Previously, reports have illustrated that at the time of transplant HLA-DP mismatching may result in an increased incidence of GvHD.[36] We hypothesize that this may be due to the upregulation of HLA-DP due to the tissue damage of the conditioning regimen in combination with activation of recipient-derived APCs. T cell depletion of the graft followed by postponed administration of HLA-DP-specific T cells for the treatment of residual disease may allow a more specific antitumor response in the absence of GvHD. These results illustrate that allo-HLA class II–specific T cell responses can also result in antitumor reactivity without GvHD.

Allo-HLA-Hematopoiesis — Restricted T Cell Responses

Since clinical and preclinical evidence has indicated that following HLA-matched allogeneic SCT T cell responses against hematopoiesis-associated antigens may result in GvL responses without GvHD, similar approaches are now being explored in the context of not only HLA class II but also HLA class I mismatches.

As with the approach following HLA-matched transplantation, a T cell response directed against a peptide derived from a hematopoiesis-specific protein that is presented in the context of HLA class I molecules can act as a hematopoiesis-specific target following HLA-mismatched (haptoidentical) SCT. Since the donor cells may express the same hematopoiesis-associated protein but not the relevant HLA restriction molecule, a donor T cell response against this hematopoiesis-associated peptide in the context of the patient-specific mismatched HLA molecule will result in eradication of recipient hematopoiesis with preservation of donor hematopoiesis.

WT1-derived peptides have been demonstrated to be presented in the context of HLA-A2 molecules in hematological malignancies, and to be potential targets for T cell therapy.[37] Several approaches are being taken to generate T cells from HLA-A2-negative individuals capable of recognizing WT1-derived peptides in the context of HLA-A2 molecules.[38] It has been demonstrated that these T cells may be capable of recognizing leukemic cells, and may therefore be used in the context of haploidentical transplantation of HLA-A2-positive patients. Similarly, other peptides derived from hematopoiesis-specific proteins presented in the context of mismatched HLA molecules may be targets for specific immune responses after haploidentical transplantation. Potential targets have been suggested to be other overexpressed self antigens but may also be peptides derived from mHags with high population frequencies, like HA-2.[39,40] Obviously, these specific T cell responses are not likely to develop *in vivo* in patients after haploidentical transplantation and DLI in the absence of codevelopment of detrimental T cell responses against allo-HLA molecules presenting more abundantly expressed peptides. Therefore, only *in vitro* selection of T cells recognizing these hematopoiesis-associated peptides in the context of allo-HLA molecules will allow treatment of patients after HLA-mismatched transplantation.

Adoptive Transfer of Alloreactive T Cells

Several approaches are being explored to isolate T cells for adoptive transfer following allogeneic SCT. First, antigen-specific T cells can be isolated using multimeric peptides/HLA complexes coupled to immunomagnetic beads.[9,41] Alternatively, antigen-specific T cells can be isolated based on specific production of interferon gamma by activated T cells stimulated with the target of interest.[43] Using the interferon gamma capture assay, high purities of antigen-specific T cells can be obtained. Both using multimeric peptide–HLA complexes and using the interferon gamma capture assay, highly purified antigen-specific T cell responses can be obtained and adoptively transferred, as demonstrated by the treatment of patients suffering from persistent CMV reactivation after transplantation with *in-vitro*-selected and expanded CMV-specific T cells.[43] Unfortunately, the frequencies of mHag-specific T cells in donor peripheral blood are a magnitude lower than those of virus-specific T cells, and therefore the isolation of large numbers of mHag-specific T cells from healthy donors has been relatively unsuccessful. Various stimulation protocols are being explored to further improve these isolation methods. The direct isolation of antigen-specific T cells recognizing peptides in the context of nonself HLA molecules has further been hampered by the coisolation of detrimental allo-HLA-specific T cells.

Alternatively, large numbers of antigen-specific T cells may be generated using T cell receptor (TCR) gene transfer. High affinity antigen-specific TCRs have been characterized and isolated from high avidity T cell responses, which have been demonstrated to cause an antitumor response *in vivo*. Transfer of the TCR alpha and beta genes to primary donor T cells allows the generation of large numbers of T cells specifically expressing the TCR of interest in addition to the endogenous TCR.[45,46] Since pathogen-specific T cells, including CMV-specific T cells, have been demonstrated to sustain an effective immune response after transplantation with control of viral infection, we proposed transferring the antigen-specific TCRs to virus-specific T cells. This will allow the transfer of T cells recognizing both the tumor target of interest and a pathogen which is persistently present in the recipient.[47,48] Due to the persistence of the pathogen, these T cells will be prolongedly present during a state of minimal residual disease. We have demonstrated that these T cells exert both virus-specific and hematopoiesis-specific reactivities, can be activated, and proliferate *in vitro*, and therefore may be used for adoptive transfer after transplantation.[49] The use of TCR-transduced T cells in the treatment of melanoma has demonstrated the feasibility of the approach, although the clinical efficacy has thus far been limited.[46] Future clinical studies will have to demonstrate which of the approaches leading to the generation of antigen-specific T cells *in vitro* will result in the most effective antitumor reactivity *in vivo*.

Summary

Hematopoiesis-restricted mHags presented by recipient cells in the context of HLA-matched transplantation, hematopoiesis-associated antigens presented in the context of HLA-mismatched transplantation, as well as HLA class II–associated targets, may be appropriate target structures for the induction of a beneficial GvL reactivity after allogeneic SCT. The tissue distribution of the antigens will determine the clinical outcome of the T cell responses, and manipulation of T cell reactivities toward hematopoietic targets in the absence of coexpression on nonhematopoietic targets may result in GvL with a low likelihood of developing GvHD. Treatment of patients with *in-vitro*-selected antigen-specific T cells may result in profound antitumor responses with preservation of donor hematopoiesis with few side effects. *In vitro* isolation and expansion of antigen-specific T cells under good manufacturing practice (GMP) conditions need to be further developed to allow the clinical evaluation of adoptive transfer of antigen-specific T cells. By redirection of T cell specificity through gene transfer of T cell receptors, large numbers of specifically targeted T cells may be generated for future treatment of resistant hematological malignancies after allogeneic SCT.

References

1. Storb R. (2003) Allogeneic hematopoietic stem cell transplantation — yesterday, today and tomorrow. *Exp Hematol* **31**: 1–10.
2. Suciu S, Mandelli F, de Witte T *et al.* (2003) Allogeneic compared with autologous stem cell transplantation in the treatment of patients younger than 46 years with acute myeloid leukemia (AML) in first complete remission (CR1): An intention to treat analysis of the EORTC/GIMEMAAML-10 trial. *Blood* **102**: 1232–1240.
3. Marmont AM, Horowitz MM, Gale RP *et al.* (1991) T cell deletion of HLA-identical transplants in leukemia. *Blood* **78**: 2120–2130.
4. Fefer A, Sullivan KM, Weiden P *et al.* (1987) Graft versus leukemia effect in man: the relapse rate of acute leukemia is lower after

allogeneic than after syngeneic marrow transplantation. *Prog Clin Biol Res* **224**: 401–408.

5. Falkenburg JHF, Willemze R. (2004) Minor histocompatibility antigens as targets of cellular immunotherapy in leukemia. *Best Pract Res Clin Haematol* **17**: 415–425.

6. Simpson E, Scott D, James E *et al.* (2002) Minor H antigens: Genes and peptides. *Transpl Immunol* **10**: 115–123.

7. Goulmy E. (2006) Minor histocompatibility antigens: From transplantation problems to therapy of cancer. *Hum Immunol* **67**(6): 433–438.

8. Bleakley M, Riddell SR. (2004) Molecules and mechanisms of the graft-versus-leukaemia effect. *Nat Rev Cancer* **4**(5): 371–380.

9. Marijt WAF, Heemskerk MH, Kloosterboer FM *et al.* (2003) Hematopoiesis-restricted minor histocompatibility antigens HA-1 or HA-2 specific T cells can induce complete remissions of relapsed leukemia. *Proc Natl Acad Sci USA* **100**: 2742–2747.

10. Falkenburg JHF, Fibbe WE, Goselink HM *et al.* (1985) Human hematopoietic progenitor cells in long-term cultures express HLA-DR antigens and lack HLA-DQ antigens. *J Exp Med* **162**: 1359–1369.

11. Amatruda TT 3rd, Bohman R, Ranyard J, Koeffler HP. (1987) Pattern of expresson of HLA-DR and HLA-DQ antigens and mRNA in myeloid differentiation. *Blood* **69**: 1225–1236.

12. Guy K, Krajewski AS, Dewar AE. (1986) Expression of MHC class II antigens in human B cell leukemia and non-Hodgkin's lymphoma. *Br J Cancer* **53**: 161–173.

13. den Haan JM, Sherman NE, Blokland E *et al.* (1995) Identification of a graft versus host disease-associated human minor histocompatibility antigen. *Science* **268**: 1476–1480.

14. den Haan JM, Meadows LM, Wang W *et al.* (1998) The minor histocompatibility antigen HA-1: A diallelic gene with a single amino acid polymorphism. *Science* **279**: 1054–1057.

15. Dolstra H, Fredrix H, Maas F *et al.* (1999) A human minor histocompatibility antigen specific for B cell acute lymphoblastic leukemia. *J Exp Med* **189**: 301.

16. Akatsuka Y, Nishida T, Kondo E *et al.* (2003) Identification of a polymorphic gene, BCL2A1, encoding two novel hematopoietic lineage-specific minor histocompatibility antigens. *J Exp Med* **197**: 1489–1500.

17. de Rijke B, van Horssen-Zoetbrood A, Beekman JM *et al.* (2005) A frameshift polymorphism in P2X5 elicits an allogeneic cytotoxic T lymphocyte response associated with remission of chronic myeloid leukemia. *J Clin Invest* **115**: 3506–3516.

18. Brickner AG, Evans AM, Mito JK *et al.* (2006) The pane1 gene encodes a novel human minor histocompatibility antigen that is selectively expressed in B-lymphoid cells and B-CLL. *Blood* **107**: 3779–3786.

19. Slager EH, Honders MW, van der Meijden ED *et al.* (2006) Identification of the angiogenic endothelial-cell growth factor-1/thymidine phospholylase as a potential target for immunotherapy of cancer. *Blood* **107**: 4950–4960.

20. Griffioen M, van der Meijden ED, Slager EH *et al.* (2008) Identification of phosphatidylinositol 4 kinase type II beta as HLA class II restricted target in graft versus leukemia reactivity. *Proc Natl Acad Sci USA* **105**: 3837–3842.

21. Shlomchik WD, Couzens MS, Tang CB *et al.* (1999) Prevention of graft versus host disease by inactivation of host antigen-presenting cells. *Science* **285**: 412–415.

22. Matte CC, Liu J, Cormier J *et al.* (2004) Donor APCs are required for maximal GvHD but not for GvL. *Nat Med* **10**: 987–992.

23. Ferrara JL, Reddy P. (2006) Pathophysiology of graft-versus-host disease. *Semin Hematol* **43**: 3–10.

24. Chakraverty R, Sykes M. (2007) The role of antigen-presenting cells in triggering graft versus host disease and graft versus leukaemia. *Blood* **110**: 9–17.

25. Jedema I, Meij P, Steeneveld E *et al.* (2007) Early detection and rapid isolation of leukemia-reactive donor T cells for adoptive transfer using the IFN-gamma secretion assay. *Clin Cancer Res* **13**: 636–643.

26. Kolb HJ, Schattenberg A, Goldman JM, European Group for Blood and Marrow transplantation Working Party Chronic Leukemia. (1995) Graft versus leukemia effect of donor lymphocyte transfusion in marrow grafted patients. *Blood* **86**: 2041–2050.

27. Mackinnon S, Papadopoulos EB, Carabasi MH *et al.* (1995) Adoptive immunotherapy evaluating escalating doses of donor leukocytes for relapse of chronic myeloid leukemia after bone marrow transplantation: Separation of graft-versus-leukemia responses from graft-versus-host disease. *Blood* **86**: 1261–1268.

28. Levine JE, Braun T, Penza SL *et al.* (2002) Prospective trial of chemotherapy and donor leukocyte infusions for relapse of advanced myeloid malignancies after allogeneic stem cell transplantation. *Clin Oncol* **20**: 405–412.

29. Posthuma EF, Marijt WAF, Barge RMY *et al.* (2004) Alpha-interferon with very-low dose donor lymphocyte infusion for hematologic or cytogenetic relapse of chronic myeloid leukemia induces rapid and durable complete remissions and is associated with acceptable graft versus host disease. *Biol Blood Marrow Transplant* **10**: 204–212.

30. Porter D, Levine JE. (2006) Graft-versus-host disease and graft-versus-leukemia after donor leukocyte infusion. *Semin Hematol* **43**: 53–61.

31. Smit WM, Rijnbeek M, van Bergen CAM *et al.* (1998) Cytotoxic T cells recognizing leukemic CD34 positive progenitor cells mediate the antileukemic reactivity of donor lymphocyte transfusions for relapsed chronic myeloid leukemia after allogeneic stem cell transplantation. *Proc Natl Acad Sci USA* **95**: 10152–10157.

32. Van Bergen CAM, Kester MGD, Jedema I *et al.* (2007) Multiple myeloma reactive T cells recognize an activation induced minor histocompatibility antigen encoded by the ATP dependent interferon responsive (ADIR) gene. *Blood* **109**: 4089–4096.

33. Janssen EM, Lemmes EE, Wolfe T *et al.* (2003) CD4[+] T cells are required for secondary expansion and memory in CD8[+] T lymphocytes. *Nature* **421**: 852–856.

34. Kennedy R, Celis E. (2006) T helper lymphocytes rescue CTL from activation-induced cell death. *J Immunol* **177**: 2862–2872.

35. Rutten CE, van Luxemburg-Heijs SA, Griffioen M *et al.* (2008) HLA-DP as specific target for cellular immunotherapy in HLA class II-expressing B-cell leukemia. *Leukemia* **22**: 1387–1394.

36. Shaw BE, Gooley TA, Malkki M *et al.* (2007) The importance of HLA-DPB1 in unrelated donor hematopoietic cell transplantation. *Blood* **110**: 4560–4566.

37. Gao L, Bellantuono I, Elsässer A *et al.* (2000) Selective elimination of leukemic CD34(+) progenitor cells by cytotoxic T lymphocytes specific for WT1. *Blood* **1**: 2198–2203.

38. Savage P, Gao L, Vento K *et al.* (2004) Use of B cell-bound HLA-A2 class I monomers to generate high-avidity, allo-restricted CTLs against the leukemia-associated protein Wilms tumor antigen. *Blood* **103**: 4613–4615.

39. Rezvani K, Yong AS, Mielke S *et al.* (2008) Leukemia-associated antigen-specific T cell responses following combined PR1 and WT1 peptide vaccination in patients with myeloid malignancies. *Blood* **111**: 236–242.

40. Oosten LE, Blokland E, Kester MG *et al.* (2007) Promiscuity of the alloHLA-A2 restricted T cell repertoire hampers in the generation of minor histocompatibility antigen specific cytotoxic T cells across HLA barriers. *Biol Blood Marrow Transplant* **13**: 151–163.

41. Gillespie G, Mutis T, Schrama E *et al.* (2000) HLA class I-minor histocompatibility antigen tetramers select cytotoxic T cells with high avidity to the natural ligand. *Hematol J* **1**: 403–410.

42. Cobbold M, Khan N, Pourgheysari B *et al.* (2005) Adoptive transfer of cytomegalovirus-specific CTL to stem cell transplant patients after selection by HLA-peptide tetramers. *J Exp Med* **202**: 379–386.

43. Kloosterboer FM, van Luxemburg-Heijs SA, van Soest RA *et al.* (2005) Minor histocompatibility antigen-specific T cells with multiple distinct specificities can be isolated by direct cloning of IFN gamma-secreting T cells from patients with relapsed leukemia responding to donor lymphocyte infusion. *Leukemia* **19**: 83–90.

44. Einsele H, Kapp M, Grigoleit GU. (2008) CMV-specific T cell therapy. *Blood Cells Mol Dis* **40**: 71–75.

45. Kessels HW, Wolkers MC, van den Boom MD *et al.* (2001) Immunotherapy through TCR gene transfer. *Nat Immunol* **2**: 957–961.

46. Morgen RA, Dudley ME, Wunderlich JR *et al.* (2006) Cancer regression in patients after transfer of genetically engineered lymphocytes. *Science* **314**: 126–129.

47. Heemskerk MHM, Hoogeboom M, de Paus RA *et al.* (2003) Redirection of antileukemic reactivity of peripheral T lymphocytes using gene transfer of minor histocompatibilty antigen HA-2 specific T cell receptor complexes expressing a conserved alpha joining region. *Blood* **102**: 3530–3540.

48. Heemskerk MHM, Hoogeboom M, Hagedoorn R *et al.* (2004) Reprogramming of virus-specific T cells into leukemia-reactive T cells using T cell receptor gene transfer. *J Exp Med* **199**: 885–894.

49. Griffioen M, van Egmond HME, Barnby-Porritt H *et al.* (2008) Genetic engineering of virus specific T cells with T cell receptors recognizing minor histocompatibility antigens for clinical applications. *Haematologica* **93**: 1535–1543.

Chapter 18

Mobilization of Hematopoietic Stem and Progenitor Cells

Kfir Lapid, Tomer Itkin*, Eike C. Buss**
and Tsvee Lapidot,†*

Mobilized peripheral blood is enriched with hematopoietic stem and progenitor cells which are essential for reconstitution in patients, and serves as a primary source for bone marrow transplantation procedures. The process, by which hematopoietic stem cells and progenitors egress out of the bone marrow to the circulation, and its enhancement by mobilization protocols, is not trivial and is regarded today as a highly regulated process involving multiple players, such as osteoblast–osteoclast interactions, the chemokine SDF-1 and its major receptor CXCR4, and a complex cross-talk between cytokines, proteolytic enzymes and adhesion molecules. In this chapter, we will review clinical stem cell mobilization in brief, discuss experimental animal models, such as immune-deficient mice transplanted with human progenitor cells, as well as promising novel mobilizing agents, such as the CXCR4 antagonist AMD3100. In addition, we will focus on the molecular mechanistic aspect of stem cell mobilization, involving dynamic regulation of hematopoietic stem cells and the bone marrow microenvironment by the nervous and immune systems. A better understanding of these mechanisms will enable improvement of clinical mobilization protocols in the future.

Introduction

Hematopoietic stem and progenitor cells (HSPCs) are defined functionally in transplantation assays by their self-renewal and multilineage differentiation

*Department of Immunology, Weizmann Institute of Science, Rehovot, Israel.
Tel: +972-89342481. Fax: +972-89344141.
†E-mail: tsvee.lapidot@weizmann.ac.il.

capacities. They mostly reside in the bone marrow (BM) at specialized niches, where they are maintained, and undergo proliferation and differentiation, giving rise to mature leukocytes and erythrocytes, which in turn are released to the blood in order to carry out their function.[1] Thus, transplantation of HSPCs is essential for hematopoietic reconstitution following myeloablative treatments in patients. In the past, BM aspirates were mostly utilized for stem cell transplantation; however, today, many protocols are practiced to harvest blood-derived HSPCs from either autologous origin or allogeneic donors, by inducing a process known as stem cell mobilization.[2] Under steady-state conditions, peripheral blood (PB) harbors minute amounts of transplantable HSPCs. Circulating HSPCs participate in homeostasis and are able to functionally re-engraft the BM, as demonstrated by murine parabiosis models, in which paired congenic mice share a common blood system.[3] In the same system, it was demonstrated that the numbers of circulating HSPCs with repopulation potential are highly increased in response to repeated cytokine administration.[4] Thus, during induced mobilization, the amount of circulating HSPCs may reach sufficient levels, suitable for transplantation. Mobilization of HSPCs to the periphery of patients in response to chemotherapy and/or cytokine stimulation was first documented in the late 1970s and early 1980s.[5] Today, the cytokine granulocyte colony-stimulating factor (G-CSF) is the most common regimen used clinically to effectively induce stem cell mobilization; however, many other mobilizing agents were shown to induce mobilization, and synergistic effects were often observed in combination with G-CSF administration (discussed in the next section). Most of these mobilizing agents have not been tested yet in clinical trials. Since G-CSF is a natural protein, one has to ask whether mobilization protocols utilized clinically actually mimic physiological processes. Repetitive daily stimulations with G-CSF could be considered as stress. Indeed, various stress-induced situations cause elevated egress levels of HSPCs, including exercise,[6] inflammation,[7] chemotherapy[8] and even psychological anxiety.[9] Notably, cytotoxic DNA-damaging chemotherapy drugs, such as cyclophosphamide (Cy), are often used clinically in autologous mobilization protocols.[10] This process can be enhanced by a combined administration with G-CSF.[11] Hence, preconditioning of patients by chemotherapy or irradiation as a prerequisite step for transplantation may cause mobilization by itself, an effect that is taken advantage of in autologous transplantations. The hallmark of Cy- and G-CSF-induced mobilization is enhanced proliferation and differentiation in the BM prior to progenitor cell egress, leading to higher cell doses for transplantation.[12] During stress situations, the increased demand for functional immune cells and tissue regeneration triggers various mechanisms that induce enhanced stem cell release, in addition to intensified *in situ* proliferation and differentiation. G-CSF administration is associated with neutrophilia, and neutrophils play a significant role in interfering with stem cell retention in the BM, by activating neutrophil-derived proteases, which cleave adhesion interactions, resulting in enhanced release of progenitors to the PB[13] (discussed under "Mechanistic Insights"). Nevertheless, mobilizing agents act via versatile mechanisms, some of which induce rapid HSPC release within a few hours. For instance, the CXCR4 antagonist AMD3100 prevents retention of HSPCs in the BM.[14] The chemokine stromal-derived factor 1 (SDF-1) (also termed CXCL12) and its major receptor, CXCR4, are important for attracting HSPCs to the BM, maintain quiescence, and trigger tight adhesion to the niches where HSPCs are located.[15,16] By interfering with SDF-1/CXCR4 interactions, AMD3100 rapidly releases HSPCs with repopulation potential to the PB[14] (discussed under "Clinical and Preclinical Aspects of Mobilization" and "Mechanistic Insights"). In fact, altering SDF-1 levels in the BM and PB is a major mechanism that enables HSPC egress and mobilization to the circulation. Many recent studies have pointed out that the dynamic regulation of the BM microenvironment plays an essential role in the mobilization process. Stimulations of the sympathetic nervous system, as well as of immune-system-originated bone-degrading osteoclasts, promote stem cell release from the BM, by detaching HSPCs from their niches, affecting bone remodeling dynamics and downregulating SDF-1 levels in the BM[17–19] (discussed under "The Involvement of the Microenvironment"). It should be noted that mobilized PB and BM cells are not the only source of transplantable HSPCs; the umbilical cord blood and additional blood from the placenta or fetal liver cells are plausible sources (not discussed). In this chapter, we will focus on mobilization of HSPCs: the current clinical practice, where mobilizing agents are used at the bedside or the bench; mechanistic insights into this process, involving dynamic regulation of HSPCs and the BM microenvironment, by the nervous and immune systems as part of host defense and repair. Finally, we discuss future directions.

Clinical and Preclinical Aspects of Mobilization

G-CSF-induced Mobilization

Mobilization of HSPCs is an established clinical procedure. During steady-state hematopoiesis, the BM contains several magnitudes of order more immature cells compared to the PB. Therefore, several methods have been used to mobilize HSPCs in order to harvest enriched fractions from the PB. Following chemotherapeutic treatment, an increase in circulating HSPCs is observed.[11] These high levels can be significantly raised by combined administration of mobilizing agents. To this end, several mobilizing agents have been applied, one of which is recombinant G-CSF, being now the standard for clinical mobilization.[20] In healthy donors, G-CSF, is typically given subcutaneously for 4–5 successive days.[21] Soon after, leukapheresis is performed and the enriched mobilized immature CD34$^+$ cells are used for allogeneic transplantations. CD34$^+$ cell content is considered as a predictive parameter for successful stem cell harvest. G-CSF-induced mobilization leads to an increase of circulating immature CD34$^+$ cells up to a factor of 25 compared to steady-state hematopoiesis,[22,23] and in comparison with BM harvests, G-CSF-mobilized blood contains 3–4 higher CD34$^+$ cell doses.[21] On the other hand, mobilization for autologous transplantations, which is mostly practiced in patients with hematological malignancies, is usually performed together with administration of chemotherapeutical drugs, such as Cy.[24] Combination of chemotherapy with G-CSF leads to a median 50-fold increase of circulating immature CD34$^+$ progenitors, but a high variation amongst individual patients is noted.[25] G-CSF is also available in a slow release pegylated version with a longer half-life *in vivo*, which is able to mobilize with a single dose alone.[26] In what terms are G-CSF-mobilized immature CD34[+] progenitors different from their steady-state BM counterparts, apart from increased motility toward the chemokine SDF-1? Gene expression array analyses show that the mobilized cells are less cycling and less differentiating,[27,28] supporting the observations that circulating stem and progenitor cells are quiescent.[29] Indeed, immature G-CSF-mobilized human CD34[+] cells demonstrate a higher short-term repopulation capacity in transplanted immune-deficient mice, when cells in the G0 state are transplanted in comparison with cells in the G1 state.[30] We reported that G-CSF also enhances the motility and homing of differentiating human progenitor cells. In addition to the more primitive quiescent human CD34[+]CD38[−] cells, the more differentiated human CD34[+]CD38[+] progenitors obtained from G-CSF-mobilized PB, or *ex vivo* cytokine-treated human CD34[+] cells, efficiently home to the murine BM, as opposed to naïve nontreated human CD34[+] cells.[31]

Mobilization Induced by Other Cytokines and Chemokines

Although many other chemokines and cytokines have been shown to induce mobilization of HSPCs in animal models, only a few were tested in humans, such as granulocyte macrophage colony-stimulating factor (GM-CSF) and stem cell factor (SCF). GM-CSF was successfully applied for HSPC mobilization and subsequent autologous transplantation in the late 1980s and early 1990s.[32] Nevertheless, in a comparative study of mobilization in healthy donors, G-CSF was superior to GM-CSF and a combined G-CSF + GM-CSF treatment resulted in a similar HSPC content compared to G-CSF alone.[22] On the other hand, studies on nonhuman primates showed that a combination of G-CSF and SCF has a synergistic effect on mobilization of HSPCs.[33] Unfortunately, mobilization trials in humans with a combined G-CSF and SCF administration led to severe mast-cell-mediated reactions.[34] Nonetheless, several studies have shown that with an appropriate comedication SCF can be used safely and, in combination with G-CSF, is able to achieve mobilization in patients who have failed to mobilize with G-CSF alone or are expected to be poor mobilizers.[35] Another promising mobilizing natural agent, which has not yet been tested clinically, is the chemokine GROβ (also known as CXCL2), a ligand for the receptor CXCR2. Pelus and colleagues (2007) examined mobilization characteristics of GROβ and GRO$\beta\Delta4$ (a more potent form *in vitro*) in mice and found that mobilization of murine HSPCs was similar to G-CSF alone.[36] Combination of GROβ or GRO$\beta\Delta4$ with G-CSF-mobilized about five times more HSPCs than each of these agents alone. Serial competitive repopulation assays in mice showed that GRO$\beta\Delta4$ produced about four times better long-term engraftment than G-CSF alone, with further improvement by combination of the two.[36] Furthermore, these cells seem to engraft better with significantly shorter times to recovery of WBCs and platelets.[36] In summary, administration of chemotherapy and cytokines is a conventional approach to mobilizing HSPCS nowadays, and new candidate agents, including chemokines, may be utilized in the near future. A different approach, employing small molecules to achieve rapid mobilization, is discussed next.

Mobilization Induced by CXCR4 Antagonists

In recent years, the field of clinical mobilization has received a new impetus with the discovery of the SDF-1/CXCR4 axis, which is pivotal for maintenance and motility of HSPCs in the BM and blood (further discussed under "Mechanistic Insights"). Since CXCR4 also serves as a coreceptor for HIV entry into human T lymphocytes, extensive research led to the development of small molecule inhibitors of CXCR4. One of the promising discoveries was the bicyclam AMD3100. This demonstrated a rapid and high yield of mobilized HSPCs even following single-dose administration within a few hours.[37,38] The mobilization potential in mice was explored systematically by Broxmeyer and colleagues.[14] AMD3100-induced rapid mobilization of HSPCs and synergistically augmented G-CSF-induced mobilization. This was assessed by competitive repopulation assays in transplanted mice. The mobilization potential of AMD3100 was tested in healthy volunteers as well, by assessing the long-term engraftment potential in a xenograft system (i.e. transplanting human HSPCs into immunodeficient mice).[14] A combination of AMD3100 with G-CSF synergistically enhanced mobilization of human HSPCs, which is in accordance with the number of mobilized CD34[+] cells determined in another study on healthy volunteers. The combination of AMD3100 with G-CSF led to successful mobilization in about 70% of patients who had failed mobilization with conventional mobilization protocols.[39] Furthermore, AMD3100 was recently reported to be successfully used alone in mobilization of allogeneic donors.[38] Due to the success of several clinical studies, AMD3100 is currently undergoing approval in the USA and Europe, and is expected to be clinically available soon. A different set of CXCR4 antagonists, based on peptide engineering, has been developed by Nobutaka Fujii and colleagues. They were developed from polyphemusin II, a naturally occurring 18-amino-acid peptide isolated from the American horseshoe crab (*Limulus polyphemus*). One of them, T-140, underwent preclinical testing by the group of Amnon Peled.[40] They found that it effectively mobilized murine HSPCs within a few hours in a dose-dependent manner and mobilized synergistically with G-CSF administration. Mobilization characterized by WBC content and CFU parameters showed similar mobilization potential for T-140 and AMD3100. Interestingly, the combination of T-140 with G-CSF resulted in higher mobilization rates of murine progenitor cells compared to the combination of AMD3100 with G-CSF. This inhibitor is intended for clinical usage in the future. In summary, due to their rapid and potent effects, lack of adverse side effects and relatively inexpensive synthesis, CXCR4 antagonists may change the concept behind clinical mobilization practice for the better.

Functional Preclinical Models

Interestingly, *in vitro* migratory ability of mobilized immature CD34[+] cells to the chemokine SDF-1 correlated with the hematopoietic recovery of autologously transplanted patients, indicating that functional *in vitro* migration assays could be helpful in predicting the success of transplantation.[41] Nevertheless, in order to evaluate the engraftment capacity of mobilized human progenitor cells or the potency of an investigated mobilizing agent, laboratory animals are utilized as preclinical models. Immunodeficient mice serve as the predominant model, due to the relative ease of colony maintenance and their ability to accept human grafts. Nonobese diabetic/severe combined immunodeficient (NOD/SCID) mice are one of the most common strains.[42] NOD/SCID mice lack mature B and T lymphocytes, as well as having reduced innate immunity. Other strains, which have impaired NK cell activity and demonstrate improved repopulation of transplanted human cells, are available, such as the NOD/SCID/β2m^{null} and NOD/SCID/IL-2γR^{null} mice.[43,44] Establishment of human/murine chimeras is useful for evaluating the homing and engraftment capacities of transplanted human HSPCs. The level of engraftment is screened by counting repopulating human HSPCs (also termed "SCID repopulating cells" — SRCs). One of the major contributions of this preclinical model is the identification of primitive long-term repopulating human SRCs, characterized mostly as CD34$^+$CD38$^-$ cells.[31] These cells efficiently home to the BM of NOD/SCID and NOD/SCID/β2m^{null} mice in a CXCR4-dependent manner and are able to provide multilineage reconstitution in both primary and secondary recipients.[31] In addition to repopulation assays, immune-deficient mice are utilized for the comparison of different mobilization protocols with human cells.[43] For example, a comparative study between cells mobilized by G-CSF alone or by combined G-CSF + SCF administration was performed in chimeric NOD/SCID mice.[45] Although SCF + G-CSF–mobilized cells exhibited enhanced repopulation compared to G-CSF-alone-mobilized cells (probably due to increased numbers), qualitatively they were inferior. BM-resident SRCs are also tested directly for their mobilization efficacy.[42] Apart from immunodeficient mice, the preimmune fetal sheep model was utilized. For example, a qualitative comparison showed that human mobilized PB HSPCs were inferior to equivalent cells from the BM, in terms of proliferation, differentiation, long-term repopulation potential and serial transplantations, in sheep fetuses.[46] Another preclinical model of laboratory animals is based on nonhuman primates, which are physiologically more similar to humans. For example, in a particular study performed in myeloablated rhesus macaques, G-CSF-mobilized immature CD34[+] cells were compared to AMD3100-mobilized CD34[+] cells.[47] AMD3100-mobilized CD34[+] progenitor cells were found to express higher levels of CXCR4 and the integrin VLA-4 in comparison with their G-CSF-mobilized counterparts, and consequently stronger migration toward SDF-1 *in vitro* and higher *in vivo* repopulation.[47] These results are supported by studies on NOD/SCID mice, showing an increased SRC capacity by AMD3100-alone or G-CSF and AMD3100–mobilized immature human CD34[+] cells in comparison with their G-CSF-mobilized counterparts.[14] The SRC capacity of human CD34[+] cells and *in vitro* migration toward SDF-1 of human CD34[+] cells were synergistically augmented when G-CSF + AMD3100 administration was performed.[14] Altogether, these findings suggest that AMD3100 leads to mobilization of HSPCs, which are more motile than G-CSF-mobilized HSPCs and therefore their engraftment capacity could be more rapid. Although xenotranplantation models can serve as predictors for clinical mobilization, they have some limitations, due to obvious genetic and molecular differences and xenogeneic barriers. Nonetheless, murine models and to a lesser degree other animal models (and not humanized chimeras) dominate as the main tool in the extensive basic research on HSPC egress and mobilization, and many of the findings contribute to the improvement of clinical mobilization protocols and the development of novel mobilizing agents (discussed below).

Mechanistic Insights

Adhesion Molecules Keep HSPCs in the Niche

HSPCs reside in specialized niches in the BM, composed of supportive stromal cells, such as osteoblasts, endothelial and reticular cells.[48] Many adhesion molecules are involved in the interactions between the HSPCs and the stromal cells. These interactions regulate various features of

HSPC behavior, such as retention and quiescence. During the mobilization process, the breakdown of these interactions, created by the adhesion molecules, is necessary for the release of HSPCs from their niches, allowing their proliferation and egress to the PB.[48] Regulation of these interactions is also necessary for entry into the cell cycle, enabling subsequent proliferation and differentiation. The important interactions which mediate HSPC retention include VCAM-1/VLA-4; the integrins VLA-4,5/fibronectin (FN); membrane-bound SCF/c-Kit; Ang-1/Tie-2; CD44/hyaluronan; β1-integrins/osteopontin (OPN), as well as the SDF-1/CXCR4 axis (this will be separately discussed).[49] VCAM-1 and VLA-4 are expressed on stromal and hematopoietic cells, respectively. *In vivo* administration of neutralizing antibodies for VCAM-1 or VLA-4 induced the egress of HSPCs to the PB in both murine and primate models.[50,51] The same phenotype was observed in inducible deletion models for VLA-4 or VCAM-1,[52,53] as well as following administration of a small molecule that inhibits VLA-4 function (called AMD15057).[54] SCF and its receptor c-Kit are essential for the self-renewal and survival of HSPCs. Deletion of one of these molecules in mice led to direct hematopoietic failure.[55] Another aspect of SCF and c-Kit interactions was demonstrated in a study showing that the cleavage and release of BM membrane-bound SCF promotes the egress of HSPCs in the mobilization process.[56] SCF/c-Kit interactions also promote retention via activation of VLA-4 itself, and the administration of soluble c-Kit resulted in the egress of HSPCs from the BM.[57] Ang-1 and Tie-2 interactions were shown to maintain the quiescence of HSPCs and induce their adherence to osteoblast cells.[58] *In vivo* administration of Ang-1 resulted in a modest mobilization, which was enhanced by combined administration of VEGF.[59] CD44 is an adhesion molecule interacting with multiple adhesion components found in the ECM, including hyaluronan.[60] It was discovered to be essential for homing of immature human CD34$^+$ cells to the BM of immune-deficient mice.[60] Moreover, its major role in retention can be deduced from the observation that CD44 is downregulated on human HSPCs upon G-CSF-induced mobilization.[23] Indeed, *in vivo* administration of CD44-neutralizing antibodies promoted the egress of HSPCs from the BM, and the combined treatment with G-CSF or anti-VLA-4 acted synergistically to increase the numbers of mobilized HSPCs.[61] Many BM stromal cell types express OPN, including bone-lining osteoblasts, and OPN was shown to negatively regulate the stem cell pool size.[62] It was also shown that OPN directs migrating primitive hematopoietic cells toward the endosteal regions via interactions with β1-integrins.[63] It is possible to speculate that neutralization or inhibition of this interaction will also result in HSPC egress into the periphery.

Proteases Release HSPCs from their Niches

In order to release HSPCs from their niches, downregulation of adhesion molecules is crucial for their egress in the mobilization process. Disrupting adhesion interactions by artificial methods, such as administration of antagonists or neutralizing antibodies, mimicks physiological mechanisms. The cleavage of different adhesion molecules and ECM components is a common mechanism by which proteases enable progenitor cell detachment.[49] During G-CSF-induced mobilization, there is robust proliferation and activation of neutrophils in the BM.[64] Neutrophils secrete serine proteases like neutrophil elastase and cathepsin G, which were shown to cleave VCAM-1,[65] c-Kit,[66] SDF-1[67] and CXCR4.[68] Indeed, inhibition of elastase activity reduced G-CSF-induced mobilization of murine HSPCs from the BM.[67] Notably, administration of various cytokines and chemokines, known to activate neutrophils (e.g. GM-CSF, IL-8, GROβ and MIP-1α), causes mobilization, pointing at a major course of action mediating release of HSPCs from their niches.[13] Another family of proteases participating in the HSPC mobilization process is the matrix metalloproteinase (MMP) family. Upon activation, MMPs cleave ECM components and other factors, promoting transendothelial migration and release of HSPCs from their niches. MMP-9, specifically, is upregulated during mobilization and was shown to cleave membrane-bound SCF and its receptor c-Kit.[56,66] Another member of the MMP family, the membranal type 1 MMP (MT1-MMP or MMP-14), promotes HSPC mobilization via CD44 cleavage.[69] CD26 (dipeptidyl peptidase IV) is expressed by hematopoietic cells and was shown to cleave SDF-1 into a truncated form, which serves in fact as an antagonist for CXCR4 signaling.[70] Inhibition of CD26 or its genetic ablation in a mouse knockout system reduces G-CSF-induced mobilization.[71] Osteoclasts, the bone-degrading cells, participate in mobilization of HSPCs by secreting proteases like MMP-9 and cathepsin K.[19] Cathepsin K, the hallmark of bone resorption, is involved in the mobilization process by promoting the cleavage of SDF-1, OPN and membrane-bound SCF in the BM endosteal region,[19] linking bone remodeling with mobilization of progenitor cells. Altogether, proteases play a key role in mediating HSPC mobilization, "clearing" the way out from the BM to the blood.

The SDF-1/CXCR4 Axis

The chemokine SDF-1 is the strongest known chemoattractant for hematopoietic stem and progenitor cells.[15,72] It was shown to be involved also in retention, homing, survival and quiescence of human and murine HSPCs.[15,16,73] In the BM, different cell types are implied to compose the stem cell niche, such as endosteal bone-lining osteoblasts,[74] endothelial cells[75] and CXCL12 (SDF-1), abundant reticular (CAR) cells.[16] These cells express high levels of SDF-1, promoting retention of CXCR4 expressing HSPCs to their niches. Human and mouse SDF-1 are cross-reactive and differ in one amino acid only, allowing human CD34$^+$ progenitors to repopulate transplanted immune-deficient mice in a CXCR4-dependent manner.[43] In an inducible knockout mouse model for CXCR4, a reduction of BM cellularity is observed by time, accompanied by increased proliferation of HSPCs, leading eventually to impaired long-term repopulating capacity.[16] In addition, these mice show more sensitivity to irradiation and myelosuppressive treatment, due to the fact that CXCR4-deficient HSPCs are continuously cycling and not quiescent. CXCR4 conditional knockout mice also exhibit increased numbers of stem and progenitor cells in the PB and in the spleen, strengthening the role of CXCR4 in HSPC BM retention and quiescence.[16] Repetitive administration of SDF-1 for five consecutive days or single-dose administration of the Met-SDF1 analog *in vivo* triggers preferential mobilization of murine progenitor cells.[19,76] During G-CSF-induced mobilization, SDF-1 levels in the BM are transiently increased, followed by their eventual reduction at mRNA and protein levels, suggesting formation of local and transient gradients of SDF-1 from the BM to the PB.[67,68,77] CXCR4 levels are increased on BM HSPCs following G-CSF treatment, enhancing their migration potential toward SDF-1.[67] Moreover, blocking either CXCR4 or SDF-1 with neutralizing antibodies during G-CSF treatment in chimeric mice reduces both human and murine HSPC–induced mobilization,[67] implying a major involvement of the SDF-1/CXCR4 pathway. Upon administration of the CXCR4 antagonist AMD3100, rapid mobilization is triggered in both mouse and human subjects.[14] A combination of G-CSF and AMD3100 administration demonstrates a synergistic effect on HSPC mobilization.[14] These observations imply that AMD3100 administration disrupts SDF-1/CXCR4 interaction, releasing HSPCs from the BM to the circulation. However, this view is simplistic, because not only does blockage of SDF-/CXCR4 signaling cause loss of retention and consequently mobilization, but also its stimulation plays a part in the mobilization process. For instance, repeated SDF-1, HGF or RANKL stimulation triggers preferential mobilization of murine progenitor cells.[19] Moreover, since AMD3100 is a good mobilizer, while neutralizing anti-CXCR4 or anti-SDF-1 antibodies are not (anti-VLA-4 antibody does mobilize), other players and mechanisms must be part of the mobilization process induced by AMD3100. Preliminary data reveal that AMD3100 does not act on hematopoietic cells only, but also on CXCR4-positive BM stromal cells.[78] In response to AMD3100, SDF-1 secretion from BM osteoblasts and endothelial cells is increased, elevating SDF-1 release to the circulation of treated mice, which the mobilized HSPCs eventually follow.[78] Importantly, neutralizing SDF-1 or CXCR4 by antibodies blocks AMD3100-induced mobilization, showing that AMD3100 effects on stromal cells are essential for this rapid mobilization. Of interest is the fact that steady state levels of BM SDF-1 are dynamic and dependent on circadian stimulation by the sympathetic nervous system in response to exposure to light. Thus, the numbers of circulating HSPCs inversely correlate with SDF-1 levels in the BM and are thereby subject to circadian oscillations.[79] These findings add to the complexity of the mobilization process, showing that the BM stromal microenvironment plays a significant role as well. The emerging involvement of the microenvironment and its dynamic regulation is discussed next.

The Involvement of the Microenvironment

Bone Remodeling: Osteoblast and Osteoclast Activities Regulate HSPC Behavior

HSPCs reside in an ever-changing dynamic BM microenvironment. Constant bone-degrading and bone-rebuilding processes occur in the BM. These processes are carried out by the mesenchymally-originated bone-forming osteoblasts and by the hematopoietic-stem-cell-derived, immune-monocyte-originated, bone-degrading osteoclasts. A subset of endosteal osteoblasts was shown to localize in proximity to quiescent HSPCs in the BM, supporting hematopoiesis.[80] Osteoblast expansion by parathyroid hormone (PTH) treatment, in a murine model, was coupled with the expansion of the HSPC pool, implying a regulatory axis between the mesenchymally derived cells and the hematopoietic compartment.[81] During G-CSF-induced mobilization of HSPCs, it was shown that there is a significant decrease in SDF-1 levels in the BM.[67,77] Examination of the osteoblast population following G-CSF treatment revealed that there is a significant reduction in the numbers of endosteal SDF-1-producing osteoblasts.[77] This reduction in endosteal osteoblast numbers was shown to be regulated by the sympathetic nervous system responding to G-CSF stimulation.[17] Interestingly, osteoblasts isolated after two days of a combined G-CSF and Cy treatment exhibited an increased capacity to expand murine HSPCs under *in vitro* conditions.[82] Moreover, following irradiation-induced stress, endosteal osteoblasts increase the secretion of interleukin-10, which in turn promotes the self-renewal of murine HSPCs.[83] These results suggest that BM niches are undergoing dynamic changes, during stress-induced mobilization, to allow proliferation and egress of HSPCs. Osteoclasts, which are counterplayers to osteoblasts, regulate HSPC mobilization as well. During G-CSF-induced mobilization, donors sometimes suffer from bone loss, implying increased bone resorption activity.[84] Osteoclasts express both SDF-1 and CXCR4, and SDF-1 is involved in recruitment of osteoclast precursors to the endosteal bone surface and promotes immature osteoclast development and survival.[85] Administration of G-CSF, SDF-1 or HGF for five consecutive days induces both activation of osteoclast numbers and preferential mobilization of HSPCs to the blood.[19] Administration of RANKL, which specifically activates osteoclasts, results in selective mobilization of HSPCs, while inhibition of osteoclast activity by the hormone calcitonin impairs both steady state egress, stress-induced recruitment and G-CSF-induced mobilization of murine progenitor cells. The mobilization induction by RANKL was abolished in PTPε young female mice that displayed a defect in osteoclast development.[19] The direct role of osteoclasts in mobilization is mediated by cathepsin K secretion. Cathepsin K, the hallmark of bone resorption, was shown to cleave endosteal SDF-1, SCF and OPN, further promoting the release and egress of progenitor cells to the blood,[19] linking bone remodeling with HSPC mobilization. Another example of the involvement of osteoclasts in the mobilization process is presented by CD45 KO mice, which demonstrate defective osteoclast activity, altered metaphysial trabecular bone structure and a reduced BM pool of primitive HSPCs.[86] RANKL and suboptimal G-CSF-induced mobilization are consequently impaired in those mice. The two cell types, osteoblasts and osteoclasts, maintain close interactions and crosstalk, demonstrated by the osteoclast ability to induce osteoblast retraction.[87] Due to this fact and since the bone and BM topography is dynamic, we believe that the BM stem cell niches, including endothelial and reticular cells, undergo a dynamic process of remodeling, which is part of bone turnover and hematopoietic stem cell regulation and host defense and repair mechanisms.

The Nervous System Regulates HSPCs and their Niches

The mammalian nervous system regulates cellular behavior under many physiological conditions, especially stress. Both in rats and in humans, administration of epinephrine (adrenaline) increases leukocyte numbers in the peripheral blood.[88,89] These observations suggest that the sympathetic nervous system is involved in regulating hematopoiesis. Sympathetic nerve endings penetrate and invade the BM and localize in the metaphysis and epiphysis, where HSPCs reside.[90] Immature hematopoietic progenitor cells, among other leukocytes, express β2 adrenergic and dopamine receptors.[18] Furthermore, the expression of these receptors on immature human CD34$^+$ cells was upregulated during G-CSF-induced mobilization.[18] Administration of epinephrine, which binds to β2 adrenergic receptors, significantly increased the numbers of immature progenitors in the PB. On the other hand, administration of propranolol, a β2 adrenergic receptor antagonist, reduced the number of circulating progenitors. *In vitro* treatment by catecholamines, such as the neurotransmitters dopamine and epinephrine, increased the motility of human CD34$^+$ HSPCs, strengthening the role of the nervous system in promoting mobilization.[18] Apart from a direct effect on HSPCs, the sympathetic nervous system also regulates the BM microenvironment. Preliminary data reveal that norepinephrine triggered murine BM stromal cells to secrete SDF-1 and actively transport it out of the BM into the PB, thereby governing HSPC egress to the periphery.[78] Interestingly, G-CSF-mediated osteoblast suppression together with SDF-1 reduction is dependent on the sympathetic nervous system.[17] The mechanism is mediated by the adrenergic system, which in response to G-CSF influences the BM environment to promote HSPC mobilization. Thereby, G-CSF is unable to cause mobilization in young mice lacking adrenergic neurons activity.[17] Adrenergic stimulation was also shown to positively affect osteoclasts, which participate in the mobilization process.[91] The involvement of the nervous system in regulating HSPC egress does not seem to end with the "fight or flight" stress-induced stimulation by the adrenergic sympathetic system. Recent findings have revealed that the central nervous system may play a role as well. For instance, newly diagnosed patients with Alzheimer's disease show reduced numbers of circulating immature CD34[+] cells and plasma SDF-1 levels.[92,93] Altogether, the involvement of the nervous system adds another layer of complexity to the mobilization process. In addition, it is possible that the nervous system control over hematopoiesis extends to other features except for mobilization, such as regulation of HSPC self-renewal and hematopoietic development.

The Endothelial Cells — Keepers of the Blood–Bone Barrier

During egress from the BM to the PB, the progenitor cell regains motility, leaves its niche, and finds the path to the nearest blood vessel, to actively transmigrate through the endothelilal cells into the lumen. In stress-induced conditions, such as following chemotherapy, irradiation or G-CSF administration, there is an increase in endothelial permeability around the BM sinuses, allowing better conditions for HSPC egress.[94,95] In response to G-CSF administration, proteases, such as MMP-9, are activated.[56] MMP-9 was shown to actively cleave components of tight junctions between endothelial cells, promoting their increased permeability.[96] It is also possible that in addition to active cleavage of tight junction components, other mechanisms disrupt endothelial integrity, during stress-induced mobilization. Another function of endothelial cells in the mobilization process is their ability to function as cellular transporters of SDF-1, using CXCR4,[97] as well as a reservoir for secreted SDF-1.[78] Thus, by altering SDF-1 levels in the BM and PB, endothelial cells may facilitate the egress of HSPCs.[78] It is possible that in a similar manner to the blood–brain barrier, the BM endothelial cells may serve as gatekeepers, selecting which cells are allowed to enter or leave the BM, under various conditions as part of host defense and repair mechanisms.

Future Directions

One of the major aims of the stem cell mobilization research field is to develop improved procedures for harvesting HSPCs from mobilized blood together with improved reconstitution capacity for clinical protocols. Translation of basic research and preclinical investigation into clinical practice takes a long time; however, understanding the molecular and cellular mechanisms that govern stem cell mobilization is crucial for the development of new regimens. For example, the promising novel mobilizing agent AMD3100 would have not been suggested as a potential drug without the discovery of the SDF-1/CXCR4 pathway and its roles in HSPC retention, migration and proliferation. Likewise, the development of small molecules that target VLA-4-mediated retention demonstrates how molecular mechanisms are translated into clinical practice. The emerging concept of the dynamic microenvironment interactions with the nervous and immune systems and their involvement in the mobilization process is of high importance. Activation of osteoclasts, suppression of osteoblasts, adrenergic stimuli and endothelial integrity dynamically regulate progenitor cell egress and recruitment to the periphery, and therefore manipulation of these regulators may assist in improving clinical protocols. For example, PTH treatment in mice, which drives bone remodeling, protects the HSPC pool from exposure to cytotoxic chemotherapy, in addition to enhancement of G-CSF-induced mobilization.[98] Mobilized HSPCs from PTH + G-CSF–treated mice have a higher engraftment capacity than mobilized HSPCs from G-CSF-only treated mice.[98] Thus, PTH has beneficial characteristics in terms of the stem cell harvest quality in addition to its quantity, and therefore might be exploited in the future. Notably, studies on mice have shown that both RANKL and nor-epinephrine mobilize selectively immature cells to the circulation,[17–19] demonstrating that not only the quantity but also the quality of the mobilized cells is important. While current clinical practice is based on increasing cell harvest for transplantation, the ability of transplanted cells to rapidly engraft and to reach a sustained hematopoietic reconstitution is as important.

Acknowledgment

We thank Dr. Abraham Avigdor for fruitful discussions on clinical mobilization protocols.

References

1. Orkin SH, Zon LI. (2008) Hematopoiesis: An evolving paradigm for stem cell biology. *Cell* **132**: 631–644.
2. Korbling M, Anderlini P. (2001) Peripheral blood stem cell versus bone marrow allotransplantation: Does the source of hematopoietic stem cells matter? *Blood* **98**: 2900–2908.
3. Wright DE, Wagers AJ, Gulati AP *et al.* (2001) Physiological migration of hematopoietic stem and progenitor cells. *Science* **294**: 1933–1936.
4. Abkowitz JL, Robinson AE, Kale S *et al.* (2003) Mobilization of hematopoietic stem cells during homeostasis and after cytokine exposure. *Blood* **102**: 1249–1253.
5. To LB, Haylock DN, Simmons PJ, Juttner CA. (1997) The biology and clinical uses of blood stem cells. *Blood* **89**: 2233–2258.
6. Barrett AJ, Longhurst P, Sneath P, Watson JG. (1978) Mobilization of CFU-C by exercise and ACTH induced stress in man. *Exp Hematol* **6**: 590–594.
7. Cline MJ, Golde DW. (1977) Mobilization of hematopoietic stem cells (CFU-C) into the peripheral blood of man by endotoxin. *Exp Hematol* **5**: 186–190.
8. To LB, Haylock DN, Kimber RJ, Juttner CA. (1984) High levels of circulating haemopoietic stem cells in very early remission from acute nonlymphoblastic leukaemia and their collection and cryopreservation. *Br J Haematol* **58**: 399–410.
9. Elsenbruch S *et al.* (2006) Public speaking stress-induced neuroendocrine responses and circulating immune cell redistribution in irritable bowel syndrome. *Am J Gastroenterol* **101**: 2300–2307.
10. Verma UN *et al.* (1999) Paclitaxel vs. cyclophosphamide in peripheral blood stem cell mobilization: Comparative studies in a murine model. *Exp Hematol* **27**: 553–560.

11. Schwartzberg LS *et al.* (1992) Peripheral blood stem cell mobilization by chemotherapy with and without recombinant human granulocyte colony-stimulating factor. *J Hematother* **1**: 317–327.

12. Morrison SJ, Wright DE, Weissman IL. (1997) Cyclophosphamide/granulocyte colony-stimulating factor induces hematopoietic stem cells to proliferate prior to mobilization. *Proc Natl Acad Sci USA* **94**: 1908–1913.

13. Levesque JP, Winkler IG, Larsen SR, Rasko JE. (2007) Mobilization of bone marrow-derived progenitors. In *Handb Exp Pharmacol* pp. 3–36.

14. Broxmeyer HE *et al.* (2005) Rapid mobilization of murine and human hematopoietic stem and progenitor cells with AMD3100: A CXCR4 antagonist. *J Exp Med* **201**: 1307–1318.

15. Peled A *et al.* (1999) Dependence of human stem cell engraftment and repopulation of NOD/SCID mice on CXCR4. *Science* **283**: 845–848.

16. Sugiyama T, Kohara H, Noda M, Nagasawa T. (2006) Maintenance of the hematopoietic stem cell pool by CXCL12–CXCR4 chemokine signaling in bone marrow stromal cell niches. *Immunity* **25**: 977–988.

17. Katayama Y *et al.* (2006) Signals from the sympathetic nervous system regulate hematopoietic stem cell egress from bone marrow. *Cell* **124**: 407–421.

18. Spiegel A *et al.* (2007) Catecholaminergic neurotransmitters regulate migration and repopulation of immature human CD34[+] cells through Wnt signaling. *Nat Immunol* **8**: 1123–1131.

19. Kollet O *et al.* (2006) Osteoclasts degrade endosteal components and promote mobilization of hematopoietic progenitor cells. *Nat Med* **12**: 657–664.

20. Sheridan WP *et al.* (1992) Effect of peripheral-blood progenitor cells mobilised by filgrastim (G-CSF) on platelet recovery after high-dose chemotherapy. *Lancet* **339**: 640–644.

21. Cashen AF, Lazarus HM, Devine SM. (2007) Mobilizing stem cells from normal donors: Is it possible to improve upon G-CSF? *Bone Marrow Transplant* **39**: 577–588.

22. Lane TA *et al.* (1995) Harvesting and enrichment of hematopoietic progenitor cells mobilized into the peripheral blood of normal donors by granulocyte-macrophage colony-stimulating factor (GM-CSF) or G-CSF: Potential role in allogeneic marrow transplantation. *Blood* **85**: 275–282.

23. Lee S *et al.* (2000) Mobilization kinetics of CD34(+) cells in association with modulation of CD44 and CD31 expression during continuous intravenous administration of G-CSF in normal donors. *Stem Cells* **18**: 281–286.

24. Jantunen E, Kuittinen T. (2008) *Blood* stem cell mobilization and collection in patients with lymphoproliferative diseases: Practical issues. *Eur J Haematol* **80**: 287–295.

25. Seggewiss R *et al.* (2003) Kinetics of peripheral blood stem cell mobilization following G-CSF-supported chemotherapy. *Stem Cells* **21**: 568–574.

26. Fruehauf S *et al.* (2007) Efficient mobilization of peripheral blood stem cells following CAD chemotherapy and a single dose of pegylated G-CSF in patients with multiple myeloma. *Bone Marrow Transplant* **39**: 743–750.

27. Graf L, Heimfeld S, Torok-Storb B. (2001) Comparison of gene expression in CD34$^+$ cells from bone marrow and G-CSF-mobilized peripheral blood by high-density oligonucleotide array analysis. *Biol Blood Marrow Transplant* **7**: 486–494.

28. Steidl U *et al.* (2002) Gene expression profiling identifies significant differences between the molecular phenotypes of bone marrow-derived and circulating human CD34$^+$ hematopoietic stem cells. *Blood* **99**: 2037–2044.

29. Roberts AW, Metcalf D. (1995) Noncycling state of peripheral blood progenitor cells mobilized by granulocyte colony-stimulating factor and other cytokines. *Blood* **86**: 1600–1605.

30. Gothot A, van der Loo JC, Clapp DW, Srour EF. (1998) Cell cycle-related changes in repopulating capacity of human mobilized peripheral blood CD34(+) cells in non-obese diabetic/severe combined immune-deficient mice. *Blood* **92**: 2641–2649.

31. Kollet O *et al.* (2001) Rapid and efficient homing of human CD34(+)CD38(-/low)CXCR4(+) stem and progenitor cells to the bone marrow and spleen of NOD/SCID and NOD/SCID/B2m(null) mice. *Blood* **97**: 3283–3291.

32. Gianni AM *et al.* (1989) Granulocyte-macrophage colony-stimulating factor to harvest circulating haemopoietic stem cells for autotransplantation. *Lancet* **2**: 580–585.

33. Andrews RG *et al.* (1995) Rapid engraftment by peripheral blood progenitor cells mobilized by recombinant human stem cell factor and recombinant human granulocyte colony-stimulating factor in nonhuman primates. *Blood* **85**: 15–20.

34. Stiff P *et al.* (2000) A randomized phase 2 study of PBPC mobilization by stem cell factor and filgrastim in heavily pretreated patients with Hodgkin's disease or non-Hodgkin's lymphoma. *Bone Marrow Transplant* **26**: 471–481.

35. To LB *et al.* (2003) Successful mobilization of peripheral blood stem cells after addition of ancestim (stem cell factor) in patients who had failed a prior mobilization with filgrastim (granulocyte colony-stimulating factor) alone or with chemotherapy plus filgrastim. *Bone Marrow Transplant* **31**: 371–378.

36. Fukuda S, Bian H, King AG, Pelus LM. (2007) The chemokine GROβ mobilizes early hematopoietic stem cells characterized by enhanced homing and engraftment. *Blood* **110**: 860–869.

37. Liles WC *et al.* (2005) Augmented mobilization and collection of CD34[+] hematopoietic cells from normal human volunteers stimulated with granulocyte-colony-stimulating factor by single-dose administration of AMD3100, a CXCR4 antagonist. *Transfusion* **45**: 295–300.

38. Devine SM *et al.* (2008) Rapid mobilization of functional donor hematopoietic cells without G-CSF using plerixafor, an antagonist of the CXCR4/SDF-1 interaction. *Blood.*

39. Calandra G *et al.* (2008) AMD3100 plus G-CSF can successfully mobilize CD34[+] cells from non-Hodgkin's lymphoma, Hodgkin's disease and multiple myeloma patients previously failing mobilization

with chemotherapy and/or cytokine treatment: Compassionate use data. *Bone Marrow Transplant* **41**: 331–338.

40. Abraham M *et al.* (2007) Enhanced unique pattern of hematopoietic cell mobilization induced by the CXCR4 antagonist 4F-benzoyl-TN14003. *Stem Cells* **25**: 2158–2166.

41. Voermans C *et al.* (2001) *In vitro* migratory capacity of CD34$^+$ cells is related to hematopoietic recovery after autologous stem cell transplantation. *Blood* **97**: 799–804.

42. van der Loo JC *et al.* (1998) Nonobese diabetic/severe combined immunodeficiency (NOD/SCID) mouse as a model system to study the engraftment and mobilization of human peripheral blood stem cells. *Blood* **92**: 2556–2570.

43. Lapidot T, Petit I. (2002) Current understanding of stem cell mobilization: The roles of chemokines, proteolytic enzymes, adhesion molecules, cytokines, and stromal cells. *Exp Hematol* **30**: 973–981.

44. Ishikawa F *et al.* (2005) Development of functional human blood and immune systems in NOD/SCID/IL2 receptor {gamma} chain(null) mice. *Blood* **106**: 1565–1573.

45. Hess DA *et al.* (2002) Functional analysis of human hematopoietic repopulating cells mobilized with granulocyte colony-stimulating factor alone versus granulocyte colony-stimulating factor in combination with stem cell factor. *Blood* **100**: 869–878.

46. Verfaillie CM, Almeida-Porada G, Wissink S, Zanjani ED. (2000) Kinetics of engraftment of CD34(-) and CD34(+) cells from mobilized blood differs from that of CD34(-) and CD34(+) cells from bone marrow. *Exp Hematol* **28**: 1071–1079.

47. Larochelle A *et al.* (2006) AMD3100 mobilizes hematopoietic stem cells with long-term repopulating capacity in nonhuman primates. *Blood* **107**: 3772–3778.

48. Yin T, Li L. (2006) The stem cell niches in bone. *J Clin Invest* **116**: 1195–1201.

49. Mendez-Ferrer S, Frenette PS. (2007) Hematopoietic stem cell trafficking: Regulated adhesion and attraction to bone marrow microenvironment. *Ann NY Acad Sci* **1116**: 392–413.

50. Papayannopoulou T, Craddock C, Nakamoto B *et al.* (1995) The VLA4/VCAM-1 adhesion pathway defines contrasting mechanisms of lodgement of transplanted murine hemopoietic progenitors between bone marrow and spleen. *Proc Natl Acad Sci USA* **92**: 9647–9651.

51. Papayannopoulou T, Nakamoto B. (1993) Peripheralization of hemopoietic progenitors in primates treated with anti-VLA4 integrin. *Proc Natl Acad Sci USA* **90**: 9374–9378.

52. Scott LM, Priestley GV, Papayannopoulou T. (2003) Deletion of alpha4 integrins from adult hematopoietic cells reveals roles in homeostasis, regeneration, and homing. *Mol Cell Biol* **23**: 9349–9360.

53. Ulyanova T *et al.* (2005) VCAM-1 expression in adult hematopoietic and nonhematopoietic cells is controlled by tissue-inductive signals and reflects their developmental origin. *Blood* **106**: 86–94.

54. Ramirez P, Holt M, Rettig M *et al.* (2007) Mobilization of normal mouse progenitors and acute promyelocytic leukemia (APL) cells with inhibitors of CXCR4 and VLA-4 in splenectomized and unsplenectomized mice. *ASH Annual Meeting Abstracts* **110**.

55. Bernstein A, Forrester L, Reith AD *et al.* (1991) The murine W/c-kit and Steel loci and the control of hematopoiesis. *Semin Hematol* **28**: 138–142.

56. Heissig B *et al.* (2002) Recruitment of stem and progenitor cells from the bone marrow niche requires MMP-9 mediated release of kit-ligand. *Cell* **109**: 625–637.

57. Nakamura Y *et al.* (2004) Soluble c-kit receptor mobilizes hematopoietic stem cells to peripheral blood in mice. *Exp Hematol* **32**: 390–396.

58. Arai F *et al.* (2004) Tie2/angiopoietin-1 signaling regulates hematopoietic stem cell quiescence in the bone marrow niche. *Cell* **118**: 149–161.

59. Hattori K *et al.* (2001) Vascular endothelial growth factor and angiopoietin-1 stimulate postnatal hematopoiesis by recruitment of vasculogenic and hematopoietic stem cells. *J Exp Med* **193**: 1005–1014.

60. Avigdor A *et al.* (2004) CD44 and hyaluronic acid cooperate with SDF-1 in the trafficking of human CD34$^+$ stem/progenitor cells to bone marrow. *Blood* **103**: 2981–2989.

61. Christ O, Kronenwett R, Haas R, Zoller M. (2001) Combining G-CSF with a blockade of adhesion strongly improves the reconstitutive capacity of mobilized hematopoietic progenitor cells. *Exp Hematol* **29**: 380–390.

62. Stier S *et al.* (2005) Osteopontin is a hematopoietic stem cell niche component that negatively regulates stem cell pool size. *J Exp Med* **201**: 1781–1791.

63. Nilsson SK *et al.* (2005) Osteopontin, a key component of the hematopoietic stem cell niche and regulator of primitive hematopoietic progenitor cells. *Blood* **106**: 1232–1239.

64. Falanga A *et al.* (1999) Neutrophil activation and hemostatic changes in healthy donors receiving granulocyte colony-stimulating factor. *Blood* **93**: 2506–2514.

65. Levesque JP, Takamatsu Y, Nilsson SK *et al.* (2001) Vascular cell adhesion molecule-1 (CD106) is cleaved by neutrophil proteases in the bone marrow following hematopoietic progenitor cell mobilization by granulocyte colony-stimulating factor. *Blood* **98**: 1289–1297.

66. Levesque JP, Hendy J, Winkler IG *et al.* (2003) Granulocyte colony-stimulating factor induces the release in the bone marrow of proteases that cleave c-KIT receptor (CD117) from the surface of hematopoietic progenitor cells. *Exp Hematol* **31**: 109–117.

67. Petit I *et al.* (2002) G-CSF induces stem cell mobilization by decreasing bone marrow SDF-1 and up-regulating CXCR4. *Nat Immunol* **3**: 687–694.

68. Levesque JP, Hendy J, Takamatsu Y *et al.* (2003) Disruption of the CXCR4/CXCL12 chemotactic interaction during hematopoietic stem cell mobilization induced by GCSF or cyclophosphamide. *J Clin Invest* **111**: 187–196.

69. Avigdor A *et al.* (2009) MT1-MMP and RECK are involved in human CD34$^+$ progenitor cell retention, egress and mobilization. *J Clin Invest* **119**: 492–503.

70. Christopherson KW, 2nd, Cooper S, Broxmeyer HE. (2003) Cell surface peptidase CD26/DPPIV mediates G-CSF mobilization of mouse progenitor cells. *Blood* **101**: 4680–4686.

71. Christopherson KW, Cooper S, Hangoc G, Broxmeyer HE. (2003) CD26 is essential for normal G-CSF-induced progenitor cell mobilization as determined by CD26-/- mice. *Exp Hematol* **31**: 1126–1134.

72. Wright DE, Bowman EP, Wagers AJ *et al.* (2002) Hematopoietic stem cells are uniquely selective in their migratory response to chemokines. *J Exp Med* **195**: 1145–1154.

73. Nagasawa T *et al.* (1996) Defects of B-cell lymphopoiesis and bone-marrow myelopoiesis in mice lacking the CXC chemokine PBSF/SDF-1. *Nature* **382**: 635–638.

74. Ponomaryov T *et al.* (2000) Induction of the chemokine stromal-derived factor-1 following DNA damage improves human stem cell function. *J Clin Invest* **106**: 1331–1339.

75. Ceradini DJ *et al.* (2004) Progenitor cell trafficking is regulated by hypoxic gradients through HIF-1 induction of SDF-1. *Nat Med* **10**: 858–864.

76. Shen H *et al.* (2001) CXCR-4 desensitization is associated with tissue localization of hemopoietic progenitor cells. *J Immunol* **166**: 5027–5033.

77. Semerad CL *et al.* (2005) G-CSF potently inhibits osteoblast activity and CXCL12 mRNA expression in the bone marrow. *Blood* **106**: 3020–3027.

78. Dar A *et al.* (2006) AMD3100 signals via the nervous system, inducing release to the circulation of bone marrow SDF-1: Which is crucial for progenitor cell mobilization. *ASH Annual Meeting Abstracts* **108**: 1315.

79. Mendez-Ferrer S, Lucas D, Battista M, Frenette PS. (2008) Haematopoietic stem cell release is regulated by circadian oscillations. *Nature* **452**: 442–447.

80. Zhang J *et al.* (2003) Identification of the haematopoietic stem cell niche and control of the niche size. *Nature* **425**: 836–841.

81. Calvi LM *et al.* (2003) Osteoblastic cells regulate the haematopoietic stem cell niche. *Nature* **425**: 841–846.

82. Mayack SR, Wagers AJ. (2008) Osteolineage niche cells initiate hematopoietic stem cell mobilization. *Blood.*

83. Kang YJ *et al.* (2007) A novel function of interleukin-10 promoting self-renewal of hematopoietic stem cells. *Stem Cells* **25**: 1814–1822.

84. Stroncek DF *et al.* (1996) Treatment of normal individuals with granulocyte-colony-stimulating factor: Donor experiences and the effects on peripheral blood CD34$^+$ cell counts and on the collection of peripheral blood stem cells. *Transfusion* **36**: 601–610.

85. Wright LM *et al.* (2005) Stromal cell-derived factor-1 binding to its chemokine receptor CXCR4 on precursor cells promotes the chemotactic recruitment, development and survival of human osteoclasts. *Bone* **36**: 840–853.

86. Shivtiel S *et al.* (2008) CD45 regulates retention, motility, and numbers of hematopoietic progenitors, and affects osteoclast remodeling of metaphyseal trabecules. *J Exp Med.*

87. Kollet O, Dar A, Lapidot T. (2007) The multiple roles of osteoclasts in host defense: bone remodeling and hematopoietic stem cell mobilization. *Annu Rev Immunol* **25**: 51–69.

88. Benschop RJ, Rodriguez-Feuerhahn M, Schedlowski M. (1996) Catecholamine-induced leukocytosis: Early observations, current research, and future directions. *Brain Behav Immun* **10**: 77–91.

89. Iversen PO, Stokland A, Rolstad B, Benestad HB. (1994) Adrenaline-induced leucocytosis: recruitment of blood cells from rat spleen, bone marrow and lymphatics. *Eur J Appl Physiol Occup Physiol* **68**: 219–227

90. Artico M *et al.* (2002) Noradrenergic and cholinergic innervation of the bone marrow. *Int J Mol Med* **10**: 77–80.

91. Kondo H *et al.* (2005) Unloading induces osteoblastic cell suppression and osteoclastic cell activation to lead to bone loss via sympathetic nervous system. *J Biol Chem* **280**: 30192–30200.

92. Maler JM *et al.* (2006) Decreased circulating CD34$^+$ stem cells in early Alzheimer's disease: Evidence for a deficient hematopoietic brain support? *Mol Psychiatry* **11**: 1113–1115.

93. Laske C, Stellos K, Eschweiler GW *et al.* (2008) Decreased CXCL12 (SDF-1) plasma levels in early Alzheimer's disease: A contribution to a deficient hematopoietic brain support? *J Alzheimers Dis* **15**: 83–95.

94. Narayan K, Juneja S, Garcia C. (1994) Effects of 5-fluorouracil or total-body irradiation on murine bone marrow microvasculature. *Exp Hematol* **22**: 142–148.

95. Szumilas P *et al.* (2005) Effect of stem cell mobilization with cyclophosphamide plus granulocyte colony-stimulating factor on morphology of haematopoietic organs in mice. *Cell Prolif* **38**: 47–61.

96. Giebel SJ, Menicucci G, McGuire PG, Das A. (2005) Matrix metallo-proteinases in early diabetic retinopathy and their role in alteration of the blood-retinal barrier. *Lab Invest* **85**: 597–607.

97. Dar A *et al.* (2005) Chemokine receptor CXCR4-dependent internal-ization and resecretion of functional chemokine SDF-1 by bone marrow endothelial and stromal cells. *Nat Immunol* **6**: 1038–1046.

98. Adams GB *et al.* (2007) Therapeutic targeting of a stem cell niche. *Nat Biotechnol* **25**: 238–243.

Chapter 19

A Revolutionary BMT Method

*Susumu Ikehara**

We have recently developed a new bone marrow transplantation method consisting of a perfusion method (PM) and intrabone marrow — bone marrow transplantation (IBM-BMT). This method was found to be applicable to various otherwise intractable diseases, including autoimmune diseases, age-related diseases (emphysema, osteoporosis, etc.), and also malignant tumors. This article describes how we developed this powerful method.

Introduction

In 1985, we found that allogeneic (but not syngeneic or autologous) bone marrow transplantation (BMT) could be used to treat autoimmune diseases in autoimmune-prone mice.[1,2] Since then, using various autoimmune-prone mice, we have confirmed that allogeneic BMT can indeed be used to treat autoimmune diseases.[3–5]

Conversely, we have succeeded in inducing autoimmune diseases in normal mice by the transplantation of T cell-depleted bone marrow cells (BMCs) or partially purified hemopoietic stem cells (HSCs) from autoimmune-prone mice.[6,7] Based on these findings, we have proposed that autoimmune diseases are "stem cell disorders (SCDs)".[6–8]

*First Department of Pathology, Transplantation Center, Regeneration Research Center for Intractable Diseases, Center for Cancer Therapy, Kansai Medical University, 10–15 Fumizono-cho, Moriguchi City, Osaka 570-85506, Japan. Tel.: 81-6-6993-9429 Fax: 81-6-6994-8283 E-mail: ikehara@takii.kmu.ac.jp.

Our findings were also confirmed in humans: patients with autoimmune diseases were cured after allogeneic BMT, while autoimmune diseases were transferred to recipients after BMT from donors who were suffering from autoimmune diseases.[9]

In this article, we show that various otherwise intractable diseases (including SCDs) can be cured by our novel BMT method.

The Discovery of IBM-BMT

Using conventional BMT, we succeeded in treating a wide range of autoimmune diseases in various autoimmune-prone mice.[1–8] However, in the MRL/lpr mouse, which is radiosensitive (<8.5 Gy) and chimeric-resistant, we found that conventional intravenous BMT (IV-BMT) had a transient effect, and the autoimmune diseases were prone to recur.[10]

Using the MRL/lpr mouse, we found that the recruitment of donor stromal cells (including mesenchymal stem cells, MSCs) was essential for the success of allogeneic BMT, since there is a major histocompatibility complex (MHC) restriction between HSCs and stromal cells.[11,12] We therefore carried out three experiments to recruit donor stromal cells including MSCs: (i) conventional intravenous BMT (IV-BMT) plus bone grafts[13,14]; (ii) BMC injection from the portal vein (PV-BMT),[15] since it is well known that tolerance can easily be induced when the antigen is portal-venously (PV) injected into the liver; and (iii) IBM-BMT.[16]

As shown in Fig. 1, all recipients treated with 5.5 Gy × 2 plus IV-BMT died by 200 days after the treatment due to the recurrence of autoimmune diseases. However, the survival rate of the recipients treated with 5.5 Gy × 2 plus PV-BMT was 70%. When BMCs from which the stromal cells had been removed were injected via the PV, the survival rate of the recipients was markedly reduced (Fig. 1), indicating the crucial role of stromal cells in the success of the engraftment[17]; donor-derived stromal cells are trapped in the liver when whole BMCs are injected via the PV, and the stromal cells not only support the proliferation and differentiation of donor-derived HSCs trapped in the liver but also protect the HSCs from being attacked by the host's immunocompetent cells. They do this by

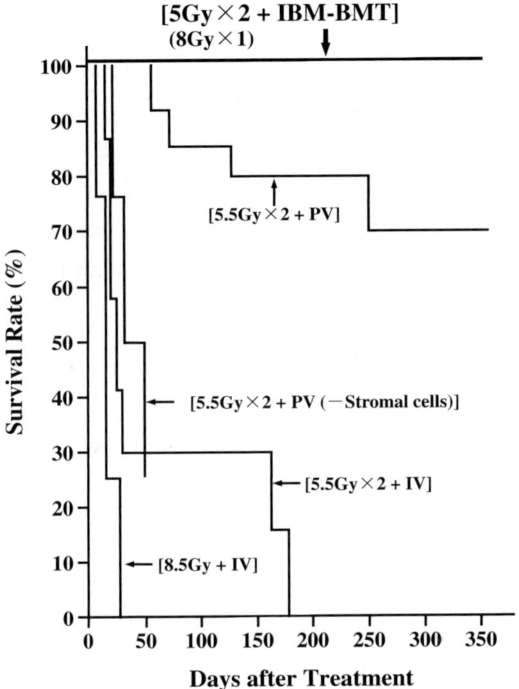

Fig. 1. Treatment of autoimmune diseases in MRL/lpr mice by IBM-BMT (5 Gy × 2). IBM-BMT can be used to treat autoimmune diseases in MRL/lpr mice even when the radiation dose is reduced to 5 Gy × 2. When stromal-cell-depleted HSCs were injected via the PV, the recipients died of graft failure.

directly embracing the HSCs[18] and/or producing immunosuppressive cytokines such as HGF and TGFβ.[19]

We next injected whole BMCs (including MSCs) directly into the bone marrow cavity (IBM-BMT), since we have found that the hemopoietic site moves from the liver to the bone marrow, even when the whole BMCs are injected via the PV. As shown in Fig. 1, IBM-BMT-treated recipients showed excellent survival rates even when the radiation dose was reduced to 5 Gy × 2.[16] These findings indicate that IBM-BMT is so far the best strategy for allogeneic BMT.

IBM-BMT for Organ Transplantation

Since we have previously found that the combination of organ allografts and conventional IV-BMT from the same donors prevents the rejection of organ allografts,[20,21] we attempted to apply IBM-BMT to organ allografts. IBM-BMT was found to be the most effective strategy as the radiation dose could be reduced to 4.0 Gy × 2 (which is equivalent to 6 G in one shot) in mouse skin allografts.[22] In addition, we found that IBM-BMT was applicable to allografts of other organs and tissues, such as the pancreatic islet,[23] leg,[24] lung,[25] and heart.[26]

IBM-BMT for Regeneration Therapy

Since it was apparent that donor stromal cells could be effectively recruited by IBM-BMT, we next attempted to treat osteoporosis in SAMP6 mice; the SAMP6 mouse (a substrain of senescence-accelerated mice) spontaneously develops osteoporosis early in life and is therefore a useful model for examining the mechanisms underlying osteoporosis. After IBM-BMT, the hematolymphoid system was completely reconstituted with donor-type cells. Thus-treated SAMP6 mice (8 months after IBM-BMT) showed marked increases in trabecular bone even at 20 months of age (Fig. 2), and the bone mineral density (BMD) remained similar to that of normal B6 mice. Bone marrow stromal cells in IBM-BMT-treated SAMP6 mice were replaced by donor stromal cells.[27,28] Thus, we succeeded in curing osteoporosis in SAMP6 mice by IBM-BMT, which can recruit both donor HSCs and MSCs.

Since IBM-BMT appeared to be a powerful strategy in regeneration therapy, we next used tight-skin (Tsk) mice (an animal model for emphysema) to examine whether emphysema could be cured by IBM-BMT.

IBM-BMT was carried out from C3H mice into Tsk mice (8–10 weeks old) that had already shown emphysema. Eight months after the transplantation, the lungs of all the Tsk mice treated with IBM-BMT [C3H → Tsk] showed structures similar to those of normal mice, whereas the [Tsk → Tsk] mice showed emphysema, as seen in age-matched Tsk

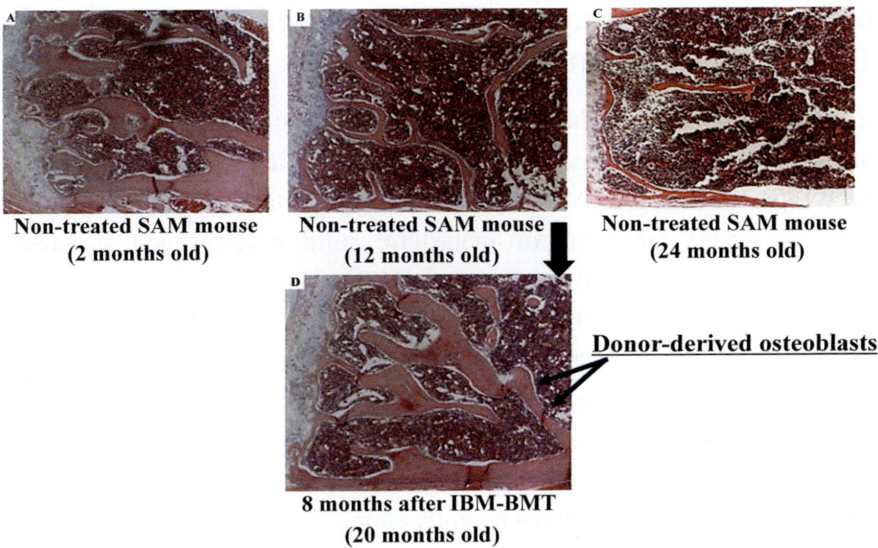

Fig. 2. Prevention and treatment of osteoporosis in SAMP6 mice by IBM-BMT from normal B6 mice.

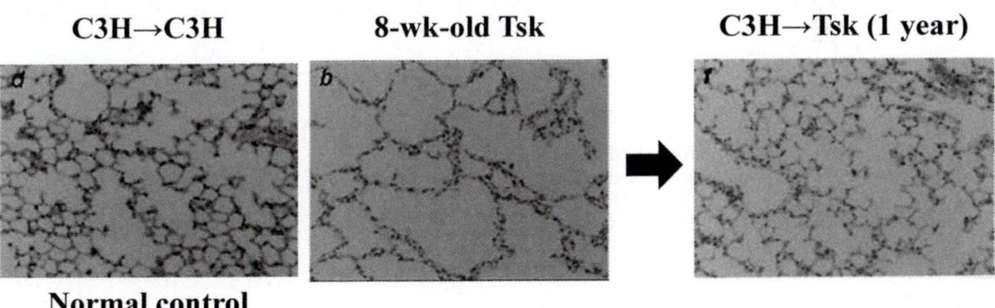

Fig. 3. Amelioration of emphysema in Tsk/+ mice by IBM-BMT.

mice (Fig. 3). Next, we attempted to transfer emphysema from Tsk mice to C3H mice by IBM-BMT. Six months after IBM-BMT, the [Tsk → C3H] mice showed emphysema.[29] These results strongly suggest that emphysema in Tsk mice originates from defects in the stem cells (probably MSCs) in the bone marrow.[29]

IBM-BMT + Donor Lymphocyte Infusion (DLI) for Treatment of Malignant Tumors

It is well known that the graft-vs-leukemia reaction (GvLR) can cure patients of a variety of hematological malignancies.[30,31] Recently, it has been reported that graft-vs-tumor (GvT) effects can induce partial (complete in some) remission of metastatic solid tumors such as breast cancer[32–34] and renal cell carcinoma.[35–40] Based on these findings, donor lymphocyte infusion (DLI) has recently been used for the treatment of malignant solid tumors even in humans. However, it is very difficult to completely eradicate the tumors, since extensive DLI induces graft-vs-host disease (GvHD). We therefore attempted to establish a new method for the treatment of malignant tumors, this method consisting of IBM-BMT plus DLI, since we have recently found that IBM-BMT can allow a reduction in radiation doses as a conditioning regimen and prevent GvHD in mice.[16,41] Using the Meth-A cell line (BALB/c-derived fibrosarcoma), we found that IBM-BMT plus the injection of CD4$^+$ T cell-depleted (but not CD8$^+$ T cell-depleted) spleen cells (as DLI) could prevent GvHD while suppressing tumor growth (Fig. 4). In addition, we have found that

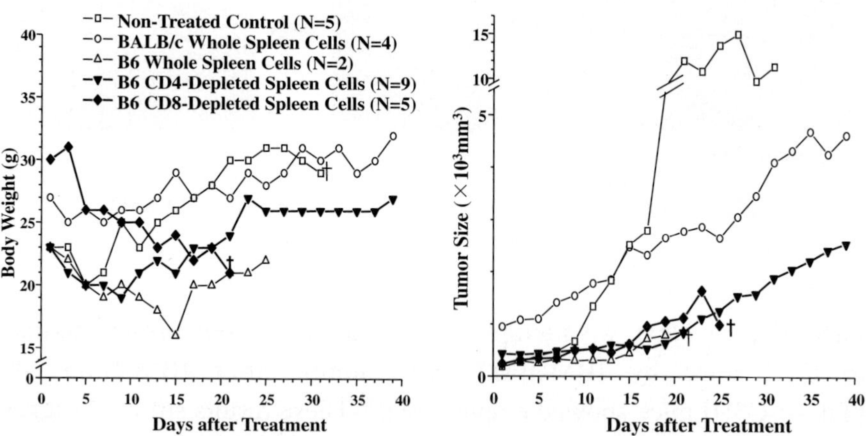

Fig. 4. Prevention of GvHD and suppression of tumor growth by IBM-BMT+DLI (CD4$^-$).

IBM-BMT plus extensive DLI (3 times every 2 weeks) leads to the complete rejection of the tumor, although the success rate (3/50) has not been high so far.[42]

In addition, we have examined whether this strategy (IBM-BMT+ DLI) is applicable to other tumors in other animals. We have obtained similar results in another system (colon cancer: ACL-15 in rats).[43] We are now establishing more efficient strategies to eradicate malignant tumors.

Novel BMT (PM+IBM-BMT) is Superior to Conventional BMT

Conventional BMT is carried out as follows: bone marrow needles are inserted into the iliac bones more than 100 times, and the BMCs are collected by the aspiration method (AM) (Fig. 5). Contamination with peripheral blood (particularly T cells) is therefore inevitable. When

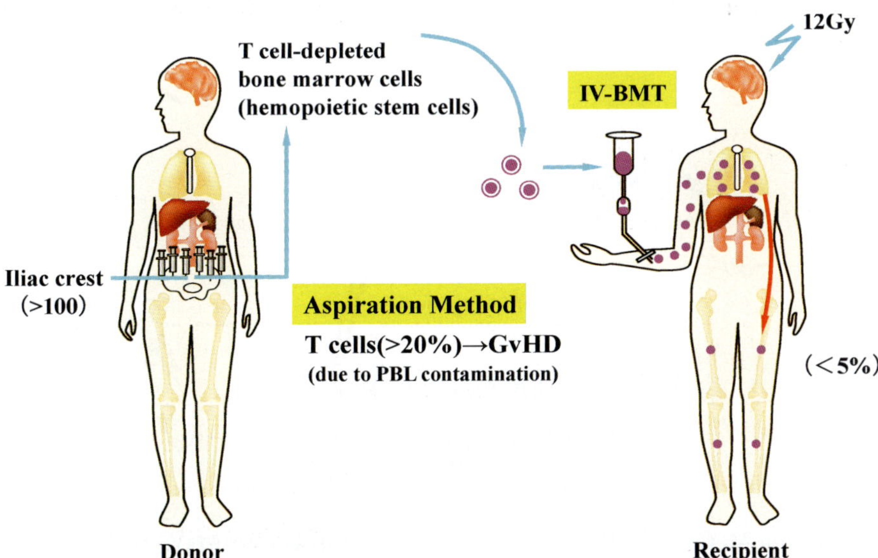

Fig. 5. Conventional BMT for allogeneic BMT. Conventional BMT is carried out using an aspiration method (AM), followed by the intravenous injection of HSCs (IV-BMT).

thus-collected cells are intravenously injected, most become trapped in the lung and only a few cells (<5%) migrate into the bone marrow (Fig. 5).

To apply our new BMT methods to humans, we established, using cynomolgus monkeys, a perfusion method (PM), which minimizes the contamination of BMCs with T cells. As shown in Fig. 6, two needles are inserted into a long bone such as the humerus, femur, or tibia. One end of the extension tube is connected to one needle. The other end is placed in a syringe containing 0.5 ml heparin. The other needle is connected to a syringe containing 30 ml of saline, and the saline is then pushed gently from the syringe into the medullary cavity to flush out the bone marrow. The saline containing the bone marrow fluid is then collected.

There is significantly less contamination with T cells using the PM (<10%) than the conventional AM (>20%). Therefore, T cell depletion is unnecessary with the PM, and whole BMCs can be used. In contrast, in

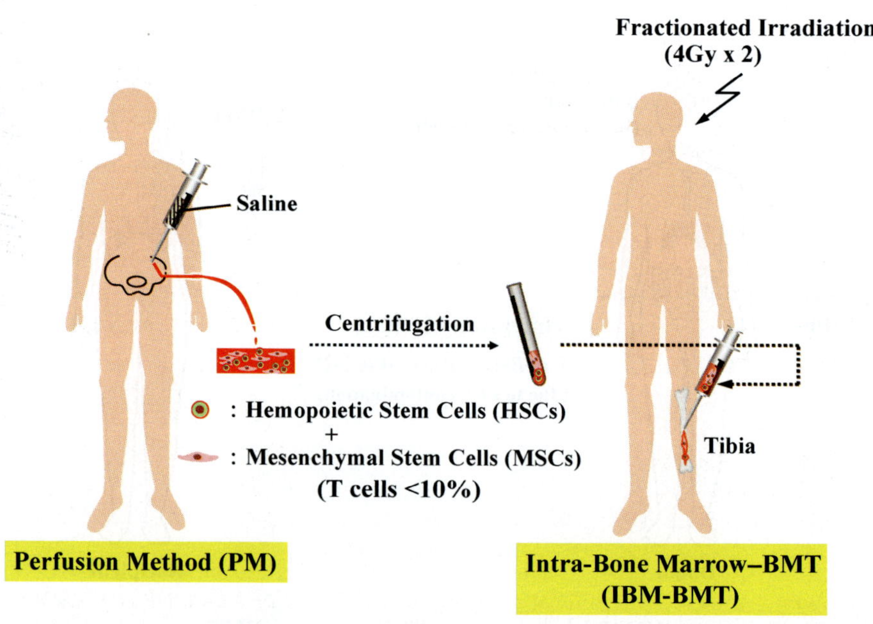

Fig. 6.　A new BMT method for allogeneic BMT. It consists of PM+IBM-BMT.

the case of the conventional AM, T cell depletion is necessary, and the loss of some important cells, such as MSCs, during the process of T cell depletion is inevitable. Furthermore, the number and progenitor activities of the cells harvested using the PM are greater than when using the conventional AM.[44,45]

We have also found that the PM is applicable to the iliac bones as well as the long bones not only in monkeys but also in humans.[45,46]

Conclusions and Future Directions

As described here, the new BMT method (PM+IBM-BMT) can be used to treat various otherwise intractable diseases, including (i) autoimmune diseases, (ii) age-associated diseases (osteoporosis, emphysema, etc.), (iii) diseases curable by organ transplantation, and (iv) malignant tumors (including solid tumors). The PM can efficiently be used to collect whole BMCs (including HSCs and MSCs) without their being contaminated with T cells, and therefore no GvHD develops. IBM-BMT can efficiently recruit donor whole BMCs (both HSCs and MSCs) into recipients. Therefore, this method can be used to quickly replace not only HSCs but also MSCs with donor-derived cells.

From the findings to date, it is conceivable that all the body's cells originate in the bone marrow, and that all diseases might therefore originate from defects in the bone marrow. One paper already suggests that gastric cancer originates from bone-marrow-derived cells.[47]

We believe that the development of our BMT method heralds a revolution in the field of transplantation (BMT and organ transplantation) and regeneration therapy.

Acknowledgments

I thank Mr. Hilary Eastwick-Field and Ms. K. Ando for their help in the preparation of the manuscript. These studies were mainly supported by the 21st Century Center of Excellence (COE) program of the Ministry of Education, Culture, Sports, Science and Technology. They were also supported by a grant from the Haiteku Research Center of the Ministry of Education, Health and Labor Sciences Research Grants, a grant from the Science Frontier program of the Ministry of Education, Culture, Sports, Science and Technology, and a grant from the Department of Transplantation for Regeneration Therapy (sponsored by Otsuka Pharmaceutical Co., Ltd.), a grant from the Molecular Medical Science Institute, Otsuka Pharmaceutical Co., Ltd., and a grant from Japan Immunoresearch Laboratories Co., Ltd. (JIMRO).

References

1. Ikehara S, Good RA, Nakamura T *et al.* (1985) Rationale for bone marrow transplantation in the treatment of autoimmune diseases. *Proc Natl Acad Sci USA* **82**: 2483–2487.

2. Ikehara S, Ohtsuki H, Good RA *et al.* (1985) Prevention of type I diabetes in nonobese diabetic mice by allogeneic bone marrow transplantation. *Proc Natl Acad Sci USA* **82**: 7743–7747.

3. Oyaizu S, Yasumizuy R, Miyama-Inaba M *et al.* (1988) (NZW × BXSB) F$_1$ mouse: A new animal model of idiopathic thrombocytopenic purpura. *J Exp Med* **167**: 2017–2022.

4. Than S, Ishida H, Inaba M *et al.* (1992) Bone marrow transplantation as a strategy for treatment of non-insulin-dependent diabetes mellitus in KK-Ay mice. *J Exp Med* **176**: 1233–1238.

5. Nishimura M, Toki J, Sugiura K *et al.* (1994) Focal segmental glomerular sclerosis, a type of intractable chronic glomerulonephritis, is a stem cell disorder. *J Exp Med* **179**: 1053–1058.

6. Ikehara S, Kawamura M, Takao F *et al.* (1990) Organ-specific and systemic autoimmune diseases originate from defects in hematopoietic stem cells. *Proc Natl Acad Sci USA* **87**: 8341–8344.

7. Kawamura M, Hisha H, Li Y *et al.* (1997) Distinct qualitative differences between normal and abnormal hematopoietic stem cells *in vivo* and *in vitro*. *Stem Cells* **15**: 56–62.

8. Ikehara S. (2003) A new concept of stem cell disorders and their new therapy. *J Hematother Stem Cell Res* **12**: 643–653.

9. Marmont AM. (1994) Immune ablation followed by allogeneic or autologous bone marrow transplantation: A new treatment for severe autoimmune diseases? *Stem Cells* **12**: 125–135.

10. Ikehara S, Yasumizu R, Inaba M *et al.* (1989) Long-term observations of autoimmune-prone mice treated for autoimmune disease by allogeneic bone marrow transplantation. *Proc Natl Acad Sci USA* **86**: 3306–3310.

11. Hashimoto F, Sugiura K, Inoue K *et al.* (1997) Major histocompatibility complex restriction between hematopoietic stem cells and stromal cells *in vivo*. *Blood* **89**: 49–54.

12. Sugiura K, Hisha H, Ishikawa J *et al.* (2001) Major histocompatibility complex restriction between hematopoietic stem cells and stromal cells *in vitro*. *Stem Cells* **19**: 46–58.

13. Ikehara S, Inaba M, Ishida S *et al.* (1991) Rationale for transplantation of both allogeneic bone marrow and stromal cells in the treatment of autoimmune diseases. In: Champlin RE, Gale RP (eds.), *New Strategies in Bone Marrow Transplantation*. UCLA Symposia on Molecular and Cellular Biology, New Series, Vol. 137, pp. 251–257. Wiley-Liss, New York, Chichester, Brisbane, Toronto, Singapore.

14. Ishida T, Inaba M, Hisha H *et al.* (1994) Requirement of donor-derived stromal cells in the bone marrow for successful allogeneic bone marrow transplantation: Complete prevention of recurrence of autoimmune diseases in MRL/MP-lpr/lpr mice by transplantation of bone marrow plus bones (stromal cells) from the same donor. *J Immunol* **152**: 3119–3127.

15. Kushida T, Inaba M, Takeuchi K *et al.* (2000) Treatment of intractable autoimmune diseases in MRL/lpr mice using a new strategy for allogeneic bone marrow transplantation. *Blood* **95**: 1862–1868.

16. Kushida T, Inaba M, Hisha H *et al.* (2001) Intra-bone marrow injection of allogeneic bone marrow cells: A powerful new strategy for treatment of intractable autoimmune diseases in MRL/lpr mice. *Blood* **97**: 3292–3299.

17. Kushida T, Inaba M, Hisha H *et al.* (2001) Crucial role of donor-derived stromal cells in successful treatment for intractable autoimmune diseases in MRL/lpr mice by BMT via portal vein. *Stem Cells* **19**: 226–235.

18. Ikehara S. (1998) Autoimmune diseases as stem cell disorders: Normal stem cell transplant for their treatment. *Int J Mol Med* **1**: 5–16.

19. Nicola MD, Stella-Carlo C, Magn M *et al.* (2002) Human bone marrow stromal cells suppress T-lymphocyte proliferation induced by cellular or nonspecific mitogenic stimuli. *Blood* **99**: 3838–3843.

20. Nakamura T, Good RA, Inoue S *et al.* Successful liver allografts in mice by combination with allogeneic bone marrow transplantation. *Proc Natl Acad Sci USA* **83**: 4529–4532.

21. Yasumizu R, Sugiura K, Iwai H *et al.* (1987) Treatment of type I diabetes mellitus in non-obese diabetic mice by transplantation of allogeneic bone marrow and pancreatic tissue. *Proc Natl Acad Sci USA* **84**: 6555–6557.

22. Ikehara S. (2008) A novel method of bone marrow transplantation (BMT) for intractable autoimmune diseases. *J Autoimmun* **30**: 108–115.

23. Ikebukuro K, Adachi Y, Suzuki Y *et al.* (2006) Synergistic effects of induction in transplantation of allogeneic pancreatic islets. *Bone Marrow Transplantation* **38**: 657–664.

24. Esumi T, Inaba M, Ichioka N *et al.* (2003) Successful allogeneic leg transplantation in rats by combination of intra-bone marrow (IBM) injection of donor bone marrow cells. *Transplantation* **76**: 1543–1548.

25. Kaneda H, Adachi Y, Saiyo Y *et al.* (2005) Long-term observation after simultaneous lung and intra-bone marrow–bone marrow transplantation. *J Heart Lung Transplant* **24**: 1415–1423.

26. Guo K, Inaba M, Li M *et al.* (2008) Long-term donor-specific tolerance in rat cardiac allografts by intra-bone marrow injection of donor bone marrow cells. *Transplantation* **85**: 93–101.

27. Ichioka N, Inaba M, Kushida T *et al.* (2002) Prevention of senile osteoporosis in SAMP6 mice by intra-bone marrow injection of allogeneic bone marrow cells. *Stem Cells* **20**: 542–551.

28. Takada K, Inaba M, Ichioka N *et al.* (2006) Treatment of senile osteoporosis in SAMP6 mice by intra-bone marrow injection of allogeneic bone marrow cells. *Stem Cells* **24**: 399–405.

29. Adachi Y, Oyaizu H, Taketani S *et al.* (2006) Treatment and transfer of emphysema by a new bone marrow transplantation method from normal mice to Tsk mice and vice versa. *Stem Cells* **24**: 2071–2077.

30. Thomas ED, Blume KG. (1999) Historical markers in the development of allogeneic hematopoietic cell transplantation. *Biol Blood Marrow Transplant* **5**: 341–346.

31. Weiden PL, Flournoy N, Thomas ED *et al.* (1979) Antileukemic effect of graft-versus-host diseases in human recipients of allogeneic-marrow grafts. *N Engl J Med* **300**: 1068–1073.

32. Ben-Yosef R, Or R, Nagker A *et al.* (1996) Graft-versus-tumor and graft-versus-leukaemia effect in patient with concurrent breast cancer and acute myelocytic leukaemia. *Lancet* **348**:1242–1243.

33. Eibi B, Schwaigofer H, Nachbaur D *et al.* (1996) Evidence for a graft-versus-tumor effect in a patient treated with marrow ablative chemotherapy and allogeneic bone marrow transplantation for breast cancer. *Blood* **88**: 1501–1508.

34. Ueno NT, Rondon G, Mirza NQ *et al.* (1998) Allogeneic peripheral-blood progenitor-cell transplantation for poor-risk patients with metastatic breast cancer. *J Clin Oncol* **16**: 986–993.

35. Childs RW, Clave E, Tisdale J *et al.* (1999) Successful treatment of metastatic renal cell carcinoma with a nonmyeloablative allogeneic peripheral-blood progenitor-cell transplant: Evidence for a graft-versus-tumor effect. *J Clin Oncol* **17**: 2044–2049.

36. Childs R, Chernoff A, Contentin N *et al.* (2000) Regression of metastatic renal-cell carcinoma after nonmyeloablative allogeneic peripheral-blood stem-cell transplantation. *N Engl J Med* **343**: 750–758.

37. Appelbaum FR, Sandmaier B. (2002) Sensitivity of renal cell cancer to nonmyeloablative allogeneic hematopoietic cell transplantation: Unusual or unusually important? *J Clin Oncol* **20**:1965–1967.

38. Bregni M, Dodero A, Peccatori J *et al.* (2002) Nonmyeloablative conditioning followed by hematopoietic cell allografting and donor lymphocyte infusions for patients with metastatic renal and breast cancer. *Blood* **99**: 4234–4236.

39. Hentschke P, Barkholt L, Uzunel M *et al.* (2003) Low-intensity conditioning and hematopoietic stem cell transplantation in patients with renal and colon carcinoma. *Bone Marrow Transplant* **31**: 253–261.

40. Rini BI, Zimmerman T, Stadler WM *et al.* (2002) Allogeneic stem-cell transplantation of renal cell cancer after nonmyeloablative chemotherapy: Feasibility, engraftment, and clinical results. *J Clin Oncol* **20**: 2017–2024.

41. Nakamura K, Inaba M, Sugiura K *et al.* (2004) Enhancement of allogeneic hematopoietic stem cell engraftment and prevention of GvHD by intra-bone marrow–bone marrow transplantation plus donor lymphocyte infusion. *Stem Cells* **22**:125–134.

42. Suzuki Y, Adachi Y. Minamino K *et al.* (2005) A new strategy for treatment of malignant tumor: Intra-bone marrow–bone marrow transplantation plus CD4$^-$ donor lymphocyte infusion. *Stem Cells* **23**: 365–370.

43. Koike Y, Adachi Y, Suzuki Y *et al.* (2007) Allogeneic intra-bone marrow–bone marrow transplantation plus donor lymphocyte infusion suppresses growth of colon cancer cells implanted in skin and liver of rats. *Stem Cells* **25**: 385–391.

44. Inaba M, Adachi Y, Hisha H *et al.* (2007) Extensive studies on perfusion method plus intra-bone marrow–bone marrow transplantation using cynomolgus monkeys. *Stem Cells* **25**: 2098–2103.

45. Kushida T, Inaba M, Ikebukuro K *et al.* (2002) Comparison of bone marrow cells harvested from various bones of cynomolgus monkeys of various ages by perfusion or aspiration methods: A preclinical study for human BMT. *Stem Cells* **20**: 155–162.

46. Li C, He Y, Feng X *et al.* (2007) An innovative approach to bone marrow collection and transplantation in a patient with β-thalassemia major: Marrow collection using a perfusion method followed by intra-bone marrow injection of collected bone marrow cells. *Int J Hematol* **85**: 73–77.

47. Houghton J, Stoicov C, Nomura S *et al.* (2004) Gastric cancer originating from bone marrow-derived cells. *Science* **306**: 1568–1571.

Chapter 20

Hematopoietic Cell Transplantation for Induction of Transplantation Tolerance: From Animal Models to Clinical Trials

*Megan Sykes**

Introduction

Immune tolerance denotes a state in which the immune system accepts donor organs or tissues but is capable of responding normally to foreign antigens. While recent improvements in immunosuppressive drugs have greatly augmented early organ allograft survival rates, these improvements have had little impact on late graft loss, which is due in large part to chronic rejection. Moreover, a high incidence of malignancies and opportunistic infections as well as drug-specific metabolic and other toxicities severely limit the tolerability of long-term chronic immunosuppressive therapy. The induction of donor-specific immune tolerance would avoid these complications while also preventing chronic rejection. However, any approach to tolerance induction in humans would be a radical departure from the standard of care, as immunosuppressive therapy would be withdrawn, exposing the patient to the risk of rejection.

*Bone Marrow Transplantation Section, Transplantation Biology Research Center, Surgical Service, Massachusetts General Hospital/Harvard Medical School, MGH East, Building 149-5102, 13th Street, Boston, MA 02129, USA. Tel.: 617/726-4070 Fax: 617/724-9892. E-mail: megan.sykes@tbrc.mgh.harvard.edu.

Thus, the expected efficacy of any tolerance approach to be considered in humans must be very high on the basis of animal data before it is evaluated in clinical trials. Fortunately, organ transplant studies on large animals can mimic clinical transplantation quite well, allowing relevant safety and efficacy evaluations to be performed. Many strategies reported to induce tolerance in rodent models either have failed to achieve tolerance in large animals[1-4] or have not been evaluated. In order to move from rodent models to clinical trials of tolerance induction, it is important to first demonstrate efficacy in stringent rodent models such as MHC-mismatched skin grafts, which are among the most immunogenic and least tolerogenic grafts in these species. Next, both efficacy and safety should be demonstrated in large animal models.

Tolerance Induction by Allogeneic Hematopoietic Cell Transplantation

Allogeneic hematopoietic cell transplantation (HCT) provides a potent means of inducing donor-specific tolerance. Allogeneic hematopoietic chimerism was first associated with tolerance when Freemartin cattle (fraternal twins sharing a placental circulation) were shown to be chimeric and tolerant of one another.[5] However, achievement of this state in adult recipients with already-established immune systems has presented a major challenge. The major immune barrier to allogeneic hematopoietic cell engraftment is imposed by recipient T cells.[6,7] This barrier can be overcome by host conditioning that either eliminates mature host immune cells, creating an immunological "clean slate," or permits pre-existing T cells to be rendered tolerant by the donor hematopoietic cells. Since newly developing T and B lymphocytes are tolerized by antigens which they encounter during their maturation, especially those expressed by hematopoietic cells, HCT can educate T and B cells to recognize an engrafted donor and host antigens as "self," resulting in donor- and host-specific tolerance. When both peripheral and intrathymic alloresistance are overcome by conditioning therapy, both donor- and host-reactive T cells arising *de novo* in the thymus do so in the presence of donor and recipient antigen-presenting cells (APCs), and both donor- and host-reactive T cells are specifically deleted.[8–12] An advantage of mixed chimerism over full allogeneic chimerism induced across extensive MHC barriers is that, in the former, a continuous source of host-type hematopoietic cells insures that host-reactive T cell clones will not emerge from the thymus,[8] whereas such cells can emerge in animals reconstituted with fully mismatched allogeneic marrow alone.[13]

However, reliable, nontoxic methods of achieving allogeneic hematopioetic stem cell (HSC) engraftment across major histocompatibility complex (MHC) barriers will be required before HCT can be routinely used for the induction of organ or tissue allograft tolerance. These regimens must be nonmyeloabaltive, so that recipient hematopoiesis can protect the recipient from marrow failure should the donor graft be rejected. Nevertheless, these methodologies must be sufficiently potent to overcome the T cell barrier to HLA-mismatched HSC grafts, allowing their engraftment. While NK cells also impose a barrier to HSC engraftment when cell doses are limiting, administration of higher HSC numbers quite readily overcomes NK cell barriers in rodent models.[14] Nevertheless, NK cells pose a more serious barrier to HSC engraftment when T cell suppression is incomplete,[15] resulting in reductions in the number of donor stem cells that survive.

Engraftment of allogeneic (and syngeneic) HSCs can also be promoted by making "space" in the hematopoietic system using myelosuppressive treatments such as a low dose of total body irradiation (TBI) or busulfan. The mechanism by which myelosuppressive host treatment promotes marrow engraftment is not fully understood, and could include both the creation of physical niches and the upregulation of cytokines and other molecules that transmit signals to promote hematopoiesis. However, the creation of space is not an absolute requirement, as it can be circumvented by the administration of very high doses of HSCs.[16–18] Nevertheless, some degree of myelosuppression is required for the achievement of mixed chimerism with HSC doses that are currently obtainable in humans.

If the above conditions are met, then donor HSC engraftment will result in a permanent state of multilineage mixed hematopoietic chimerism, which is known to be associated with lifelong central, deletional T cell tolerance[8–12] with the acceptance of any donor allograft without immunosuppression.[19–21] B cells[22,23] and NK cells[24] are also tolerized by the induction of mixed chimerism, permitting long-term stability of chimerism once it is achieved. However, to be applicable for the induction of organ allograft tolerance, the state of mixed chimerism must be achieved without the complication of GvHD, which is an unacceptable risk if HCT is being performed purely for this purpose. Since, unlike HCT for the the treatment of hematologic malignancies, solid organ transplantation is routinely performed across extensive HLA barriers, it would be desirable to achieve this GvHD-free state of mixed chimerism across HLA barriers. Clearly, this represents a major challenge.

Experimental Approaches to Achieving Mixed Chimerism

A number of experimental HCT protocols have been developed that involve myelotoxic and/or immunosuppressive, but not myeloablative, conditioning regimens. Since host HSCs survive, mixed chimerism develops when allogeneic marrow is administered. Such regimens include TLI,[25] sublethal TBI,[26] administration of cyclophosphamide following sensitization with allogeneic donor antigens,[27] and the use of mAbs against host T cells in combination with other modalities.[28] *In vivo* depletion of host $CD4^+$ and $CD8^+$ T cells along with TBI (at least 6 Gy) permitted engraftment of allogeneic marrow and induction of skin graft tolerance across complete MHC barriers.[29] Adding local thymic irradiation (7 Gy) to the regimen permitted engraftment of fully MHC-mismatched allogeneic marrow in animals receiving only 3 Gy TBI.[19] Thymic irradiation is needed because thymocytes, unlike T cells in the peripheral lymphoid compartment, are not eliminated by mAbs.[19] The low dose (3 Gy) of TBI is necessary for the creation of marrow "space." Permanent mixed chimerism and donor- and host-specific tolerance are reliably induced across complete MHC barriers using this regimen (reviewed in Ref. 30). Intrathymic clonal deletion is the major mechanism inducing and maintaining long-term donor-specific tolerance. Consistently, donor class II[high] cells are detectable in the recipient thymi throughout life, beginning as early as including 10 days post-BMT, when the first wave of thymopoiesis is underway. Furthermore, tolerance can be broken by depleting donor cells with donor class I MHC–specific MAbs after stable chimerism has been established and this loss of tolerance correlates with the *de novo* appearance in the periphery of T cells bearing donor-reactive TCR.[11] However, if the host thymus is removed before depletion of donor cells, or if donor-depleted spleen cells from chimeras are transferred to syngeneic athymic mice, donor-specific tolerance is maintained, and cells with donor-reactive TCR do not appear in the periphery.[11] These results demonstrate that intrathymic chimerism is essential and sufficient to maintain ongoing deletional tolerance in long-term mixed allogeneic chimeras, whereas peripheral chimerism plays no significant role in maintaining tolerance. Since persistent antigen is required to maintain anergy, tolerance cannot be explained by a peripheral anergy mechanism. Moreover, the ease with which new thymic emigrants break tolerance after donor cell depletion by MAb or with infusion of nontolerant recipient lymphocytes[11] indicates that suppressive cell populations do not play a significant role in maintaining long-term tolerance. Thus, in this relatively simple model, ablation of pre-existing peripheral and intrathymic mature T cells is followed by lifelong central, deletional tolerance.

Less T cell ablative conditioning regimens have subsequently been developed in murine models. Both thymic irradiation and T cell-depleting MAbs in the conditioning regimen discussed above can be replaced by costimulatory blockade.[31] Recipient preconditioning can be eliminated altogether by giving a high dose of fully MHC-mismatched donor marrow followed by a single injection of each of two costimulatory blockers[32] or repeated injections of anti-CD154 mAb.[33] This ability to replace recipient T cell depletion with costimulatory blockade to allow bone marrow engraftment is important, as it has been difficult to achieve T cell depletion with antibodies in large animals and humans that is as exhaustive as that achieved in the above rodent models. Moreover, if sufficiently exhaustive T cell depletion could be achieved in humans, T cell recovery from the thymus might be dangerously slow, especially in older patients, since thymic function diminishes with age (reviewed in Ref. 34). The ability to minimize the degree and duration of T cell depletion by replacing some[35] or all[31–33] of the T cell-depleting antibodies with costimulatory blockers is therefore encouraging.

As with other protocols achieving sustained mixed chimerism, long-term tolerance is maintained by intrathymic deletion in mixed chimeras prepared with costimulatory blockade.[31,32,35] However, since alloreactive T cells present in the peripheral repertoire at the time of BMT are not globally depleted by these regimens, these peripheral T cells must be rendered tolerant. Initial tolerance involves specific deletion of pre-exisiting peripheral donor-reactive CD4[36] and CD8[37] T cells. In recipients of BMT with anti-CD154 and 3 Gy TBI, specific donor-reactive CD8 deletion occurs within 1–2 weeks and requires CD4 cells that do not have the characteristics associated with "natural" Tregs.[37] Also, arguing against a role for "adaptive" or "induced" Tregs, CD4 cells are not required for maintenance of tolerance after this initial 2-week period.[37] Thus, while CD4 cells are clearly required for CD8 tolerance in this model, the evidence does not implicate a specific subset of CD4 cells that is differentiated to mediate suppression. Deletion of donor-reactive CD4 cells occurs more slowly, over 4–5 weeks in chimeras induced with anti-CD154 mAb, and is preceded by a state of anergy.[36,38] Regulatory cells do not appear to play a major role in inducing or maintaining the tolerance induced by anti-CD154 with BMT.[36] Since HSC engraftment ensures complete central deletional tolerance in these long-term chimeras,[31,32,35,39] and specific peripheral deletion is quite complete, there may be insufficient donor-reactive T cells present to promote the expansion and maintenance of specific regulatory cells. However, several allogeneic BMT models using CTLA4Ig and anti-CD154 as conditioning may be associated with less complete deletion of pre-exisiting donor-reactive T cells and seem to involve long-term regulatory mechanisms.[40,41]

A nonhuman primate model for mixed chimerism and renal allograft tolerance induction across MHC barriers has been developed. Cynomolgus monkeys are given 3 Gy TBI and 7 Gy thymic irradiation. Since effective

T cell-depleting MABs are not available for use in primates, polyclonal ATG and a short (28-day) course of cyclosporine are employed in their place. A high percentage of splenectomized cynomolgus monkeys receiving class I and II–mismatched marrow with this protocol develop transient mixed chimerism and donor kidney allograft acceptance.[42] The splenectomy is required to avoid antidonor antibody responses and can be replaced by the use of anti-CD154 mAb.[43]

Role for Mixed Chimerism in the Treatment of Hematologic Malignancies

In recent years, a variety of clinical HCT protocols have been developed for the treatment of hematologic malignanices in which nonmyeloablative conditioning is used. While mixed chimerism may be achieved initially in these protocols, the goal is full donor chimerism, and the complication of GvHD often occurs in association with the development of full chimerism, either spontaneously or following donor leukocyte infusion (DLI). In contrast to HCT for the induction of organ allograft tolerance, a mild-to-moderate level of GvHD is considered acceptable when hematologic malignancies are treated, as GvHD is associated with enhanced antitumor effects.[44] However, the frequency and severity of GvHD observed when extensive HLA barriers are transgressed has essentially precluded the routine use of extensively HLA-mismatched HCT.

Based on observations in animal models, we have attempted to overcome the above limitations on HLA-mismatched HCT for the treatment of hematologic malignancies. We have developed a series of clinical protocols using nonmyeloablative conditioning that includes recipient and donor graft T cell depletion and aims to achieve initial mixed chimerism without any graft-vs-host response from the initial transplant. The key observation leading to these trials is that conditioning-induced tissue inflammation plays an important role in promoting GvHD. We have found that MHC-directed alloreactivity can be confined to the lymphohematopoietic system when nontolerant donor T cells are given to mixed chimeras after host recovery from the initial conditioning regimen has occurred. As discussed above, established mixed chimeras produced with either lethal TBI or nonmyeloablative conditioning regimens are immunologically tolerant of their original marrow donor. Therefore, GvH reactions occurring after administration of nontolerant T cells in DLI are not opposed by any host-vs-graft response. The unopposed GvH response results in conversion of mixed hematopoietic chimerism to full donor chimerism and strong graft-vs-leukemia/lymphoma (GvL) effects.[45,46] However, this powerful GvH alloresponse against lymphohematopoietic cells is not associated with clinical or histological GvHD, even though the T cell numbers given cause rapidly lethal GvHD in freshly conditioned recipients.[45,47]

Antihost MHC alloreactivity mediates the most potent GvL effects[46,48] and GvH-reactive T cells in DLI become activated and proliferate in established mixed chimeras receiving DLI.[48,49] The presence of recipient hematopoietically derived APCs expressing both class I and class II MHC plays a critical role in inducing this antihost reactivity and maximal GvL. In contrast, full allogeneic chimeras, which lack host APCs, do not induce activation or expansion of T cells in DLI, and thereby fail to achieve GvL effects.[46,48]

Despite converting to the "effector/memory" phenotype following activation in established mixed chimeras, DLI-derived T cells do not migrate to the GvHD target tissues, which include epithelial tissues such as the skin, intestines and liver. This failure to traffic is due to the absence of inflammatory signals in those tissues.[49] Such inflammatory signals, including chemokines and probably adhesion molecules, are induced in GvHD target tissues by conditioning treatment and subside over time.[50]

In attempts to apply this approach to separating GvHD from GvL clinically, proof of principle has been obtained that GvH responses can be confined to the lymphohematopoietic system and thereby fail to induce GvHD in patients receiving nonmyeloablative HCT with an initially T cell-depleted product, followed by delayed DLI, even across extensive HLA barriers.[51] However, some patients who are mixed chimeras and show no evidence for GvHD prior to receiving DLI do develop GvHD after receiving the DLI. One major difference between these patients and the mouse model is that T cell recovery in patients is generally poor at the time when DLIs are given,[52] resulting in bacterial, viral and fungal infections. In contrast, mice have excellent T cell recovery due to robust thymopoiesis by the time DLIs are given. Additionally, these animals are maintained in a specific pathogen-free facility, making the likelihood of infection at the time of DLI administration very low. This freedom from infection may play an important role in the observed failure of DLI-derived activated T cells to migrate to GvHD target tissues. In agreement with this notion, even in such "quiescent" established mixed chimeras, activation of toll-like receptors (TLRs), as occurs in infection, promotes the trafficking of DLI-derived T cells to the GvHD target tissues.[49] If the TLR stimulus is provided systemically (mimicking a systemic infection), systemic GvHD develops. In contrast, when a TLR stimulus is applied locally to the skin, the GvHD resulting from DLI administration is confined to the treated area of the skin.[49] These results have several important implications: (1) they indicate that regulatory cells, which are present in mixed chimeras by the time of DLI administration, are insufficient to prevent the development of GvHD when an inflammatory stimulus is provided by TLR activation; (2) they show that local inflammatory stimuli in the skin play a critical role in promoting the trafficking of GvH-reactive T cells into that tissue and hence the induction of GvHD; this "inflammatory checkpoint" confines GvHD to the inflamed tissue; (3) they suggest that improved immune recovery, which would lead to better control of posttransplant infections and prevent TLR-dependent immune activation, might improve the ability to separate GvHD and GvL with this approach in patients.

Convergence of Mixed Chimerism Induction for Tolerance Induction and Treatment of Hematologic Malignancies

The successful achievement of renal allograft tolerance in a primate model using nonmyeloablative conditioning for mixed chimerism induction,[42] combined with clinical results using the approach described above for achieving GvL without GvHD by inducing mixed chimerism and later giving DLI,[53,54] allowed the first successful trial of organ allograft tolerance induction to be carried out in humans. The clinical experience with our relatively nontoxic nonmyeloablative HCT protocol provided an opportunity to evaluate the potential of this approach to induce transplantation tolerance in patients with a hematologic malignancy, multiple myeloma, and consequent renal failure. Six patients received a simultaneous nonmyeloablative bone marrow transplant and renal allograft from an HLA-identical sibling, and have accepted their kidney graft without any immunosuppression for followups for as long as ten years. Three of the six patients achieved prolonged complete remissions of their myelomas. This was especially surprising, since chimerism in four of these six patients (including two with prolonged CRs of their myelomas) was only transient.[55] These data raised the possibility that transient chimerism followed by marrow rejection, which was evidenced by sensitized antidonor T cell responses in some patients,[55] could lead to antitumor responses. This hypothesis has been supported by data obtained subsequently in a mouse model.[56–59] In view of the sensitization to antigens on hematopoietic cells observed in some patients who lost their chimerism,[55] the renal allograft tolerance that was nevertheless achieved suggests that the kidney graft itself may participate in tolerance induction and/or maintenance. These patients demonstrated unresponsiveness to donor renal tubular epithelial cells,[55] raising the possibility that tolerance may be specific to minor antigens expressed on the kidney graft itself. In the primate model described above, chimerism is also transient, but both BMT and early renal transplantation have been shown to be required for achievement of tolerance.[42] Because T cell depletion is only partial in these models, the pure central, deletional tolerance described above in murine models is unlikely to be the major mechanism of allograft tolerance.

Recently, this approach has been extended to a pilot study on patients without malignant disease who have renal failure from other causes, who received HLA-mismatched combined kidney and bone marrow transplantation. Safety data in a trial involving HLA-mismatched BMT in patients with hematologic malignancies, again using the approach of nonmyeloablative mixed chimerism induction followed by delayed DLI, provided the impetus to extend this approach to the HLA-mismatched kidney transplant setting.[51] Four patients with hematologic malignancies received haploidentical related bone marrow grafts following conditioning with cyclophosphamide, thymic irradiation and peritransplant treatment with a humanized anti-CD2 mAb, a more potent T cell-depleting agent than the equine ATG used in the above HLA-identical studies in myeloma patients. Only transient chimerism was achieved in the HLA-mismatched study, and loss of chimerism was associated with robust recipient hematopioesis, documenting that the regimen was truly nonmyeloablative. Although loss of chimerism was not the desired outcome in efforts to achieve antitumor effects, an important observation was that none of these patients developed GvHD. Thus, we had made several observations that justified a second combined kidney-BMT clinical tolerance trial, this time using haploidentical related donors in recipients without malignant disease: (1) the achievement of initial mixed chimerism without GvHD, a critical safety parameter, in the setting of HLA-mismatched HCT; (2) the demonstration in nonhuman primates that transient chimerism was associated with renal allograft tolerance when combined MHC-mismatched bone marrow and kidney transplantation was performed; and (3) the demonstration in multiple myeloma patients that transient chimerism was associated with renal allograft tolerance in recipients of combined kidney–BMT. The HLA-mismatched combined kidney-BMT trial in patients without malignant disease involved five patients, with followup now from about three to more than six years. Four of the five patients were successfully taken off their initial immunosuppressive monotherapy with the calcineurin inhibitor, and have had stable graft function off immunosuppression for more than two to five years. One patient lost his graft early due to acute humoral rejection.[60] This trial is the first to intentionally achieve tolerance to an organ allograft across HLA barriers.

In vitro analyses of these patients revealed the progressive development of donor-specific unresponsiveness in both MLR and CML assays in the four patients who achieved renal allograft tolerance. Robust third party alloresponses recovered in all of them,[60] suggesting that a systemic state of donor-specific tolerance developed. The contrast of these observations with those in recipients of HLA-identical transplants, who sometimes showed sensitization to donor hematopoietic antigens in association with loss of chimerism, raises the unsatisfying possibility that the mechanisms of tolerance may differ between the HLA-identical and the HLA-mismatched setting. A more unifying (and hence satisfying) hypothesis is that in both groups tolerance is restricted to antigens expressed by the kidney. In recipients of HLA-mismatched transplants, the pre-existing bulk antidonor response may disappear after transplant because most allogeneic MHC/peptide complexes responsible for the strong direct alloresponse *in vitro* are shared by the kidney and the hematopoietic cells. This may preclude the existence of a significant number of T cells recognizing antigens expressed only on hematopoietic cells, and tolerance to those expressed on the kidney would thereby lead to loss of the bulk MLR and CML response. The loss of chimerism in these patients occurs very early, when T cells are markedly depleted by the conditioning, and there is no direct evidence that the loss of chimerism is due to a T cell-mediated immune response. Loss of chimerism might reflect inadequate HSC engraftment and competition from surviving host hematopoietic cells. Comparison of the *in vitro* results for combined haploidentical kidney–BMT patients with those for patients with hematologic malignancies who received a similar haploidentical BMT regimen without a kidney transplant suggests a role for the kidney in the tolerance achieved. In contrast to the combined transplant recipients, the patients who received BMT alone showed generally weak alloresponses but tended to have stronger antidonor than anti-third-party responses following the loss of chimerism.[52]

Regardless of the actual mechanism of tolerance in the recipients of HLA-mismatched combined kidney–BMT, it is unlikely that central deletion mediates long-term tolerance in these patients, given the transient nature of the chimerism. Moreover, initial T cell recovery in these patients appears to be mainly from the residual peripheral T cell pool rather than from the thymus[55] (G. Andreola *et al.*, manuscript in preparation).

Intragraft levels of FoxP3 relative to Granzyme B mRNA were increased in tolerant patients compared to patients on immunosuppression, raising the possibility that regulatory T cells might play a role in tolerance.[60] Regulatory cells are enriched among the T cells initially present in recipients of this regimen with (G. Andreola *et al.*, manuscript in preparation) or without[52] a kidney transplant, and *in vitro* assays to assess the possible role of such cells are in progress.

Future Directions

It is clear that HCT has not yet met its full potential to achieve organ allograft tolerance in humans. Advances in the ability to achieve engraftment of hematopoietic cells without ablative host treatment across HLA barriers without increasing host toxicity should further broaden the applicability of this approach. In order to overcome the existing organ allograft shortage, it will be desirable to extend this ability to xenogeneic marrow and organ transplantation, which presents additional immunological and physiological hurdles. A better understanding of the mechanisms by which tolerance is induced and maintained in rodent model systems will aid in the exploitation of these mechanisms in large animals and humans.

References

1. Kirk AD, Harlan DM, Armstrong NN *et al.* (1997) CTLA4-Ig and anti-CD40 ligand prevent renal allograft rejection in primates. *Proc Natl Acad Sci USA* **94**: 8789–8798.
2. Kirk AD, Burkly LC, Batty DS *et al.* (1999) Treatment with humanized monoclonal antibody against CD154 prevents acute renal allograft rejection in nonhuman primates. *Nat Med* **5**: 686–693.
3. Kirk AD, Tadaki DK, Celniker A *et al.* (2001) Induction therapy with monoclonal antibodies specific for CD80 and CD86 delays the onset of acute renal allograft rejection in non-human primates. *Transplantation* **72**: 377–384.

4. Elster EA, Xu H, Tadaki DK *et al.* (2001) Treatment with the humanized CD154-specific monoclonal antibody, hu5C8, prevents acute rejection of primary skin allografts in nonhuman primates. *Transplantation* **72**: 1473–1478.

5. Owen RD. (1945) Immunogenetic consequences of vascular anastomoses between bovine twins. *Science* **102**: 400–401.

6. Sharabi Y, Sachs DH, Sykes M. (1992) T cell subsets resisting induction of mixed chimerism across various histocompatibility barriers. In: Gergely J, Benczur M, Falus A *et al.* (eds.), *Progress in Immunology VIII: Proc. Eighth International Congress of Immunology (Budapest, 1992)*. Springer-Verlag, Heidelberg, pp. 801–805.

7. Hayashi H, LeGuern C, Sachs DH, Sykes M. (1996) Alloresistance to K locus mismatched bone marrow engraftment is mediated entirely by CD4$^+$ and CD8$^+$ T cells. *Bone Marrow Transplant* **18**: 285–292.

8. Tomita Y, Khan A, Sykes M. (1994) Role of intrathymic clonal deletion and peripheral anergy in transplantation tolerance induced by bone marrow transplantation in mice conditioned with a nonmyeloablative regimen. *J Immunol* **153**: 1087–1098.

9. Tomita Y, Sachs DH, Khan A, Sykes M. (1996) Additional mAb injections can replace thymic irradiation to allow induction of mixed chimerism and tolerance in mice receiving bone marrow transplantation after conditioning with anti-T cell mAbs and 3 Gy whole body irradiation. *Transplantation* **61**: 469–477.

10. Tomita Y, Khan A, Sykes M. (1996) Mechanism by which additional monoclonal antibody injections overcome the requirement for thymic irradiation to achieve mixed chimerism in mice receiving bone marrow transplantation after conditioning with anti-T cell mAbs and 3 Gy whole body irradiation. *Transplantation* **61**: 477–485.

11. Khan A, Tomita Y, Sykes M. (1996) Thymic dependence of loss of tolerance in mixed allogeneic bone marrow chimeras after depletion of donor antigen: Peripheral mechanisms do not contribute to maintenance of tolerance. *Transplantation* **62**: 380–387.

12. Manilay JO, Pearson DA, Sergio JJ *et al.* (1998) Intrathymic deletion of alloreactive T cells in mixed bone marrow chimeras prepared with a nonmyeloablative conditioning regimen. *Transplantation* **66**: 96–102.

13. Ramsdell F, Fowlkes BJ. (1990) Clonal deletion versus clonal anergy: The role of the thymus in inducing self tolerance. *Science* **248**: 1342–1348.

14. Lee LA, Sachs DH, Sykes M. (1992) Effect of NK cell depletion on long-term, multilineage allogeneic bone marrow engraftment. *Transplant Proc* **25**: 1246–1247.

15. Kean LS, Hamby K, Koehn B *et al.* (2006) NK cells mediate costimulation blockade-resistant rejection of allogeneic stem cells during nonmyeloablative transplantation. *Am J Transplant* **6**: 292–304.

16. Tomita Y, Sachs DH, Sykes M. (1994) Myelosuppressive conditioning is required to achieve engraftment of pluripotent stem cells contained in moderate doses of syngeneic bone marrow. *Blood* **83**: 939–948.

17. Ramshaw HS, Crittenden RB, Dooner M *et al.* (1995) High levels of engraftment with a single infusion of bone marrow cells into normal unprepared mice. *Biol Blood Marrow Transplant* **1**: 74–80.

18. Sykes M, Szot GL, Swenson K *et al.* (1997) Separate regulation of hematopietic and thymic engraftment. *Exp Hematol* **26**: 457–465.

19. Sharabi Y, Sachs DH. (1989) Mixed chimerism and permanent specific transplantation tolerance induced by a non-lethal preparative regimen. *J Exp Med* **169**: 493–502.

20. Guo Z, Wang J, Dong Y *et al.* (2003) Long-term survival of intestinal allografts induced by costimulation blockade, busulfan and donor bone marrow infusion. *Am J Transplant* **3**: 1091–1098.

21. Shirasugi N, Adams AB, Durham MM *et al.* (2002) Prevention of chronic rejection in murine cardiac allografts: A comparison of chimerism- and nonchimerism-inducing costimulation blockade-based tolerance induction regimens. *J Immunol* **169**: 2677–2684.

22. Yang Y-G, de Goma E, Ohdan H *et al.* (1998) Tolerization of anti-galα1-3gal natural antibody-forming B cells by induction of mixed chimerism. *J Exp Med* **187**: 1335–1342.

23. Ohdan H, Yang Y-G, Shimizu A *et al.* (1999) Mixed bone marrow chimerism induced without lethal conditioning prevents T cell and anti-Galα1,3Gal-mediated graft rejection. *J Clin Invest* **104**: 281–290.

24. Zhao Y, Ohdan H, Manilay JO, Sykes M. (2003) NK cell tolerance in mixed allogeneic chimeras. *J Immunol* **170**: 5398–5405.

25. Slavin S. (1987) Total lymphoid irradiation. *Immunol Today* **3**: 88–92.

26. Pierce GE. (1990) Allogeneic versus semiallogeneic F1 bone marrow transplantation into sublethally irradiated MHC-disparate hosts: Effects on mixed lymphoid chimerism, skin graft tolerance, host survival, and alloreactivity. *Transplantation* **49**: 138–144.

27. Eto M, Mayumi H, Tomita Y *et al.* (1990) Intrathymic clonal deletion of V beta 6$^+$ T cells in cyclophosphamide-induced tolerance to H-2-compatible, Mls-disparate antigens. *J Exp Med* **171**: 97–113.

28. Mayumi H, Good RA. (1989) Long-lasting skin allograft tolerance in adult mice induced across fully allogeneic (multimajor H-2 plus multiminor histocompatibility) antigen barriers by a tolerance-inducing method using cyclophosphamide. *J Exp Med* **169**: 213–238.

29. Cobbold SP, Qin S, Waldmann H. (1990) Reprogramming the immune system for tolerance with monoclonal antibodies. *Sem Immunol* **2**: 377–387.

30. Sykes M. (2007) Mechanisms of tolerance induced via mixed chimerism. *Front Biosci* **12**: 2922–2934.

31. Wekerle T, Sayegh MH, Hill J *et al.* (1998) Extrathymic T cell deletion and allogeneic stem cell engraftment induced with costimulatory blockade is followed by central T cell tolerance. *J Exp Med* **187**: 2037–2044.

32. Wekerle T, Kurtz J, Ito H *et al.* (2000) Allogeneic bone marrow transplantation with costimulatory blockade induces macrochimerism and tolerance without cytoreductive host treatment. *Nat Med* **6**: 464–469.

33. Durham MM, Bingaman AW, Adams AB *et al.* (2000) Cutting edge: Administration of anti-CD40 ligand and donor bone marrow leads to hemopoietic chimerism and donor-specific tolerance without cytoreductive conditioning. *J Immunol* **165**: 1–4.

34. Haynes BF, Markert ML, Sempowski GD *et al.* (2000) The role of the thymus in immune reconstitution in aging, bone marrow transplantation, and HIV-1 infection. *Annu Rev Immunol* **18**: 529–560.

35. Ito H, Kurtz J, Shaffer J, Sykes M. (2001) CD4 T cell-mediated alloresistance to fully MHC-mismatched allogeneic bone marrow engraftment is dependent on CD40-CD40L interactions, and lasting T cell tolerance is induced by bone marrow transplantation with initial blockade of this pathway. *J Immunol* **166**: 2981.

36. Kurtz J, Shaffer J, Anosova N *et al.* (2004) Mechanisms of early peripheral CD4 T cell tolerance induction by anti-CD154 monoclonal antibody and allogeneic bone marrow transplantation: Evidence for anergy and deletion, but not regulatory cells. *Blood* **103**: 4336–4343.

37. Fehr T, Takeuchi Y, Kurtz J, Sykes M. (2005) Early regulation of CD8 T cell alloreactivity by CD4$^+$CD25$^-$ T cells in recipients of anti-CD154 antibody and allogeneic BMT is followed by rapid peripheral deletion of donor-reactive CD8$^+$ T cells, precluding a role for sustained regulation. *Eur J Immunol* **35**: 2679–2690.

38. Kurtz J, Ito H, Wekerle T *et al.* (2001) Mechanisms involved in the establishment of tolerance through costimulatory blockade and BMT: Lack of requirement for CD40L-mediated signaling for tolerance or deletion of donor-reactive CD4$^+$ cells. *Am J Transplant* **1**: 339–349.

39. Wekerle T, Sayegh MH, Chandraker A *et al.* (1999) Role of peripheral clonal deletion in tolerance induction with bone marrow transplantation and costimulatory blockade. *Transplant Proc* **31**: 680.

40. Bigenzahn S, Blaha P, Koporc Z *et al.* (2005) The role of non-deletional tolerance mechanisms in a murine model of mixed chimerism with costimulation blockade. *Am J Transplant* **5**: 1237–1247.

41. Domenig C, Sanchez-Fueyo A, Kurtz J *et al.* (2005) Roles of deletion and regulation in creating mixed chimerism and allograft tolerance using a nonlymphoablative irradiation-free protocol. *J Immunol* **175**: 51–60.

42. Kawai T, Cosimi AB, Colvin RB *et al.* (1995) Mixed allogeneic chimerism and renal allograft tolerance in cynomologus monkeys. *Transplantation* **59**: 256–262.

43. Kawai T, Sogawa H, Boskovic S *et al.* (2004) CD154 blockade for induction of mixed chimerism and prolonged renal allograft survival in nonhuman primates. *Am J Transplant* **4**: 1391–1398.

44. Weiden PL, Flournoy N, Thomas ED *et al.* (1979) Antileukemic effect of graft-versus-host disease in human recipients of allogeneic marrow grafts. *New Engl J Med* **300**: 1068–1073.

45. Sykes M, Sheard MA, Sachs DH. (1988) Graft-versus-host-related immunosuppression is induced in mixed chimeras by alloresponses against either host or donor lymphohematopoietic cells. *J Exp Med* **168**: 2391–2396.

46. Mapara MY, Kim Y-M, Wang S-P *et al.* (2002) Donor lymphocyte infusions mediate superior graft-versus-leukemia effects in mixed compared to fully allogeneic chimeras: A critical role for host antigen-presenting cells. *Blood* **100**: 1903–1909.

47. Pelot MR, Pearson DA, Swenson K *et al.* (1999) Lymphohematopoietic graft-vs-host reactions can be induced without graft-vs-host disease in murine mixed chimeras established with a cyclophosphamide-based non-myeloablative conditioning regimen. *Biol Blood Marrow Transplant* **5**: 133–143.

48. Chakraverty R, Eom HS, Sachs J *et al.* (2006) Host MHC Class II[+] antigen-presenting cells and CD4 cells are required for CD8-mediated graft-versus-leukemia responses following delayed donor leukocyte infusions. *Blood* **108**: 2106–2113.

49. Chakraverty R, Cote D, Buchli J *et al.* (2006) An inflammatory checkpoint regulates recruitment of graft-versus-host-reactive T cells to peripheral tissues. *J Exp Med* **203**: 2021–2031.

50. Mapara MY, Leng C, Kim YM *et al.* (2006) Expression of chemokines in GVHD target organs is influenced by conditioning and genetic factors and amplified by GVHR. *Biol Blood Marrow Transplant* **12**: 623–634.

51. Spitzer TR, McAffee S, Dey BR *et al.* (2003) Non-myeloablative haploidentical stem cell transplantation using anti-CD2 monoclonal antibody (MEDI-507)–based conditioning for refractory hematologic malignancies. *Transplantation* **75**: 1748–1751.

52. Shaffer J, Villard J, Means TK *et al.* (2007) Regulatory T cell recovery in recipients of haploidentical nonmyeloablative hematopoietic cell transplantation with a humanized anti-CD2 mAb, MEDI-507, with or without fludarabine. *Exp Hematol* **35**: 1140–1152.

53. Sykes M, Preffer F, McAffee S *et al.* (1999) Mixed lymphohematopoietic chimerism and graft-vs-lymphoma effects are achievable in adult humans following non-myeloablative therapy and HLA-mismatched donor bone marrow transplantation. *Lancet* **353**: 1755–1759.

54. Spitzer TR, McAffee S, Sackstein R *et al.* (2000) The intentional induction of mixed chimerism and achievement of anti-tumor responses following non-myeloablative conditioning therapy and HLA-matched and mismatched donor bone marrow transplantation for refractory hematologic malignancies. *Biol Blood Marrow Transplant* **6**: 309–320.

55. Fudaba Y, Spitzer TR, Shaffer J *et al.* (2006) Myeloma responses and tolerance following combined kidney and nonmyeloablative marrow transplantation: *In vivo* and *in vitro* analyses. *Am J Transplant* **6**: 2121–2133.

56. Rubio MT, Kim YM, Sachs T *et al.* (2003) Antitumor effect of donor marrow graft rejection induced by recipient leukocyte infusions in mixed chimeras prepared with nonmyeloablative conditioning: Critical role for recipient-derived IFN-{gamma}. *Blood* **102**: 2300–2307.

57. Rubio MT, Saito TI, Kattelman K *et al.* (2005) Mechanisms of the anti-tumor responses and host-versus graft reactions induced by

recipient leukocyte infusions in mixed chimeras prepared with non-myeloablative conditioning: A critical role for recipient CD4$^+$ T cells and recipient leukocyte infusion-derived IFN-gamma-producing CD8$^+$ T cells. *J Immunol* **175**: 665–676.

58. Rubio MT, Zhao G, Buchli J *et al.* (2006) Role of indirect allo- and autoreactivity in anti-tumor responses induced by recipient leukocyte infusions (RLI) in mixed chimeras prepared with nonmyeloablative conditioning. *Clin Immunol* **120**: 33–44.

59. Saito TI, Rubio MT, Sykes M. (2006) Clinical relevance of recipient leukocyte infusion as antitumor therapy following nonmyeloablative allogeneic hematopoietic cell transplantation. *Exp Hematol* **34**: 1271–1277.

60. Kawai T, Cosimi AB, Spitzer TR *et al.* (2008) HLA-mismatched renal transplantation without maintenance immunosuppression. *New Engl J Med* **358**: 353–361.

Index